Cardiac Resynchronization - A Reappraisal

Editors

JAGMEET P. SINGH
GOPI DANDAMUDI

CARDIAC ELECTROPHYSIOLOGY CLINICS

www.cardiacEP.theclinics.com

Consulting Editors
RANJAN K. THAKUR
ANDREA NATALE

March 2019 • Volume 11 • Number 1

ELSEVIER

1600 John F. Kennedy Boulevard • Suite 1800 • Philadelphia, Pennsylvania, 19103-2899

http://www.theclinics.com

CARDIAC ELECTROPHYSIOLOGY CLINICS Volume 11, Number 1
March 2019 ISSN 1877-9182, ISBN-13: 978-0-323-66098-3

Editor: Stacy Eastman
Developmental Editor: Donald Mumford

Cardiac Electrophysiology Clinics (ISSN 1877-9182) is published quarterly by Elsevier Inc., 360 Park Avenue South, New York, NY 10010-1710. Months of issue are March, June, September, and December. Subscription prices are $224.00 per year for US individuals, $366.00 per year for US institutions, $249.00 per year for Canadian individuals, $413.00 per year for Canadian institutions, $303.00 per year for international individuals, $442.00 per year for international institutions and $100.00 per year for US, Canadian and international students/residents. To receive student/resident rate, orders must be accompanied by name of affilliated institution, date of term, and the signature of program/residency coordinator on institution letterhead. Orders will be billed at individual rate until proof of status is received. Foreign air speed delivery is included in all Clinics subscription prices. All prices are subject to change without notice. **POSTMASTER:** Send address changes to Cardiac Electrophysiology Clinics, Elsevier Health Sciences Division, Subscription Customer Service, 3251 Riverport Lane, Maryland Heights, MO 63043. **Customer Service: 1-800-654-2452 (US and Canada). From outside of the US and Canada, call 314-477-8871. Fax: 314-447-8029. E-mail: JournalsCustomerService-usa@elsevier.com (for print support); JournalsOnlineSupport-usa@elsevier.com (for online support).**

Reprints. For copies of 100 or more of articles in this publication, please contact the Commercial Reprints Department, Elsevier Inc., 360 Park Avenue South, New York, NY 10010-1710. Tel.: 212-633-3874; Fax: 212-633-3820; E-mail: reprints@elsevier.com.

Cardiac Electrophysiology Clinics is covered in *MEDLINE/PubMed (Index Medicus).*

Contributors

CONSULTING EDITORS

RANJAN K. THAKUR, MD, MPH, MBA, FHRS
Professor of Medicine and Director, Arrhythmia Service, Thoracic and Cardiovascular Institute, Sparrow Health System, Michigan State University, Lansing, Michigan, USA

ANDREA NATALE, MD, FACC, FHRS
Executive Medical Director, Texas Cardiac Arrhythmia Institute, St. David's Medical Center, Austin, Texas; Consulting Professor, Division of Cardiology, Stanford University, Palo Alto, California; Adjunct Professor of Medicine, Heart and Vascular Center, Case Western Reserve University, Cleveland, Ohio; Director, Interventional Electrophysiology, Scripps Clinic, San Diego, California; Senior Clinical Director, EP Services, California Pacific Medical Center, San Francisco, California

EDITORS

GOPI DANDAMUDI, MD
Medical Director, Cardiovascular Service Line, Cardiology, CHI-Franciscan Health System, Tacoma, Washington, USA

JAGMEET P. SINGH, MD, PhD
Associate Chief, Cardiology, Massachusetts General Hospital, Boston, Massachusetts, USA

AUTHORS

CHONYANG ALBERT, MD
Department of Cardiovascular Medicine, Heart and Vascular Institute, Cleveland Clinic, Cleveland, Ohio, USA

MAYA H. BARGHASH, MD
Assistant Professor, Department of Medicine, Division of Cardiology, Zena and Michael A. Wiener Cardiovascular Institute, Mount Sinai Hospital, Icahn School of Medicine at Mount Sinai, New York, New York, USA

ULRIKA BIRGERSDOTTER-GREEN, MD
Director, Pacemaker and ICD Services, Cardiac Electrophysiology Section, Division of Cardiology, Professor, Department of Medicine, University of California, San Diego, La Jolla, California, USA

JOSEP BRUGADA, MD, PhD
Pediatric Arrhythmia Unit, Hospital Sant Joan de Deu, Cardiovascular Clinical Institute, Hospital Clínic, Universitat de Barcelona, Barcelona, Spain

JULIA CADRIN-TOURIGNY, MD
Institut de Cardiologie de Montréal, Université de Montréal, Montreal, Quebec, Canada

YONG-MEI CHA, MD
Department of Cardiovascular Medicine, Mayo Clinic, Rochester, Minnesota, USA

SUNIT-PREET CHAUDHRY, MD
Advanced Heart Failure and Transplant, St. Vincent Heart Center, Indianapolis, Indiana, USA

MARC DUBUC, MD
Institut de Cardiologie de Montréal,
Université de Montréal, Montreal, Quebec,
Canada

JERRY D. ESTEP, MD
Department of Cardiovascular Medicine, Heart
and Vascular Institute, Kaufman Center for
Heart Failure, Cleveland Clinic, Cleveland,
Ohio, USA

DANIEL J. FRIEDMAN, MD
Fellow, Clinical Cardiac Electrophysiology,
Electrophysiology Section, Duke University
Hospital, Durham, North Carolina, USA

ALAN HANLEY, MB, MSc
Electrophysiology Fellow, Cardiac Arrhythmia
Service, Massachusetts General Hospital,
Boston, Massachusetts, USA

E. KEVIN HEIST, MD, PhD
Associate Professor of Medicine,
Cardiac Arrhythmia Service, Massachusetts
General Hospital, Boston, Massachusetts,
USA

NATALIA HERNANDEZ, MD
Fellow in Cardiac Electrophysiology,
Department of Cardiology, University of
Rochester Medical Center, Rochester,
New York, USA

DAVID T. HUANG, MD
Professor of Medicine, Director of
Cardiac Electrophysiology, Department
of Cardiology, University of Rochester
Medical Center, Rochester, New York,
USA

KEVIN P. JACKSON, MD
Assistant Professor of Medicine,
Electrophysiology Section, Duke
University Hospital, Durham, North
Carolina, USA

PAUL KHAIRY, MD, PhD
Institut de Cardiologie de Montréal, Université
de Montréal, Montreal, Quebec, Canada

LAURENT MACLE, MD
Institut de Cardiologie de Montréal,
Université de Montréal, Montreal, Quebec,
Canada

THEOFANIE MELA, MD
Cardiac Arrhythmia Service, Massachusetts
General Hospital, Boston, Massachusetts,
USA

SUNEET MITTAL, MD
Director, Electrophysiology Laboratory, The
Valley Hospital, Valley Health System, Snyder
Center for Comprehensive Atrial Fibrillation,
Ridgewood, New Jersey, USA

BLANDINE MONDÉSERT, MD
Institut de Cardiologie de Montréal,
Université de Montréal, Montreal, Quebec,
Canada

SAMAN NAZARIAN, MD, PhD
Associate Professor, Department of
Medicine, Cardiovascular Division,
Clinical Cardiac Electrophysiology Section,
Perelman School of Medicine at the University
of Pennsylvania, Philadelphia, Pennsylvania,
USA

MARIN NISHIMURA, MD
Fellow, Cardiovascular Diseases, Division of
Cardiovascular Medicine, Department of
Medicine, UC San Diego Medical Center,
University of California, San Diego, La Jolla,
California, USA

EDMOND OBENG-GYIMAH, MD
Department of Medicine, Cardiovascular
Division, Clinical Cardiac Electrophysiology
Section, Perelman School of Medicine at the
University of Pennsylvania, Philadelphia,
Pennsylvania, USA

SEAN P. PINNEY, MD
Professor, Department of Medicine, Division of
Cardiology, Zena and Michael A. Wiener
Cardiovascular Institute, Mount Sinai Hospital,
Icahn School of Medicine at Mount Sinai,
New York, New York, USA

NIELS RISUM, MD, PhD
Rigshospitalet, Copenhagen University
Hospital, Copenhagen, Denmark

**PARIKSHIT S. SHARMA, MD, MPH, FACC,
FHRS**
Assistant Professor of Medicine, Division of
Cardiology, Rush University Medical Center,
Chicago, Illinois, USA

DAVID SNIPELISKY, MD
Advanced Heart Disease Fellow, Division of Cardiovascular Medicine, Brigham and Women's Hospital, Boston, Massachusetts, USA

PETER SOGAARD, MD, DMSc
Department of Cardiology, Aalborg University Hospital, Aalborg, Denmark

JONATHAN S. STEINBERG, MD
Professor of Medicine (adj), Heart Research Follow-up Program, University of Rochester School of Medicine and Dentistry, Rochester, New York, USA; Professor of Cardiology and Internal Medicine, Hackensack Meridian School of Medicine at Seton Hall University, Nutley, New Jersey, USA; Director, SMG Arrhythmia Center, Summit Medical Group, Short Hills, New Jersey, USA

GARRICK C. STEWART, MD
Associate Physician, Division of Cardiovascular Medicine, Brigham and Women's Hospital, Boston, Massachusetts, USA

BHUPENDAR TAYAL, MD, PhD
Department of Cardiology, Aalborg University Hospital, Aalborg, Denmark

BERNARD THIBAULT, MD
Institut de Cardiologie de Montréal, Université de Montréal, Montreal, Quebec, Canada

JOSE MARÍA TOLOSANA, MD, PhD
Cardiovascular Clinical Institute, Arrhythmia Section, Hospital Clínic, Universitat de Barcelona, Barcelona, Spain

PUGAZHENDHI VIJAYARAMAN, MD, FACC, FHRS
Professor of Medicine, Geisinger Commonwealth School of Medicine, Geisinger Heart Institute, Wilkes-Barre, Pennsylvania, USA

CHANCE M. WITT, MD
Department of Cardiovascular Medicine, Mayo Clinic, Rochester, Minnesota, USA

SETH J. WORLEY, MD, FHRS, FACC
Director of the Interventional Implant Program, MedStar Heart & Vascular Institute, Washington, DC, USA

Contents

Heart Failure and Why it Matters

Heart failure is a global pandemic that is becoming an increasingly common diagnosis due to aging of the population and increased longevity. Understanding the scope and costs of current heart failure management will lead to improved health economic decision making. Interventions to reduce spending in heart failure care have been centered on reduction of readmissions, improvement in transitions of care, and innovations in technology that have further improved quality of life. Technological advancements in outpatient monitoring offers the hope of further reducing morbidity, mortality, and cost in heart failure.

Heart failure is a heterogeneous clinical syndrome stemming from cardiac overload and injury that leads to considerable morbidity and mortality. This review highlights the many faces of heart failure, a major and growing public health problem, including its causes, classification, underlying pathophysiology, and variable progression. An individualized, patient-centered treatment approach that focuses on guideline-directed pharmacologic and device therapies is required for optimal management of this complex syndrome.

Heart failure (HF) affects 2.4% of the adult population in the United States and is associated with high health care costs. Medical and device therapy delay disease progression and improve survival in HF with reduced ejection fraction. Stage D HF is characterized by significant functional limitation, frequent HF hospitalization for decompensation, intolerance of medical therapy, use of inotropes, and high diuretic requirement. Advanced therapies with left ventricular assist devices and cardiac transplantation reduce mortality and improve quality of life, and early referral to specialized centers is imperative for patient selection and success with these therapies.

CRT Role in HF Management and Implant Techniques

Cardiac resynchronization therapy (CRT) is an electrical therapy to resolve an electrical problem. Any method to predict CRT response must specifically reflect the electrical substrate. Time-to-peak dyssynchrony is too unspecific for prediction of response because dyssynchrony by this approach may reflect the presence of scar or fibrosis even in the absence of conduction delay. New methods are based on the actual physiology of activation delay–induced heart failure (HF) and are superior to time-to-peak methods in predicting CRT response. Time-to-peak dyssynchrony may be used for prognosis in HF patients without signs of delayed ventricular activation and for monitoring CRT response.

Cardiac resynchronization therapy (CRT) improves cardiac mechanics and quality of life in many patients with evidence of electromechanical cardiac dyssynchrony. However, up to 30% of patients receiving CRT do not respond to therapy. The mediator for poor response likely varies among patients; however, careful evaluation of mechanical dyssynchrony may inform management strategies. In this article, some of the methods and supporting evidence for dyssynchrony assessment with MRI as a predictor for CRT response are presented. The case is made for pre-implant assessment with MRI because of its ability to characterize scar, coronary venous distribution, and regional strain patterns.

Investigative works of the past 20 years have compiled extensive data on the effectiveness and implications of cardiac resynchronization therapy (CRT) in patients with heart failure. Since then, CRT has become a well-accepted and widely adapted adjunctive therapy for patients with heart failure with ventricular dyssynchrony. This overview discusses the updated knowledge on the benefits afforded with CRT and reviews the major clinical trials that have established CRT at its current practice. Based on the data, the indications of CRT and the timing of appropriate implant of CRT devices with respect to heart failure status will be presented.

Implantation of cardiac resynchronization therapy devices represents one of the more challenging and time-consuming procedures for the clinical electrophysiologist. This article reviews several strategies used to improve efficiency, safety, and effectiveness of cardiac resynchronization therapy implantation. The cornerstone of our strategy to improve efficiency, safety, and quality of cardiac resynchronization therapy implantation is the use of a telescoping guide system with high-quality venography. Competency in subclavian venoplasty and snaring techniques are essential to maintain efficiency and effectiveness during difficult cases.

The EP Clinics article "How to implant CRT devices in a busy clinical practice" describes the basics of the "interventional telescoping technique". This article focuses on specific circumstances where the tools and techniques are invaluable: (1) inability to locate the coronary sinus (CS), (2) inability to advance a catheter into the CS, (3) patients with CS atresia, (4) unstable CS access, (4) angulated target veins, (5) small and/or tortuous target veins, (6) target veins into which a wire cannot be advanced, (7) target veins with a drain pipe takeoff, (8) target veins close to the CS ostium.

Following CRT Patients Long-term

Although cardiac resynchronization therapy (CRT) will improve symptoms and survival in selected heart failure patients, there still remains a high percentage of CRT recipients who do not obtain benefit from the therapy. During CRT follow-up, an effort should be made to identify and to treat reversible causes of nonresponse to CRT. This effort includes optimization of medical therapy, checking for appropriate and effective biventricular pacing, and treatment of arrhythmias and other reversible causes of CRT malfunction.

This article provides a general overview of the underlying mechanisms that support pacing from more discrete points and/or a wider vector (multisite and multipoint pacing) to improve left ventricular resynchronization. We performed a critical overview of the current literature and to identify some remaining knowledge gaps to spur further research. It was not our goal to provide a systematic review with a comprehensive bibliography, but rather to focus on selected publications that, in our opinion, have either expertly reviewed a specific aspect of cardiac resynchronization therapy or have been landmark studies in the field.

Cardiac resynchronization therapy (CRT) has been shown to have a multitude of beneficial effects in select patients with systolic heart failure, by enhancing reverse remodeling, improving quality of life and functional status, reducing risk of heart failure admission, and most importantly, improving survival. Although women were underrepresented in the clinical trials, they were demonstrated to derive greater therapeutic benefit from CRT compared with men. Importantly, women were noted to derive benefit at a lesser degree of QRS prolongation than men, well below the now generally accepted cutoff of QRS ≥ 150 milliseconds.

Remote monitoring has become an essential component of the care of patients with a cardiac implantable electronic device, including those undergoing cardiac resynchronization therapy–defibrillator implantations. It allows for earlier detection of battery- and lead-related issue, atrial and ventricular arrhythmias, and may facilitate early identification of patients at risk for developing an exacerbation of heart failure. The data for the clinical utility of remote monitoring have been mixed. Additional studies are ongoing to determine how best to detect heart failure in these patients and how best to manage these patients based on the information.

Cardiac resynchronization therapy (CRT) has become the gold standard for patients with systolic left ventricular function, left ventricular ejection fraction less than or equal to 35%, wide complex QRS, and symptomatic heart failure. Annual implantation volume has steadily increased because of expanding indications for CRT. Improved survival resulted in many of these patients having their CRT devices for many years and eventually requiring an increased number of device-related procedures, including coronary sinus lead revisions and replacements following a coronary sinus lead extraction.

CRT in Special Populations

Cardiac resynchronization therapy has been proven to be clearly beneficial for patients with heart failure, a prolonged QRS duration, and a left ventricular ejection fraction ≤35%. Ejection fraction cutoff, however, is arbitrary and very likely excludes many patients who could benefit from cardiac resynchronization. This article describes the major detrimental effects of left bundle branch block and summarizes the data regarding the potential beneficial effects of cardiac resynchronization in patients with a left ventricular ejection fraction greater than 35%.

There remains a great deal of uncertainty whether general application of cardiac resynchronization therapy (CRT) to patients with atrial fibrillation (AF) provides any benefit assuming all other eligibility criteria are met. Preliminary observations suggest that performing atrioventricular junction ablation can improve the results of CRT in patients with AF by rendering the patient pacemaker dependent. Ongoing randomized clinical trials may provide more definitive answers in the future.

Emerging Pacing Technologies in Heart Failure

Alan Hanley and E. Kevin Heist

Several clinical trials have established the role of cardiac resynchronization therapy in patients with heart failure, impaired left ventricular function and dyssynchrony. Challenges to traditional therapy include coronary sinus anatomy and failure to respond. Left ventricular endocardial pacing could overcome anatomic constraints, provide more flexibility, and allow for more physiologic activation. Cases and case series have demonstrated the promise of the approach. Preclinical studies support the superior hemodynamic effects of left ventricular endocardial pacing. Leadless left ventricular endocardial pacing is a recent innovation that is undergoing prospective testing. Successful delivery may be associated with clinical response and positive cardiac structural remodeling.

Parikshit S. Sharma and Pugazhendhi Vijayaraman

Permanent His bundle pacing (PHBP) has shown significant clinical benefits in patients requiring ventricular pacing compared with conventional right ventricular pacing. There is an emerging role for PHBP in patients with interventricular dyssynchrony. This article reviews the mechanisms and the available data on the use of PHBP in overcoming dyssynchrony.

CARDIAC ELECTROPHYSIOLOGY CLINICS

Foreword
Cardiac Resynchronization Therapy

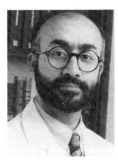
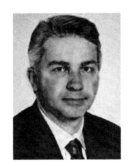

Ranjan K. Thakur, MD, MPH, MBA, FHRS   Andrea Natale, MD, FACC, FHRS

Consulting Editors

Heart failure (HF) incidence and prevalence are rising with associated morbidity, mortality, and health care costs. The mix of HF is changing as well; HF with preserved ejection fraction (EF) is increasing, for which there is no specific treatment. Health care costs for HF management is a huge issue, and new approaches to avoid hospitalizations by early detection and intervention are being evaluated.

Over the last three decades, tremendous progress has been made to establish evidence-based, optimal medical therapy (OMT) for HF with reduced EF. However, OMT is often not enough, and cardiac resynchronization therapy (CRT) has been established in patients who are not well controlled with pharmacologic therapy.

Technological advances have paved the way for increasing implantation success rates. However, there are many lacunae in our understanding, and newer approaches are being investigated to select patients so that CRT can be more effective. His-bundle pacing is emerging as a new approach, which may prove to be very promising in HF patients.

We want to congratulate Drs Singh and Dandamudi for editing this issue of *Cardiac Electrophysiology Clinics*, providing a contemporary review of what we know, the future challenges, and new frontiers in CRT for HF. They have assembled experts in this field to provide state-of-the-art reviews to explore these ideas, which the readers will find useful.

Ranjan K. Thakur, MD, MPH, MBA, FHRS
Sparrow Thoracic and Cardiovascular Institute
Michigan State University
1440 East Michigan Avenue, Suite 400
Lansing, MI 48912, USA

Andrea Natale, MD, FACC, FHRS
Texas Cardiac Arrhythmia Institute
Center for Atrial Fibrillation at
St. David's Medical Center
1015 East 32nd Street, Suite 516
Austin, TX 78705, USA

E-mail addresses:
thakur@msu.edu (R.K. Thakur)
andrea.natale@stdavids.com (A. Natale)

Preface

Evolving Strategies in Heart Failure Management: An Eye Toward Cardiac Resynchronization Therapy

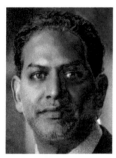 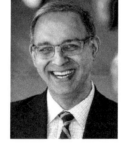

Gopi Dandamudi, MD   Jagmeet P. Singh, MD, PhD
Editors

Over the years, the economic pressures related to access and cost of care for heart failure (HF) patients have started to strain medical practices globally. Stringent criteria, such as length of stay and 30-day readmission rates, have become ubiquitous in the medical jargon. Reimbursements have been specifically tied to such measures, resulting in significant cost pressures on health care systems. As the global population ages, the incidence of HF has continued to rise, and this has forced medical communities to concoct innovative solutions to try to curb the rising health care costs. Such innovations have included programs such as the medical home, where care has shifted from the hospital to the outpatient setting and specifically into patients' homes, and the use of multidisciplinary teams, such as social workers, health care providers, and nurse navigators, to coordinate complex care to avoid hospital admissions, reduce morbidity, and ultimately, conserve expensive medical resources.

The role of cardiac resynchronization therapy (CRT) has also evolved over the years. Earlier attempts had resulted in less than ideal success rates in achieving clinically meaningful ventricular synchrony and improved outcomes. Over time, with better understanding of the substrate and also with increasing investments, we have improved our success rates dramatically. With the introduction of quadripolar leads, success rates have approached 96% in some publications. Also, the role of CRT in reducing both morbidity and mortality in patients with left ventricular (LV) systolic dysfunction and wide left bundle branch block is unquestioned. However, the majority of patients with HF do not qualify for CRT therapy based on current evidence and clinical criteria.

In this issue we have had the privilege of enlisting preeminent leaders in the management of HF. The topics are aligned in a systematic fashion. We start out by describing the complexity of HF and its current toll on medical costs and contemporary treatment strategies. The role of CRT is discussed in detail along with strategies on how to achieve a successful implant in a busy clinical

Card Electrophysiol Clin 11 (2019) xv–xvi
https://doi.org/10.1016/j.ccep.2019.01.001
1877-9182/19/© 2019 Published by Elsevier Inc.

practice. A detailed discussion is also provided on how to manage patients with CRT and emphasizes the growing role of remote monitoring. The role of cardiac magnetic resonance in assessing dyssynchrony is also discussed. CRT in special populations (near preserved LV systolic function and chronic atrial fibrillation) is addressed in subsequent articles. Finally, emerging pacing technologies in HF, such as leadless pacing and permanent His bundle pacing, are highlighted at the end of the issue to inform the readers of the exciting technologies that are on the horizon.

We want to thank all the authors who have contributed with genuine enthusiasm to this issue and also the editors for granting us the opportunity to serve as guest editors. Finally, no contribution is possible without the patience and the sacrifice of our families, who continue to support our clinical and research endeavors.

Sincerely,

Gopi Dandamudi, MD
Medical Director, Cardiovascular Service Line
Cardiology
CHI-Franciscan Health System
Tacoma, WA, USA

Jagmeet P. Singh, MD, PhD
Cardiology
Massachusetts General Hospital
Boston, MA 02114, USA

E-mail addresses:
gdandamu@iu.edu (G. Dandamudi)
JSINGH@mgh.harvard.edu (J.P. Singh)

Heart Failure and Why it Matters

Economic Impact of Chronic Heart Failure Management in Today's Cost-Conscious Environment

Chonyang Albert, MD[a], Jerry D. Estep, MD[b,c],*

KEYWORDS

- QALY • Cost-effectiveness • CMS • Readmissions

KEY POINTS

- It is projected 1 in 33 Americans will have heart failure by 2030.
- Heart failure with preserved ejection fraction is nearly as common and as morbid as heart failure with reduced ejection fraction.
- Cost reduction in heart failure management has been focused on reduction of readmissions and streamlining transitions of care.
- Innovations in device therapy such as defibrillators and ventricular assist devices continue to demonstrate promising improvements in cost-effectiveness.
- Understanding the complex interplay of patient factors, health care utilization, and cost-effectiveness of various interventions will enable the clinic to deliver high-quality, cost-effective care.

DEFINING THE SCOPE

Heart failure (HF) is a global pandemic that affects an estimated 26 million people worldwide.[1] In the United States, the prevalence of HF has increased from 5.7 million to 6.5 million in the past 5 years,[2] and there are 670,000 new cases per year.[3] Of those newly diagnosed with HF, approximately half (53%) have HF with reduced ejection fraction (HFrEF), whereas 47% are diagnosed with HF with preserved ejection fraction (HFpEF).[2] Because of increased longevity, it has been projected that by 2030, more than 8 million people in the United States (1 in 33) will have HF.[4,5] Accordingly, between 2012 and 2030, the total projected medical cost of HF is expected to increase from $21 billion to $53 billion annually (**Fig. 1**). Despite advancement in care, mortality remains high, especially after the first sentinel admission for HF management. The 5-year mortality after HF diagnosis remains at approcimately 50%.[6,7] Implementation of evidence-based HF therapies including medications and implantable cardioverter defibrillators has the potential to significantly reduce HF mortality.[8] This review provides an overview of the cost of HF management, discusses strategies for reducing cost with a focus on readmissions and transitions of care, and explores innovative strategies for reducing cost.

[a] Section of Heart Failure and Transplantation, Tomsich Family Department of Cardiovascular Medicine, Sydell and Arnold Miller Family Heart & Vascular Institute, Cleveland Clinic Foundation, Mail Code J3-4 9500 Euclid Avenue, Cleveland, OH 44195, USA; [b] Department of Cardiovascular Medicine, Cleveland Clinic, 9500 Euclid Avenue, Cleveland, OH 44106, USA; [c] Heart and Vascular Institute, Kaufman Center for Heart Failure, Cleveland Clinic, 9500 Euclid Avenue, Cleveland, OH 44106, USA
* Corresponding author. Department of Cardiovascular Medicine, Cleveland Clinic, 9500 Euclid Avenue, Cleveland, OH 44106, USA.
E-mail address: estepj@ccf.org

Card Electrophysiol Clin 11 (2019) 1–9
https://doi.org/10.1016/j.ccep.2018.11.002

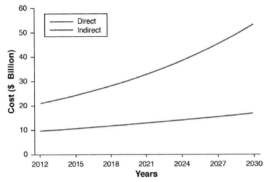

Fig. 1. Projected increase in both direct and indirect costs of HF from 2012 to 2030. (*Adapted from* Heidenreich PA, Albert NM, Allen LA, et al. Forecasting the impact of heart failure in the United States: a policy statement from the American Heart Association. Circ Heart Fail 2013;6(3):608; with permission.)

OVERALL COSTS

The cost of HF is multifaceted and encompasses direct cost of care with regard to inpatient admissions, outpatient care, and transitions of care, as well as indirect costs to individuals including opportunity costs of work days lost while ill or hospitalized or early mortality. In the United States and European countries, the cost of HF is composed of the following avenues: hospital care (60%), nursing home (13%), home health care (9%), medications (9%), and physicians (7%)[9,10] (**Fig. 2**). Several economic models have been proposed to evaluate the economics of health care.[11] Quality-adjusted life year (QALY), is a calculation of the economic value or impact of a medical intervention (**Table 1**). QALY is both a function of the quantity (or length) of life as well as the perceived quality of life. A year of life lived in perfect health is defined as 1 QALY (1 year of life × 1 utility value). Conversely, death is defined as zero QALY, and it is possible to have negative QALY for quality of life deemed to be "worse than death."[12] QALY analysis is often used for cost-effectiveness analysis in health care economics. Cost-utility ratio is another proposed model for evaluation of HF interventions.[13]

Inpatient Costs

HF is the leading cause of hospitalizations in the United States, representing 1% to 2% of all hospitalizations, amounting to more than 1 million admissions per year.[3,14] An actuarial analysis of the burden of HF in the Medicare Fee for Service Population reveals the average cost per HF admission to be $11,840 compared with $1208 for an emergency room visit without admission and $3189

for an admission to the observation unit.[15] Not only does hospitalization for HF significantly add to the costs of caring for this patient population, it also predicts higher risk of mortality.[16–18] Compared with patients with uncomplicated treatment course, those who experience inpatient worsening of HF are at the highest risk of mortality and increased health care utilization.[19] A lifetime analysis that followed newly discharged patients with HF enrolled in the Enhanced Feedback for Effective Cardiac Treatment phase 1 (EFFECT) study found the 10-year mortality rate to be 98.8% without significant differences in rate of rehospitalizations between the HFpEF and HFrEF cohorts.[20] In addition, 52.3% of cardiovascular readmissions in these cohorts occurred during the last decile of cohort survival duration, indicating high utilization of health care resources near the end of life.

A study of national trends in HF hospitalization and mortality rates for Medicare beneficiaries from 1998 to 2008 revealed a relative decline of HF admissions of 29.5% after adjusting for age, sex, and race.[21] Risk-adjusted 1-year mortality also demonstrated a modest relative decline of 6.6% from 31.7% to 29.6% in the 10-year study period. However, this study also unveiled racial disparities, with black men demonstrating the lowest rate of decline in HF hospitalizations. A corroborating finding from the 2017 American Heart Association (AHA) Heart Disease and Stroke Statistics update indicates black men encompass the highest proportion of hospitalized patients with HFrEF (70%), whereas white women constitute the highest proportion of those hospitalized with HFpEF (59%).[2] An analysis of 78,801 patients participating in the AHA's Get with the Guidelines-HF program found that although hospitalized black and Hispanic patients tended to be younger and have more comorbidities, the in-hospital mortality rate was actually lower in these 2 populations.[22] In a study comparing Hispanic patients with preserved versus reduced ejection fraction (EF) when compared with a non-Hispanic white cohort, Hispanic patients with preserved EF fared better than their non-Hispanic white counterparts, but this difference was not seen in patients with reduced EF.[23] Further exploring these discrepant findings may lead to improvement in outcomes in all patients with HF, in particular for those patients who face socioeconomic barriers to care.

Readmissions

Annually, Medicare pays $17.4 billion in unplanned readmissions, most of which are HF related.[24] In

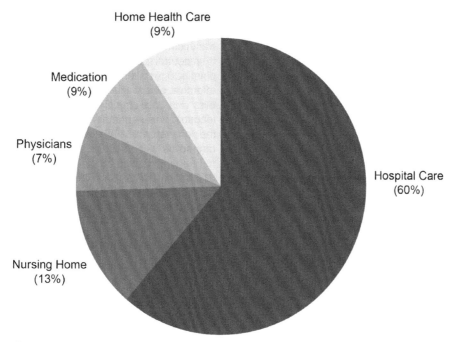

Fig. 2. Distribution of costs for HF management in the United States. (*Adapted from* Braunschweig F, Cowie MR, Auricchio A. What are the costs of heart failure. Europace 2011;13 Suppl 2:ii15; with permission.)

an effort to improve quality of care and curb health care cost, there has been a national effort to reduce 30-day admissions in a variety of diagnoses, including HF. Effective October 1, 2012, Section 3025 of the Affordable Care Act was addended with section 1886(q), establishing the Hospital Readmissions Reduction Program and requiring the Centers for Medicare and Medicare Services (CMS) to reduce payments to inpatient prospective payment system hospitals with excess of readmissions for HF. In response, health systems have implemented a variety of initiatives

to attempt to curb 30-day readmissions, these interventions are further discussed in the section "Reducing Readmissions" under "Cost-saving measures."

Several studies have failed to demonstrate a link between reducing length of stay and increasing HF readmissions, which suggest that these are not mutually competing objectives. A large study of 129 veterans hospitals during a 14-year span found that during the study period, hospital length of stay was reduced simultaneously as 30-day hospital readmission rate.[25] Another large,

Table 1
Comparison of select interventions in heart failure and estimated quality-adjusted life years in US dollars

Interventions	Estimated Dollars per QALY	Source
Cardiac rehabilitation	$668–$16,118	Papadakis et al,[67] 2005
CardioMEM PA monitor device	$12, 262	Martinson et al,[75] 2017
Ivabradine	$24,920	Kansal et al,[80] 2016
Sacubitril-Valsartan	$50,915	Ollendorf et al[33]
Implantable cardioverter defibrillators	$37,031–$138,458	Sanders et al,[81] 2010
Addition of CRT to ICD	$61,700	Woo et al,[82] 2015
Orthotopic heart transplantation	<$100,000	Long et al[29]
LVAD destination therapy	$202,000	Long et al[29]
Bridge-to-transplant LVAD	$266,000	Long et al[29]

Abbreviations: CRT, cardiac resynchronization therapy; ICD, implantable cardioverter defibrillator; LVAD, left-ventricular assist device; PA, pulmonary artery; QALY, quality-adjusted life year.

multicenter cohort study of length of stay corroborated that long length of stay is associated with increased rates of all-cause readmission and mortality.[26] These findings suggest reducing hospital length of stay does not compromise patient care by subsequently increasing 30-day readmissions.

Special Populations

Advanced heart failure and therapeutics

Patients with HF with circulatory collapse and cardiogenic shock require rapid escalation of care, which may include intravenous inotropes, vasopressors, and temporary or durable mechanical circulatory support. In hospital, worsening HF requiring escalation of care to inotropes or mechanical support portends a poor prognosis with increased mortality and/or cardiovascular/renal events.[27] A cost analysis of advanced therapies with sensitivity analysis found orthotopic heart transplantation to be most cost-effective with <$100,000 QALY, versus bridge-to-transplantation left-ventricular assist device (LVAD) ($266,000 QALY), and destination LVAD ($202,000 QALY) assuming average survival of 4.4 years with destination LVAD, 8.5 years with cardiac transplantation, and 12.3 years with bridge-to-transplant strategy.[28] Although bridge-to-transplantation LVAD is estimated to offer more than 3.8 additional life-years for patients waiting ≥6 months, it does not currently meet conventional cost-effectiveness thresholds. Because cardiac transplantation yields the longest survival advantage, it is deemed the most cost-effective.

Several studies have sought to evaluate the cost-effectiveness of mechanical circulatory support (MCS) in the advanced HF population; however, they may not account for advances in technology with development of pulsatile-flow devices and magnetically elevated impellers. A 2006 study of older generation devices including Heart-Mate (Thoratec Corp, Pleasanton, CA), MicroMed Debakey (Micromed, Houston, Texas), and Jarvik Device (Jarvik Heart, New York, New York, Inc.) failed to demonstrate cost-effectiveness of these ventricular assist devices as a bridge to transplantation.[29] A Dutch meta-analysis of cost-effectiveness using older generation continuous-flow LVADs as well as pulsatile-flow HeartMate II (Thoratec Corp) LVAD as destination therapy failed to demonstrate cost-effectiveness ratio below established cutoffs.[30] A willingness to pay threshold of roughly $59,000 per QALY has been used for cost-effective analysis.[31] As a comparison, the cost-effective analysis of sacubitril-valsartan, a novel medication combining valsartan with a neprilysin inhibitor, is estimated to be $50,915 per QALY.[32]

A systemic review of the cost-effectiveness of MCS including 7 studies of MCS as bridge to transplantation, 3 studies of MCS as destination therapy, and one study that evaluated both strategies suggested that MCS is likely not cost-effective when analyzed using accepted thresholds of cost-effectiveness.[33] Nunes and colleagues[33] found incremental cost-effectiveness ratios between MCS and medical management ranged between $85,025 and $200,166 for bridge to transplantation and between $87,622 and $1,257,946 for destination therapy in 2012 Canadian dollars per QALY. Furthermore, sensitivity analysis suggest that improving quality of life and reductions in device and initial hospital-stay costs may improve the cost-effectiveness of MCS. The HeartMate III (Thoratec) has demonstrated innovations in LVAD durability and reduction in stroke, which may improve cost-effectiveness.[34,35] Emerging data from cost-effectiveness analysis of the HeartMate III ventricular assist device suggests superiority of this device from the older generation HeartMate II at reduction of rehospitalizations, hospital days spent during rehospitalizations leading to a 51% cost savings of VAD implant.[35] The 2-year outcomes of the MOMENTUM 3 trial of the HeartMate III VAD also demonstrate superiority of the HeartMate III with regard to survival free of disabling stroke or reoperations for pump malfunction.[36]

Elderly patients and end-of-life care

Elderly patients with HF provide special challenges. More than 80% of Medicare beneficiaries with HF are hospitalized within the last 6 months of life, with nearly 40% of patients ultimately using Hospice care.[37,38] Transition of care may be especially important in the aging population of patients with HF, and a study of 6 Philadelphia academic and community hospitals found that discharge planning intervention with advanced practice nurses with home follow-up protocol effectively reduced health care costs and readmissions.[39] Optimization of care plan, especially near the end of life, may present an opportunity to further improve care and reduce cost.

COST-SAVING MEASURES
Inpatient Cost Reduction

Inpatient escalation of care of the treatment of HF can be costly.[40] To reduce costs of inpatient care, focus should be placed on early identification of patients at highest risk of decompensation, streamlining the delivery of care, and adherence to national HF guidelines. Renal failure is one of the strongest predictors of HF mortality and morbidity, including readmissions.[41] The PRO-TECT 7-day risk model has been proposed to identify inpatients admitted with acute HF with highest risk of 7-day death, HF rehospitalization, or worsening HF.[42] The strongest clinical predictor in the PROTECT 7 model is elevated blood urea nitrogen concentration. There is ample evidence that target doses of guideline-directed medications in the HFrEF population is both cost-effective and improves patient survival.[8,43,44] Thus, initiatives such as "Get with the Guidelines" have been promoted by the AHA to improve adherence to national HF recommendations.

Reducing Readmissions

Readmissions for HF are common and are costly, thus making it a major area of focus in HF care improvement. The National Strategy for Quality Improvement in Health Care of CMS identifies readmissions from HF as major priority for improvement, and the Affordable Care Act have launched major initiatives aimed reducing readmissions and improving health care delivery.[45] As a result, data from 3387 hospitals between 2007 and 2015 have demonstrated significant reductions in readmissions in target and nontarget conditions.[46]

A study of Medicare patients indicates that prior all-cause admissions within 12 months of an index admission for HF is a strong predictor of 30-day all-cause readmission.[47] A 3-phase terrain of readmission risk after index HF hospitalization has been proposed by Chun and colleagues[20] with the highest risk of readmissions the first 4 months after discharge and the last months of life.[48] However, validated risk-standardized statistical models to predict readmissions after HF hospitalization are lacking.[49] Moreover, to some extent, a higher readmission rate may be a consequence of successful care based on the observation that a higher occurrence of readmissions after index admissions for HF was associated with lower adjusted 30-day mortality given the competing risk of death during the index episode of care.[50]

Nevertheless, many strategies have been proposed to reduce 30-day readmissions, such as focus on improving transitions of care, outpatient monitoring, and early identification of exacerbation.[51,52] Early physician follow-up after discharge reduces 30-day readmissions among Medicare beneficiaries.[53] A goal of follow-up appointment within 7 days of discharge has been put forth by the "Get with the Guidelines" initiative. Innovations in interdisciplinary care in the immediate postdischarge period, including nursing phone calls, discharge planning, and clinical pharmacy medication reconciliation, have demonstrated efficacy in reducing repeat hospitalizations.[54] Discharge education materials and tools are increasingly used and refined in an effort to further bridge the gap of patient education.[55]

Improving Transitions of Care

The goal of outpatient HF management is to improve quality of life, mitigate symptoms of HF, and prevent clinical deterioration that would necessitate readmission. A smooth transition from inpatient to outpatient care is essential to ensure outpatient success and includes strategies aimed at patient education and empowerment, medication reconciliation, and outpatient access to care.[56–58] Nursing lead transition of care programs have shown promise at reducing 30-day readmissions and reducing an average $227 per Medicare patient with HF in a pilot study.[59] Care Transitions Interventions have also demonstrated efficacy at reducing readmissions.[60] However, attention also should be paid to the influence of socioeconomic status (SES), as low SES has been shown to be correlated with increased risk of readmissions.[61] Special attention should be paid to provide patients with adequate social support and empower them with the knowledge to provide self-care.[62]

Improving Outpatient Adherence and Quality of Life

Strategies to improve outpatient care should involve the multidisciplinary care team, including physicians, nurses, pharmacists, social work, and family members. Patient compliance with HF medications and life-style modifications is also of paramount importance.[63] A single-center trial randomizing a clinical pharmacist to outpatient HF clinic in addition to usual care demonstrated reduction in all-cause mortality and cardiovascular events.[64] Patients randomized to the intervention arm with clinical pharmacist were more likely to be on higher doses of angiotensin-converting enzyme inhibitors, and patients on angiotensin-converting enzyme inhibitor were more likely to have been prescribed alternate vasodilators. Another single-center study randomized patients to a multidisciplinary outpatient HF approach, including an HF physician and nurse with an algorithm for medication dose titration versus standard care demonstrated 6-month reduction in combined events of hospitalization and death with similar cost of care.[65] By reducing readmissions, multidisciplinary approaches to outpatient HF management have demonstrated significant cost savings.[66] Cardiac rehabilitation also should be strongly considered, as it is a cost-effective intervention that also improves quality of life.[67]

Technologic advancements have raised the possibility of remote monitoring of patients at home to prevent HF exacerbations and readmissions.[68] The initial data with noninvasive home telemonitoring have not been very promising. The BEAT-HF trial, which randomized patients to home electronic monitoring and telephone coaching versus usual care, failed to show a significant reduction in 30-day or 180-day readmissions.[69] Several interventions, including video-based nursing visits[70] and self-management classes,[71] also have failed to show significant reductions in readmissions. Attempts have been made to use intrathoracic impedances from implantable cardioverter defibrillator/cardiac resynchronization therapy devices to guide HF management, although studies have yet to demonstrate a significant improvement in HF outcomes.[72,73] The CHAMPION trial randomized patients with both HFpEF and HFrEF to implantable wireless pulmonary artery pressure monitoring devices (CardioMEM) versus standard of care, and it demonstrated an impressive 50% reduction in hospitalization rate in patients receiving the CardioMEM device.[74] This trial highlights the possibility of device guided remote monitoring aiding outpatient titration of medications to circumvent HF exacerbation. The incremental cost-effectiveness of a CardioMEM device has been estimated to be $12,262 per QALY[75] and deemed cost-effective in the United States and United Kingdom.[76]

FUTURE DIRECTIONS

Health care reform has and will continue to focus on quality improvement and cost reduction through various complex policy initiatives that have been proposed including bundled payments, accountable care organizations, pay-for-performance, and value-based purchasing programs.[77,78] The American College of Cardiology/AHA Task Force on Performance Measures have been developed to objectively gauge hospital performance.[79] There is an increasing recognition that 30-day readmission may be an imperfect target for improvement, and better metrics of health care quality are being developed.[24] Technologic innovations in virtual-based clinic visits and remote monitoring as well as artificial intelligence–based risk stratification are in the process of development and may play an ever more prominent role in the care of patients with HF. As new technologies develop in the treatment of HF, and as prevalence of HF increases with an aging population, it is imperative we carefully consider the cost-effectiveness of new therapies. Better understanding of the complex interplay of HF economics will enable clinicians to deliver high-quality, cost-effective HF care.

REFERENCES

1. Ambrosy AP, Fonarow GC, Butler J, et al. The global health and economic burden of hospitalizations for heart failure: lessons learned from hospitalized heart failure registries. J Am Coll Cardiol 2014;63: 1123–33.
2. Benjamin EJ, Blaha MJ, Chiuve SE, et al. Heart disease and stroke statistics-2017 update: a report from the American Heart Association. Circulation 2017;135:e146–603.
3. Go AS, Mozaffarian D, Roger VL, et al. Heart disease and stroke statistic—2013 update: a report from the American Heart Association. Circulation 2013;127:e6–245.
4. Heidenreich PA, Albert NM, Allen LA, et al. Forecasting the impact of heart failure in the United States: a policy statement from the American Heart Association. Circ Heart Fail 2013;6: 606–19.
5. Barker WH, Mullooly JP, Getchell W. Changing incidence and survival for heart failure in a well-defined older population, 1970–1974 and 1990–1994. Circulation 2006;113:799–805.
6. Bui AL, Horwich TB, Fonarow GC. Epidemiology and risk profile of heart failure. Nat Rev Cardiol 2011;8: 30–41.
7. Levy D, Kenchaiah S, Larson MG, et al. Long-term trends in the incidence of and survival with heart failure. NEJM 2002;347:1397–402.
8. Fonarow GC, Yancy CW, Hernandez AF, et al. Potential impact of optimal implementation of evidence-based heart failure therapies on mortality. Am Heart J 2011;161:1024–30.e3.
9. Braunschweig F, Cowie MR, Auricchio A. What are the costs of heart failure? Europace 2011;13: ii13–7.
10. Dickstein K, Cohen-Solal A, Filippatos G, et al. ESC guidelines for the diagnosis and treatment of acute and chronic heart failure 2008: the Task Force for the diagnosis and treatment of acute and chronic heart failure 2008 of the European Society of Cardiology. Developed in collaboration with the heart failure association of the ESC (HFA) and endorsed by the European Society of Intensive care medicine (ESICM). Eur Heart J 2008;29:2388–442.
11. Goehler A, Geisler BP, Manne JM, et al. Decision-analytic models to simulate health outcomes and costs in heart failure: a systematic review. Pharmacoeconomics 2011;29:753–69.
12. Weinstein MC, Torrance G, McGuire A. QALYs: the basics. Value Health 2009;12:S5–9.

13. Capomolla S, Febo O, Ceresa M, et al. Cost/utility ratio in chronic heart failure: comparison between heart failure management program delivered by day-hospital and usual care. J Am Coll Cardiol 2002;40:1259–66.

14. Norton C, Georgiopoulou VV, Kalogeropoulos AP, et al. Epidemiology and cost of advanced heart failure. Prog Cardiovasc Dis 2011;54:78–85.

15. Fitch K, Engel T, Lau J. The cost burden of worsening heart failure in the medicare fee for service population: an actuarial analysis. 2017. Available at: http://us.milliman.com/uploadedFiles/insight/2017/cost-bruden-worsening-heart-failure.pdf.

16. Davison BA, Metra M, Cotter G, et al. Worsening heart failure following admission for acute heart failure: a pooled analysis of the PROTECT and RELAX-AHF studies. JACC Heart Fail 2015;3:395–403.

17. Setoguchi S, Stevenson LW, Schneeweiss S. Repeated hospitalizations predict mortality in the community population with heart failure. Am Heart J 2007;154:260–6.

18. Solomon SD, Dobson J, Pocock S, et al. Influence of nonfatal hospitalization for heart failure on subsequent mortality in patients with chronic heart failure. Circulation 2007;116:1482–7.

19. DeVore AD, Hammill BG, Sharma PP, et al. In-hospital worsening heart failure and associations with mortality, readmission, and healthcare utilization. J Am Heart Assoc 2014;3 [pii:e001088].

20. Chun S, Tu JV, Wijeysundera HC, et al. Lifetime analysis of hospitalizations and survival of patients newly admitted with heart failure. Circ Heart Fail 2012;5:414–21.

21. Chen J, Normand S-LT, Wang Y, et al. National and regional trends in heart failure hospitalization and mortality rates for Medicare beneficiaries: 1998–2008. JAMA 2011;306:1669–78.

22. Thomas KL, Hernandez AF, Dai D, et al. Association of race/ethnicity with clinical risk factors, quality of care, and acute outcomes in patients hospitalized with heart failure. Am Heart J 2011;161:746–54.

23. Vivo RP, Krim SR, Krim NR, et al. Care and outcomes of Hispanic patients admitted with heart failure with preserved or reduced ejection fraction: findings from Get with the Guidelines-heart failure. Circ Heart Fail 2012;5:167–75.

24. Gheorghiade M, Vaduganathan M, Fonarow GC, et al. Rehospitalization for heart failure: problems and perspectives. J Am Coll Cardiol 2013;61:391–403.

25. Kaboli PJ, Go JT, Hockenberry J, et al. Associations between reduced hospital length of stay and 30-day readmission rate and mortality: 14-year experience in 129 veterans affairs hospitals. Ann Intern Med 2012;157:837.

26. Sud M, Yu B, Wijeysundera HC, et al. Associations between short or long length of stay and 30-day readmission and mortality in hospitalized patients with heart failure. JACC Heart Fail 2017;5:578–88.

27. Mentz RJ, Metra M, Cotter G, et al. Early vs. late worsening heart failure during acute heart failure hospitalization: insights from the PROTECT trial. Eur J Heart Fail 2015;17:697–706.

28. Long EF, Swain GW, Mangi AA. Comparative survival and cost-effectiveness of advanced therapies for end-stage heart failure. Circ Heart Fail 2014;7:470–8.

29. Long EF, Swain GW, Mangi AA. Comparative Survival and Cost-Effectiveness of Advanced Therapies for End-Stage Heart Failure. Circ Heart Fail 2014;7(3):470–8.

30. Neyt M, Van den Bruel A, Smit Y, et al. The cost-utility of left ventricular assist devices for end-stage heart failure patients ineligible for cardiac transplantation: a systematic review and critical appraisal of economic evaluations. Ann Cardiothorac Surg 2014;3:439–49.

31. Hutchinson J, Scott DA, Clegg AJ, et al. Cost-effectiveness of left ventricular-assist devices in end-stage heart failure. Expert Rev Cardiovasc Ther 2008;6:175–85.

32. Ollendorf DA, Sandhu AT, Pearson SD. Sacubitril-valsartan for the treatment of heart failure: effectiveness and value. JAMA Intern Med 2016;176:249–50.

33. Ollendorf DA, Sandu AT, Pearson SD. Sacubitril-Valsartan for the treatnemtn of heart failure effectiveness and value. JAMA Intern Med 2016;176(2):249–50.

34. Uriel N, Colombo PC, Cleveland JC, et al. Hemocompatibility-related outcomes in the MOMENTUM 3 trial at 6 months: a randomized controlled study of a fully magnetically levitated pump in advanced heart failure. Circulation 2017;135:2003–12.

35. Mehra MR, Salerno C, Cleveland JC, et al. Healthcare resource use and cost implications in the MOMENTUM 3 long-term outcome study: a randomized controlled trial of a magnetically levitated cardiac pump in advanced heart failure. Circulation 2018. https://doi.org/10.1161/CIRCULATIONAHA.118.035722.

36. Mehra MR, Goldstein DJ, Uriel N, et al. Two-year outcomes with a magnetically levitated cardiac pump in heart failure. N Engl J Med 2018;378:1386–95.

37. Unroe KT, Greiner MA, Hernandez AF, et al. Resource use in the last 6 months of life among Medicare beneficiaries with heart failure, 2000-2007. Arch Intern Med 2011;171:196–203.

38. Bain KT, Maxwell TL, Strassels SA, et al. Hospice use among patients with heart failure. Am Heart J 2009;158:118–25.

39. Naylor MD, Brooten DA, Campbell RL, et al. Transitional care of older adults hospitalized with heart failure: a randomized, controlled trial. J Am Geriatr Soc 2018;52:675–84.

40. Cooper LB, DeVore AD, Felker GM. The impact of worsening heart failure in the United States. Heart Fail Clin 2015;11:603–14.

41. Patel UD, Greiner MA, Fonarow GC, et al. Associations between worsening renal function and 30-day outcomes among Medicare beneficiaries hospitalized with heart failure. Am Heart J 2010;160:132–8.e1.

42. O'Connor CM, Mentz RJ, Cotter G, et al. The PROTECT in-hospital risk model: 7-day outcome in patients hospitalized with acute heart failure and renal dysfunction. Eur J Heart Fail 2018;14:605–12.

43. Banka G, Heidenreich PA, Fonarow GC. Incremental cost-effectiveness of guideline-directed medical therapies for heart failure. J Am Coll Cardiol 2013; 61:1440–6.

44. Fonarow GC, Albert NM, Curtis AB, et al. Associations between outpatient heart failure process-of-care measures and mortality. Circulation 2011;123: 1601–10.

45. Kocher RP, Adashi EY. Hospital readmissions and the affordable care act: paying for coordinated quality care. JAMA 2011;306:1794–5.

46. Zuckerman RB, Sheingold SH, Orav EJ, et al. Readmissions, observation, and the hospital readmissions reduction program. N Engl J Med 2016. https://doi.org/10.1056/NEJMsa1513024.

47. Hummel SL, Katrapati P, Gillespie BW, et al. Impact of prior admissions on 30-day readmissions in Medicare heart failure inpatients. Mayo Clin Proc 2014; 89:623–30.

48. Desai AS. The three-phase terrain of heart failure readmissions. Circ Heart Fail 2012;5:398–400.

49. Ross JS, Mulvey GK, Stauffer B, et al. Statistical models and patient predictors of readmission for heart failure: a systematic review. Arch Intern Med 2008;168:1371–86.

50. Gorodeski EZ, Starling RC, Blackstone EH. Are all readmissions bad readmissions? N Engl J Med 2010. https://doi.org/10.1056/NEJMc1001882.

51. Bradley EH, Curry L, Horwitz LI, et al. Contemporary evidence about hospital strategies for reducing 30-day readmissions: a national study. J Am Coll Cardiol 2012;60:607–14.

52. Gorthi J, Hunter CB, Mooss AN, et al. Reducing heart failure hospital readmissions: a systematic review of disease management programs. Cardiol Res 2014;5:126–38.

53. Hernandez AF, Greiner MA, Fonarow GC, et al. Relationship between early physician follow-up and 30-day readmission among Medicare beneficiaries hospitalized for heart failure. JAMA 2010;303: 1716–22.

54. Jack BW, Chetty VK, Anthony D, et al. A reengineered hospital discharge program to decrease rehospitalization: a randomized trial. Ann Intern Med 2009;150:178–87.

55. Koelling TM, Johnson ML, Cody RJ, et al. Discharge education improves clinical outcomes in patients with chronic heart failure. Circulation 2005;111: 179–85.

56. Coleman EA, Smith JD, Raha D, et al. Posthospital medication discrepancies: prevalence and contributing factors. Arch Intern Med 2005;165:1842–7.

57. Coleman EA, Parry C, Chalmers S, et al. The care transitions intervention: results of a randomized controlled trial. Arch Intern Med 2006;166:1822–8.

58. Feltner C, Jones CD, Cené CW, et al. Transitional care interventions to prevent readmissions for persons with heart failure: a systematic review and meta-analysis. Ann Intern Med 2014;160:774.

59. Stauffer BD, Fullerton C, Fleming N, et al. Effectiveness and cost of a transitional care program for heart failure: a prospective study with concurrent controls. Arch Intern Med 2011;171:1238–43.

60. Voss R, Gardner R, Baier R, et al. The care transitions intervention: translating from efficacy to effectiveness. Arch Intern Med 2011;171:1232–7.

61. Bikdeli B, Wayda B, Bao H, et al. Place of residence and outcomes of patients with heart failure: analysis from the telemonitoring to improve heart failure outcomes trial. Circ Cardiovasc Qual Outcomes 2014; 7:749–56.

62. Gallagher R, Luttik M-L, Jaarsma T. Social support and self-care in heart failure. J Cardiovasc Nurs 2011;26:439–45.

63. van der Wal MH, van Veldhuisen DJ, Veeger NJ, et al. Compliance with non-pharmacological recommendations and outcome in heart failure patients. Eur Heart J 2010;31:1486–93.

64. Gattis WA, Hasselblad V, Whellan DJ, et al. Reduction in heart failure events by the addition of a clinical pharmacist to the heart failure management team: results of the pharmacist in heart failure assessment recommendation and monitoring (PHARM) study. Arch Intern Med 1999;159:1939–45.

65. Kasper EK, Gerstenblith G, Hefter G, et al. A randomized trial of the efficacy of multidisciplinary care in heart failure outpatients at high risk of hospital readmission. J Am Coll Cardiol 2002;39:471–80.

66. Ledwidge M, Barry M, Cahill J, et al. Is multidisciplinary care of heart failure cost-beneficial when combined with optimal medical care? Eur J Heart Fail 2003;5:381–9.

67. Papadakis S, Oldridge NB, Coyle D, et al. Economic evaluation of cardiac rehabilitation: a systematic review. Eur J Cardiovasc Prev Rehabil 2005;12:513–20.

68. Pandor A, Thokala P, Gomersall T, et al. Home telemonitoring or structured telephone support programmes after recent discharge in patients with heart failure: systematic review and economic evaluation. Health Technol Assess 2013;17:1–207, v–vi.

69. Ong MK, Romano PS, Edgington S, et al. Effectiveness of remote patient monitoring after discharge of hospitalized patients with heart failure: the better effectiveness after transition—heart failure (BEAT-HF) randomized clinical trial. JAMA Intern Med 2016;176:310–8.

70. Pekmezaris R, Mitzner I, Pecinka KR, et al. The impact of remote patient monitoring (telehealth) upon medicare beneficiaries with heart failure. Telemed J E Health 2012;18:101–8.

71. Powell LH, Calvin JE Jr, Richardson D, et al. Self-management counseling in patients with heart failure: the heart failure adherence and retention randomized behavioral trial. JAMA 2010;304:1331–8.

72. van Veldhuisen DJ, Braunschweig F, Conraads V, et al. Intrathoracic impedance monitoring, audible patient alerts, and outcome in patients with heart failure. Circulation 2011;124:1719–26.

73. Conraads VM, Tavazzi L, Santini M, et al. Sensitivity and positive predictive value of implantable intrathoracic impedance monitoring as a predictor of heart failure hospitalizations: the SENSE-HF trial. Eur Heart J 2011;32:2266–73.

74. Adamson PB, Abraham WT, Bourge RC, et al. Wireless pulmonary artery pressure monitoring guides management to reduce decompensation in heart failure with preserved ejection fraction. Circ Heart Fail 2014;7:935–44.

75. Martinson M, Bharmi R, Dalal N, et al. Pulmonary artery pressure guided heart failure management: US cost effectiveness analyses using the results of the CHAMPION clinical trial. Eur J Heart Fail 2017;19: 652–60.

76. Cowie MR, Simon M, Klein L, et al. The cost-effectiveness of real-time pulmonary artery pressure monitoring in heart failure patients: a European perspective. Eur J Heart Fail 2017;19:661–9.

77. Shih T, Chen LM, Nallamothu BK. Will bundled payments change health care? Examining the evidence thus far in cardiovascular care. Circulation 2015; 131:2151–8.

78. Eapen ZJ, Reed SD, Curtis LH, et al. Do heart failure disease management programs make financial sense under a bundled payment system? Am Heart J 2011;161:916–22.

79. Spertus JA, Eagle KA, Krumholz HM, et al. American College of Cardiology and American Heart Association methodology for the selection and creation of performance measures for quantifying the quality of cardiovascular care. Circulation 2005;111: 1703–12.

80. Kansal AR, Cowie MR, Kielhorn A, et al. Cost-effectiveness of ivabradine for heart failure in the United States. J Am Heart Assoc 2016;5 [pii:e003221].

81. Sanders GD, Kong MH, Al-Khatib SM, et al. Cost-effectiveness of implantable cardioverter defibrillators in patients > or =65 years of age. Am Heart J 2010;160:122–31.

82. Woo CY, Strandberg EJ, Schmiegelow MD, et al. Cost-effectiveness of adding cardiac resynchronization therapy to an implantable cardioverter-defibrillator among patients with mild heart failure. Ann Intern Med 2015;163:417–26.

The Many Faces of Heart Failure

David Snipelisky, MD[a], Sunit-Preet Chaudhry, MD[b], Garrick C. Stewart, MD[a],*

KEYWORDS

- Heart failure • Systolic dysfunction • Heart disease • Cardiomyopathy

KEY POINTS

- The diagnosis and treatment of heart failure require assessment of patient symptoms, physical examination, and cardiac function.
- Heart failure is a heterogeneous clinical syndrome that requires an individualized approach to treatment based on cause, ejection fraction (preserved or reduced), and symptom burden.
- Pathologic remodeling of the myocardium is a characteristic feature of heart failure with reduced ejection fraction, and evidence-based pharmacologic and device therapies can lead to its reversal.
- Complementary classification and staging schemes for heart failure have been developed to guide treatment decisions and prognosis.

Heart failure (HF) is a complex, heterogeneous syndrome that results from impairment of ventricular filling or ejection of blood associated with symptoms of dyspnea, fatigue, as well as peripheral and/or pulmonary edema.[1,2] HF is major and growing public health problem that leads to considerable morbidity and mortality, and the battle against HF is imposing an unprecedented cost burden on the health care system. Despite widespread deployment of evidence-based pharmacologic and device therapies, an unacceptable number of patients suffer impaired functional capacity, poor quality of life, and early death due to HF. The syndrome of HF can arise from cardiac lesions at any level, including the myocardium, vasculature, pericardium, heart valves, electrical system, or a combination of cardiac abnormalities. Patients with HF can experience a wide range of symptoms attributed to elevation in cardiac filling pressures and/or reduced cardiac output, ranging in severity from relatively asymptomatic to marked functional impairment.

Patients with HF are commonly stratified into 2 groups based on the contractile function of the left ventricular myocardium: HF with reduced ejection fraction (HFrEF) or HF with preserved ejection fraction (HFpEF).[3] Patients with HFrEF have a left ventricular ejection fraction (EF) less than 40% and have an inadequate stroke volume and cardiac output as the primary manifestation. In contrast, patients with HFpEF have relatively normal contractile abilities of the left ventricle (EF >50%) with pathophysiologic manifestations of the disease process defined by impaired relaxation of the left ventricle.[4,5] Patients with an EF ranging from 41% to 49% have been variably classified as either HFpEF or HFrEF but are now thought to represent a distinct entity referred to as HF with midrange ejection fraction (HFmrEF). This subset of patients, comprising between 13% and 24% of patients with HF, has clinical characteristics resembling the HFpEF population, although their incidence of coronary artery disease is similar to the cohort of patients with HFrEF.[6,7]

Conflicts of Interest/Disclosures: None of the authors have any conflicts of interest, financial or other, to disclose regarding this article.

a Division of Cardiovascular Medicine, Brigham and Women's Hospital, 75 Francis Street, Boston, MA 02115, USA; b Advanced Heart Failure and Transplant, St. Vincent Heart Center, 8333 Naab Road, Indianapolis, IN 46260, USA

* Corresponding author. Center for Advanced Heart Disease, Brigham and Women's Hospital, 75 Francis Street, Boston, MA 02115.

E-mail address: gcstewart@bwh.harvard.edu

Card Electrophysiol Clin 11 (2019) 11–20
https://doi.org/10.1016/j.ccep.2018.11.001
1877-9182/19/© 2018 Elsevier Inc. All rights reserved.

Furthermore, HFmrEF may describe a subset of patients that initially had HFrEF and then progressed to HFpEF.[8]

Other commonly used descriptors of HF include the primary chamber of involvement (left, right, biventricular), the abnormality in cardiac output (low-output or high-output HF), and the duration of onset (acute, chronic, acute on chronic). However, the predominant classification scheme endorsed by guidelines is HFrEF (systolic) and HFpEF (diastolic) because resting contractile function of the left ventricle is a key entry criterion for the clinical trials that define the evidence base for treating chronic HF.

INCIDENCE AND PREVALENCE

The incidence of HF in the United States is 2.4% and increases significantly with age, rising from 20 per 1000 people in individuals 65 to 69 years to greater than 80 per 1000 people among individuals 85 years and older.[9] Increasing rates of hypertension, diabetes mellitus, and improved survival following myocardial infarction have led to growing prevalence of patients living with chronic HF. An estimated 6.5 million Americans have been diagnosed with HF, with more than 650,000 new cases of HF identified each year. HF continues to be the leading discharge diagnosis for hospitalized patients 65 years or older.[9] The prevalence of this syndrome, which is responsible for 300,000 annual deaths with a 5-year mortality of 50%, is expected to increase by 46% by 2030, at which time 1 in 33 Americans will be living with HF.[10]

Over the past 15 years, the prevalence of HFpEF has increased and now equals that of HFrEF. Current data predict that HFpEF may become the predominant form of HF over the next decade. When compared with patients with HFrEF, patients with HFpEF are usually older, are more likely to be women, and have a higher rate of significant comorbidities, including hypertension, chronic kidney disease, pulmonary disease, and atrial fibrillation.[4] Advanced age, pulmonary hypertension, coronary artery disease, chronic kidney disease, and obesity can each impact myocardial performance and contribute to a syndrome of HFpEF.[11] For instance, despite elevated filling pressures being a pathognomonic finding in all patients with HFpEF, obese patients tend to have different cardiac filling characteristics and plasma volume expansion interactions that result in higher filling pressures compared with nonobese HFpEF patients.[12,13] Obesity and related insulin resistance appear to be more strongly associated with a risk of developing HFpEF compared with HFrEF, an effect particularly pronounced among women, which may in part underlie sex differences in HF subtypes.[14]

CLINICAL PRESENTATION

The clinical spectrum of HF is variable and is based on the specific underlying pathologic condition. Patients with HF may initially be asymptomatic for some time until functional remodeling of the heart has taken place. Alternatively, there can be injuries to the heart leading to acute HF, such as coronary ischemia, myocarditis, or acute valvular regurgitation. Once an initial insult to the myocardium occurs, various compensatory physiologic alterations take place to preserve cardiac output and function. Alterations in the renin-angiotensin-aldosterone system, natriuretic peptide system, and sympathetic tone result in an overall catabolic, proinflammatory state of oxidative stress that, over time, results in cardiac dysfunction and onset of symptoms. Prolonged hormonal and cytokine alterations result in skeletal and respiratory muscle atrophy and weakness, which further contribute to fatigue, dyspnea, and reduced exercise capacity[15] (**Fig. 1**).

The most common HF symptoms result from an increase in plasma volume, colloquially referred to as "congestion." However, it can be difficult to discern which symptoms experienced by a patient are primarily a result of HF, because many can overlap with other comorbid conditions. The most common symptom of left ventricular failure is shortness of breath, or dyspnea, which is usually associated with activity, although patients with either marked congestion or advanced stages of HF may experience dyspnea at rest. Another cardinal symptom is orthopnea, which is dyspnea when supine, or paroxysmal nocturnal dyspnea, in which patients wake at night and must sit upright to breathe comfortably. Orthopnea has been strongly associated with a markedly elevated pulmonary capillary wedge pressure.[16] Shortness of breath when bending over, or bendopnea, may occur as a result of increased preload to a heart with already elevated filling pressures. Patients with bendopnea have a 2-fold increase in orthopnea.[17] Right-sided HF symptoms, such as lower-extremity edema, abdominal distention, and worsening renal function, occur predominantly due to systemic venous congestion and/or low cardiac output, with the most common cause of increased right ventricular afterload being long-standing left-sided HF.[18]

DIAGNOSIS

HF is primarily a clinical diagnosis, encompassing patient symptoms, physical examination findings,

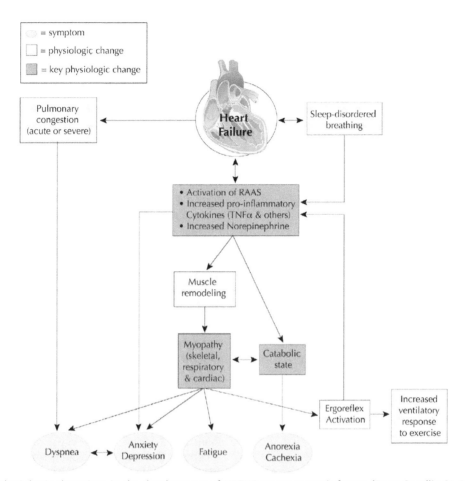

Fig. 1. Physiologic alterations in the development of HF. TNF, tumor necrosis factor. (*From* Goodlin SJ. Palliative care in congestive heart failure. J Am Coll Cardiol 2009;54:389; with permission.)

and diagnostic testing[1,5] (**Box 1**). Although almost half of patients with either severe systolic or diastolic dysfunction may not have overt evidence of HF, the diagnosis is generally entertained in the context of presenting symptoms of congestion.[19] The diagnosis of HF is made when a degree of heart dysfunction constructs a pathophysiologic state in which the heart is unable to provide sufficient output to maintain the body's metabolic demands.

Physical examination is crucial to the diagnosis of HF, because it provides evidence regarding the degree of volume overload, the extent of perfusion deficits, and the presence of concomitant circulatory pathologic conditions. On visual examination, patients may demonstrate evidence of congestion, including lower-extremity edema and abdominal ascites. Elevated jugular venous distension is a valuable indicator for HF but may not be present if an increase in right-sided pressures is absent.[20] An S3 gallop is highly specific for

reduced EF and elevated left-sided filling pressures. In patients with HFrEF, the presence of an audible S3 gallop and elevated jugular venous pressure on physical examination have been independently associated with adverse outcomes, including progression of HF.[21] Other important diagnostic findings include a displaced point of maximal impulse, palpable S3, and pulsus alternans.

Once a clinical diagnosis of HF is suspected based on history and physical examination, additional diagnostic evaluations are indicated. All patients should receive an electrocardiogram (ECG), which can identify arrhythmia, QRS prolongation indicative of dyssynchrony, elevated voltages, which can indicate chronic pressure overload, or underlying cardiomyopathy, leading to an increased ventricular mass, reduced QRS voltages suggestive of an infiltrative process, or pathologic Q waves or ST segment–T-wave abnormalities that can be indicative of coronary artery disease.

Box 1
Framingham criteria for the diagnosis of heart failure (to establish a diagnosis of heart failure, 2 major or 1 major and 2 minor criteria are required)

Major criteria

Paroxysmal nocturnal dyspnea or orthopnea

Neck-vein distension

Rales

Cardiomegaly

Acute pulmonary edema

S3 gallop

Increased venous pressure greater than 16 cm of water

Circulation time ≥25 seconds

Hepatojugular reflex

Minor criteria

Ankle edema

Night cough

Dyspnea on exertion

Hepatomegaly

Pleural effusion

Vital capacity ↓1/3 from maximum

Tachycardia (rate ≥120/min)

Major or minor criterion

Weight loss ≥4.5 kg in 5 days in response to treatment

---

as diabetes, hypertension, dyslipidemia, tobacco use, or family history of premature coronary artery disease, should undergo invasive or noninvasive evaluation for coronary disease.

Cardiac biomarkers, such as natriuretic peptides, high-sensitivity troponin, galectin-3, and cystatin-C, are also helpful in the diagnosis and prognostication in patients with HF.[26] Serial measurements of natriuretic peptides are often useful in assessing degree of response to therapies and prognosis after an HF hospitalization.[27,28] Biomarkers are not necessary to make the clinical diagnosis of HF, but can be a helpful adjunct when the physical examination is challenging or the clinical presentation is confounded by other comorbid conditions.[29] Other important evaluations include cardiac MRI, PET, and endomyocardial biopsy. These advanced diagnostic evaluations are more helpful in elucidating a cause for HF rather than establishing the diagnosis of the clinical syndrome.

CLASSIFICATION SCHEMES FOR HEART FAILURE

Considering symptoms of HF reflect the degree of mismatch between the heart's ability to pump blood and the body's metabolic needs, the syndrome is described in terms of a spectrum rather than as a single physiologic state.[30,31] The American College of Cardiology/American Heart Association (ACC/AHA) and New York Heart Association (NYHA) (**Table 1**) have established the 2 most commonly used classification systems. The NYHA classification system uses symptoms

In addition to routine ECG, echocardiographic parameters are integral in assessing the degree of ventricular dysfunction, extent of ventricular enlargement or dilatation, and presence of other structural abnormalities.[22,23] The left ventricular end-diastolic diameter is an important marker of cardiac remodeling and is independently related to the degree of HF.[24,25] Functional (secondary) mitral regurgitation may be produced by dilatation of the mitral annulus as a result of a dilated left ventricle and can improve with HF treatment. Collectively, these progressive maladaptive alterations in the size, shape, and contractile function of the ventricular myocardium are referred to as cardiac remodeling. Serial echocardiographic assessments are useful in quantifying therapeutic response because treatments shown to improve mortality in systolic HF have been linked to reverse remodeling of the left ventricle. Patients presenting with HF without established coronary artery disease but with atherosclerotic risk factors, such

Table 1
New York Heart Association classification of patients with heart failure

Class	Patient Symptoms
I	No limitation of physical activity; ordinary physical activity does not cause undue fatigue, palpitation, dyspnea
II	Slight limitation of physical activity; comfortable at rest; ordinary physical activity results in fatigue, palpitation, dyspnea
III	Marked limitation of physical activity; comfortable at rest; less than ordinary activity causes fatigue, palpitation, or dyspnea
IV	Unable to carry on any physical activity without discomfort; symptoms of HF at rest; if any physical activity is undertaken, discomfort increases

and exercise capacity to classify patients based on a simple history. NYHA functional class has been linked to prognosis and serves as a benchmark for entry into clinical trials of HF therapeutics.

In contrast, the ACC/AHA classification system places emphasize on the staging and development of disease, similar to the approach commonly used in oncology.[32] These HF stages progress from antecedent risk factors (stage A) to the development of subclinical cardiac dysfunction (stage B), then symptomatic HF (stage C), and finally, end-stage refractory disease (stage D). The NYHA functional class is labile in response to disease progression or HF treatments such as diuretics, whereas the ACC/AHA stages are progressive from stage A to stage D. Most recently, the Interagency Registry of Mechanically Assisted Circulatory Support patient profiles were developed to substratify patients with advanced HF who are undergoing consideration of durable mechanical support devices.[33] The profiles range from profile 1 (critical cardiogenic shock) to profile 7 (advanced ambulatory HF) and have been linked to outcomes after mechanical support as well as with medical therapy.[34,35] These complementary classification systems of HF are the basis for guideline-directed medical and device-based treatment strategies.[36,37]

ACUTE DECOMPENSATED HEART FAILURE

In addition to symptom burden and stage of HF, terminology is often deployed related to the tempo of clinical presentation. Chronic HF refers to patients with previous symptoms that have either resolved or may be ongoing. Such patients are at risk for decompensations, which often lead to hospitalizations, events of considerable prognostic importance. In contrast, acute HF can present de novo from acute myocardial dysfunction (eg, ischemia, myocarditis, valve insufficiency) and is a medical emergency. More commonly, however, acute HF episodes are a decompensation of chronic HF that can be triggered by one or more factors, such as concurrent infection, arrhythmia, uncontrolled hypertension, and nonadherence with drugs or dietary recommendations (**Box 2**). Patients with HF can be described as either "warm" or "cold," alluding to the ability to maintain appropriate perfusion, and "wet" or "dry," referring to their volume status[38] (**Fig. 2**). This simple bedside categorization of acute decompensated HF can be an important guide to initial therapy.

CAUSES OF CARDIOMYOPATHY

HF stems from an underlying cardiomyopathic insult that results in a heterogenous disease

---

Box 2
Factors triggering an episode of acute heart failure

Acute coronary syndromes

Tachyarrhythmias (eg, atrial fibrillation, ventricular tachycardia)

Excessive increase in blood pressure

Infection (eg, pneumonia, endocarditis, sepsis)

Nonadherence with salt/fluid intake or medications

Bradyarrhythmias

Toxic substances (alcohol, recreational drugs)

Drugs (eg, NSAIDs, corticosteroids, cardiotoxic chemotherapies, negative inotropes)

Exacerbations of chronic obstructive pulmonary disease

Pulmonary embolism

Surgery and perioperative complications

Increased sympathetic drive

Metabolic/hormonal derangements (eg, thyroid disturbance, pregnancy, adrenal insufficiency)

Cerebrovascular insult

Acute mechanical cause: myocardial rupture complicating ACS, chest trauma, cardiac intervention, acute valvular incompetence, aortic dissection or thrombosis

Abbreviations: ACS, acute coronary syndrome; NSAIDs, nonsteroidal anti-inflammatory drugs.
  Adapted from 2016 ESC guidelines for the diagnosis and management of acute and chronic heart failure. Eur Heart J 2016;37:2171; with permission.

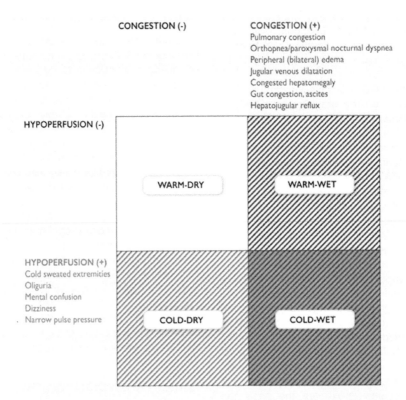

CONGESTION (-)

CONGESTION (+)
Pulmonary congestion
Orthopnea/paroxysmal nocturnal dyspnea
Peripheral (bilateral) edema
Jugular venous dilatation
Congested hepatomegaly
Gut congestion, ascites
Hepatojugular reflux

HYPOPERFUSION (-)

WARM-DRY   WARM-WET

HYPOPERFUSION (+)
Cold sweated extremities
Oliguria
Mental confusion
Dizziness
Narrow pulse pressure   COLD-DRY   COLD-WET

Hypoperfusion is not synonymous with hypotension, but often hypoperfusion is accompanied by hypotension.

Fig. 2. Bedside clinical profiles of HF. This bedside clinical classification highlights the degree of congestion (volume status) and perfusion (cardiac output) and can serve as a guide for initial therapy. Patients categorized as either dry (euvolemic) or wet (congested), warm (adequately perfused) or cold (underperfused). Most patients admitted with acute decompensated HF are in profile B and require diuresis. In contrast, those patients who are congested with reduced output require vasodilator, inotropic, or mechanical support to improve perfusion to facilitate decongestion. Patients who are in a low-output state despite optimal volume status are the most challenging to manage and often require mechanical circulatory support. (*From* 2016 ESC Guidelines for the diagnosis and management of acute and chronic heart failure. Eur Heart J 2016;37:2171; with permission.)

process triggered by a variety of causes and is broadly described as either ischemic or nonischemic in origin.[39] Both ischemic and nonischemic causes can result in HFpEF or HFrEF. Coronary artery disease is the most common cause of HFrEF. In patients with ischemic HF, the initial insult to the myocardium occurs secondary to a lack of adequate perfusion, followed by myocyte necrosis and remodeling. Compared with nonischemic causes, patients with ischemic cardiomyopathy generally have worse outcomes and may respond differently to pharmacologic and device therapies. Patients are classified as having an ischemic cause based on noninvasive and invasive testing. It is important to note that angina-like symptoms and regional wall motion abnormalities on echocardiogram may also be present in patients with nonischemic causes.[40] Quantification of the presence and extent of underlying coronary artery disease by angiography remains the gold standard, yet this may not be ideal in all patients, particularly those with underlying renal dysfunction. In these patients, noninvasive measures can be used as a safer alternative.

Nonischemic causes of HF encompass an extensive grouping of underlying pathologic conditions (**Box 3**). Patients in this category generally have intrinsic myocardial abnormalities or have suffered insults to the myocardium from abnormalities in hemodynamic loading conditions as a result of either structural abnormalities or elevation in vascular resistance, such as hypertension, over a prolonged period of time. Potentially reversible forms of systolic dysfunction include myocarditis, peripartum, stress, and tachycardia-induced and drug-induced cardiomyopathy. Idiopathic causes of nonischemic cardiomyopathies are common yet should

---

Box 3
Causes of cardiomyopathy with reduced ejection fraction

Ischemic heart disease

Valvular heart disease

Genetic/familial

    Titin mutation

    Lamin A/C mutation

    Arrhythmogenic/desmosome mutation

    "Burnt-out" hypertrophic cardiomyopathy

Idiopathic (diagnosis of exclusion)

Toxin related

    Substance abuse (alcohol, cocaine)

    Chemotherapy (anthracyclines)

    Radiation

Infectious

    Chagas disease

    Influenza

    Coxsackie

    Adenovirus

    Human immunodeficiency virus

Inflammatory/connective tissue diseases

    Lupus

    Scleroderma

    Giant cell myocarditis

Peripartum

Endocrine

    Thyroid

    Obesity

Stress induced

Tachycardia induced

    Rate related

    Premature ventricular contractions

Hypertension

Infiltrative

    Amyloid

    Sarcoid

    Hemochromatosis

---

remain a diagnosis of exclusion.[41] As the understanding and ability to identify pathogenic mutations continue to develop, previously delineated "idiopathic" cardiomyopathies are now increasingly classified as genetic/familial.[42,43] Recent data have demonstrated that patients with alcohol-induced cardiomyopathies may have underlying titin mutations with the second insult of alcoholic cardiotoxicity unmasking an underlying myopathic process.[44] Another important subset of nonischemic cardiomyopathies to recognize is infiltrative disorders, such as amyloidosis. These aberrant proteins deposit within the myocardium and result in fibrosis and dysfunction over time and can arise from a plasma cell dyscrasia (AL amyloid) or transthyretin accumulation from wild-type or mutant transthyretin (TTR amyloid).

PROGNOSIS IN HEART FAILURE

Deaths related to HF may be sudden from ventricular arrhythmia or due to progressive hemodynamic deterioration from pump failure. In milder forms of HF, the proportion of deaths that are sudden is higher, although the absolute risk of sudden death increases with HF severity. Before the advent of contemporary neurohormonal therapies, more than a third of deaths in HF were classified as sudden cardiac death. The sequential introduction of evidence-based neurohormonal therapies has reduced the risk of sudden death by more than 40% in patients enrolled in clinical trials who did not have a defibrillator at enrollment, highlighting the cumulative benefit of pharmacologic therapies.[45] In addition to improved medical therapy, widespread use of primary prevention defibrillators has dramatically reduced the risk of sudden death in systolic HF.[46] With declining sudden death rates in HF, there has been a shift in cause of death to pump failure and noncardiac causes, particularly in older patients with HF.

Considering the progressive and variable nature of HF, clinicians need to advise their patients of prognosis to assist them in making informed decisions on management. Despite the complexity of this syndrome, readily available clinical markers can flag patients at high risk for adverse prognosis (**Table 2**). A higher symptom burden often reflects the multisystem effects of HF, which lead to worsening outcomes. One of the strongest predictors of mortality in HF patients is the number of HF-related hospitalizations, which stems from the inability to maintain appropriate compensatory mechanisms.[47] Progressive cardiac remodeling as reflected by reducing EF, greater left ventricular end-diastolic dimension, and secondary mitral regurgitation is also an important marker of adverse prognosis. Underlying conduction disease, such as left bundle branch block, can lead to dyssynchronous contraction of the left ventricle, which in turn can perpetuate cardiac remodeling and worsen prognosis.[48,49]

Table 2
Select markers of adverse prognosis in chronic heart failure

Category	Risk Marker
Demographic	Advanced age
Symptoms	NYHA class IV functional limitation, syncope
Physical signs	S3 gallop, elevated jugular venous distension, pulsus alternans, Cheyne-Stokes respirations, narrow pulse pressure
Routine laboratory tests	Hyponatremia, elevated serum creatinine, reduced GFR, anemia
Echocardiographic	EF, LV end-diastolic dimension, degree of secondary mitral regurgitation
Medications	Diuretic resistance (high loop diuretic dose), intolerance of beta-blockers or RAAS inhibitors, frequent use or dependence on intravenous inotropes
ECG	Prolonged QRS duration, burden of NSVT/VT, higher resting heart rate (if in sinus rhythm)
Hemodynamic	Reduced cardiac index, elevated wedge pressure
Exercise	Reduced peak Vo_2, elevated Ve/VCO_2 slope, short 6-min walk distance
Neurohormonal	Elevated plasma norepinephrine, elevated B-type natriuretic peptides
Resource utilization	Number of HF hospitalizations

Abbreviations: GFR, glomerular filtration rate; LV, left ventricular; NSVT, nonsustained ventricular tachycardia; RAAS, renin-angiotensin-aldosterone system; Vo_2, oxygen consumption on cardiopulmonary exercise testing; VT, ventricular tachycardia.

Risk scores can also help clinicians estimate disease burden and mortality risk in HF as well as the anticipated response to therapeutic intervention. A frequently used risk score, the Seattle Heart Failure Model, uses commonly assessed clinical variables to give the clinician an estimate of 1-, 2-, and 5-year survival.[50] This score also estimates the survival benefit of adding a new therapy and an informed decision on treatment pathways and goals of care in a patient-centered fashion.

The clinical course of patients with HF is progressive, nonlinear, and characterized by worsening quality of life despite increasing levels of care.[51,52] Conversations with patients should include discussion of prognosis, patient priorities, and care goals. Patients with HF may be candidates for advanced therapies, including cardiac transplantation and ventricular assist devices, yet these therapies may not be applicable to all patients. Recent data demonstrate a trend toward palliative care service utilization in the last year of life in patients with HF, highlighting the importance of a patient-centered approach in management that focuses on symptom relief.[53,54]

SUMMARY

HF is an increasingly prevalent clinical syndrome marked by congestion and fatigue and associated with reduced quality of life and survival. This heterogenous syndrome is most commonly separated into patients according to contractile function, with reduced EF (systolic) and preserved EF (diastolic) HF. HF, which can stem from ischemic and nonischemic causes, progresses from antecedent risk factors to structural heart disease, then to symptoms described by variable functional limitation defined by NYHA class that eventually becomes refractory. These complementary descriptors shed light on the many faces of HF and, by doing so, define groups of patients most likely to benefit from evidenced-based therapies.

REFERENCES

1. McKee PA, Castelli WP, McNamara PM, et al. The natural history of congestive heart failure: the Framingham study. N Engl J Med 1971;285(26):1441–6.
2. Yancy CW, Jessup M, Bozkurt B, et al. 2017 ACC/AHA/HFSA focused update of the 2013 ACCF/AHA guideline for the management of heart failure: a report of the American College of Cardiology/American Heart Association task force on clinical practice guidelines and the Heart Failure Society of America. J Am Coll Cardiol 2017;70(6):776–803.
3. Owan TE, Hodge DO, Herges RM, et al. Trends in prevalence and outcome of heart failure with preserved ejection fraction. N Engl J Med 2006;355(3):251–9.
4. Steinberg BA, Zhao X, Heidenreich PA, et al. Trends in patients hospitalized with heart failure and

preserved left ventricular ejection fraction: prevalence, therapies, and outcomes. Circulation 2012; 126(1):65–75.

5. Vasan RS, Levy D. Defining diastolic heart failure: a call for standardized diagnostic criteria. Circulation 2000;101(17):2118–21.

6. Nadar SK, Tariq O. What is heart failure with mid-range ejection fraction? A new subgroup of patients with heart failure. Card Fail Rev 2018;4(1):6–8.

7. Hsu JJ, Ziaeian B, Fonarow GC. Heart failure with mid-range (Borderline) ejection fraction: clinical implications and future directions. JACC Heart Fail 2017;5(11):763–71.

8. Punnoose LR, Givertz MM, Lewis EF, et al. Heart failure with recovered ejection fraction: a distinct clinical entity. J Card Fail 2011;17(7):527–32.

9. Benjamin EJ, Virani SS, Callaway CW, et al. Heart disease and stroke statistics-2018 update: a report from the American Heart Association. Circulation 2018;137(12):e67–492.

10. Heidenreich PA, Albert NM, Allen LA, et al. Forecasting the impact of heart failure in the United States: a policy statement from the American Heart Association. Circ Heart Fail 2013;6(3):606–19.

11. Shah SJ, Kitzman DW, Borlaug BA, et al. Phenotype-specific treatment of heart failure with preserved ejection fraction: a multiorgan roadmap. Circulation 2016;134(1):73–90.

12. Obokata M, Reddy YNV, Pislaru SV, et al. Evidence supporting the existence of a distinct obese phenotype of heart failure with preserved ejection fraction. Circulation 2017;136(1):6–19.

13. Samson R, Jaiswal A, Ennezat PV, et al. Clinical phenotypes in heart failure with preserved ejection fraction. J Am Heart Assoc 2016;5(1) [pii:e002477].

14. Savji N, Meijers WC, Bartz TM, et al. The association of obesity and cardiometabolic traits with incident HFpEF and HFrEF. JACC Heart Fail 2018;6(8): 701–9.

15. Goodlin SJ. Palliative care in congestive heart failure. J Am Coll Cardiol 2009;54(5):386–96.

16. Binanay C, Califf RM, Hasselblad V, et al. Evaluation study of congestive heart failure and pulmonary artery catheterization effectiveness: the ESCAPE trial. JAMA 2005;294(13):1625–33.

17. Thibodeau JT, Turer AT, Gualano SK, et al. Characterization of a novel symptom of advanced heart failure: bendopnea. JACC Heart Fail 2014;2(1):24–31.

18. Konstam MA, Kiernan MS, Bernstein D, et al. Evaluation and management of right-sided heart failure: a scientific statement from the American Heart Association. Circulation 2018;137(20):e578–622.

19. Redfield MM, Jacobsen SJ, Burnett JC Jr, et al. Burden of systolic and diastolic ventricular dysfunction in the community: appreciating the scope of the heart failure epidemic. JAMA 2003; 289(2):194–202.

20. Campbell P, Drazner MH, Kato M, et al. Mismatch of right- and left-sided filling pressures in chronic heart failure. J Card Fail 2011;17(7):561–8.

21. Drazner MH, Rame JE, Stevenson LW, et al. Prognostic importance of elevated jugular venous pressure and a third heart sound in patients with heart failure. N Engl J Med 2001;345(8):574–81.

22. Ciampi Q, Villari B. Role of echocardiography in diagnosis and risk stratification in heart failure with left ventricular systolic dysfunction. Cardiovasc Ultrasound 2007;5:34.

23. Khan SG, Klettas D, Kapetanakis S, et al. Clinical utility of speckle-tracking echocardiography in cardiac resynchronisation therapy. Echo Res Pract 2016;3(1):R1–11.

24. Pfeffer MA, Braunwald E. Ventricular remodeling after myocardial infarction. Experimental observations and clinical implications. Circulation 1990;81(4): 1161–72.

25. Yeboah J, Bluemke DA, Hundley WG, et al. Left ventricular dilation and incident congestive heart failure in asymptomatic adults without cardiovascular disease: multi-ethnic study of atherosclerosis (MESA). J Card Fail 2014;20(12):905–11.

26. Braunwald E. Biomarkers in heart failure. N Engl J Med 2008;358(20):2148–59.

27. Logeart D, Thabut G, Jourdain P, et al. Predischarge B-type natriuretic peptide assay for identifying patients at high risk of re-admission after decompensated heart failure. J Am Coll Cardiol 2004;43(4): 635–41.

28. Chow SL, Maisel AS, Anand I, et al. Role of biomarkers for the prevention, assessment, and management of heart failure: a scientific statement from the American Heart Association. Circulation 2017;135(22):e1054–91.

29. Maisel AS, Krishnaswamy P, Nowak RM, et al. Rapid measurement of B-type natriuretic peptide in the emergency diagnosis of heart failure. N Engl J Med 2002;347(3):161–7.

30. Jessup M, Brozena S. Heart failure. N Engl J Med 2003;348(20):2007–18.

31. Ammar KA, Jacobsen SJ, Mahoney DW, et al. Prevalence and prognostic significance of heart failure stages: application of the American College of Cardiology/American Heart Association heart failure staging criteria in the community. Circulation 2007; 115(12):1563–70.

32. Yancy CW, Jessup M, Bozkurt B, et al. 2013 ACCF/AHA guideline for the management of heart failure: a report of the American College of Cardiology Foundation/American Heart Association task force on practice guidelines. J Am Coll Cardiol 2013;62(16): e147–239.

33. Stevenson LW, Pagani FD, Young JB, et al. INTERMACS profiles of advanced heart failure: the current picture. J Heart Lung Transplant 2009;28(6):535–41.

34. Kirklin JK, Pagani FD, Kormos RL, et al. Eighth annual INTERMACS report: special focus on framing the impact of adverse events. J Heart Lung Transplant 2017;36(10):1080–6.

35. Samman-Tahhan A, Hedley JS, McCue AA, et al. INTERMACS profiles and outcomes among non-inotrope-dependent outpatients with heart failure and reduced ejection fraction. JACC Heart Fail 2018;6(9):743–53.

36. Yancy CW, Jessup M, Bozkurt B, et al. 2017 ACC/AHA/HFSA focused update of the 2013 ACCF/AHA guideline for the management of heart failure: a report of the American College of Cardiology/American Heart Association Task Force on Clinical Practice Guidelines and the Heart Failure Society of America. J Card Fail 2017;23(8):628–51.

37. McMurray JJ, Adamopoulos S, Anker SD, et al. ESC guidelines for the diagnosis and treatment of acute and chronic heart failure 2012: the task force for the diagnosis and treatment of acute and chronic heart failure 2012 of the European Society of Cardiology. Developed in collaboration with the Heart Failure Association (HFA) of the ESC. Eur Heart J 2012;33(14):1787–847.

38. Ponikowski P, Voors AA, Anker SD, et al. 2016 ESC guidelines for the diagnosis and treatment of acute and chronic heart failure: the task force for the diagnosis and treatment of acute and chronic heart failure of the European Society of Cardiology (ESC). Developed with the special contribution of the Heart Failure Association (HFA) of the ESC. Eur J Heart Fail 2016;18(8):891–975.

39. Felker GM, Shaw LK, O'Connor CM. A standardized definition of ischemic cardiomyopathy for use in clinical research. J Am Coll Cardiol 2002;39(2):210–8.

40. Wallis DE, O'Connell JB, Henkin RE, et al. Segmental wall motion abnormalities in dilated cardiomyopathy: a common finding and good prognostic sign. J Am Coll Cardiol 1984;4(4):674–9.

41. Felker GM, Thompson RE, Hare JM, et al. Underlying causes and long-term survival in patients with initially unexplained cardiomyopathy. N Engl J Med 2000;342(15):1077–84.

42. Lakdawala NK, Winterfield JR, Funke BH. Dilated cardiomyopathy. Circ Arrhythm Electrophysiol 2013;6(1):228–37.

43. Hershberger RE, Siegfried JD. Update 2011: clinical and genetic issues in familial dilated cardiomyopathy. J Am Coll Cardiol 2011;57(16):1641–9.

44. Schafer S, de Marvao A, Adami E, et al. Titin-truncating variants affect heart function in disease cohorts and the general population. Nat Genet 2017;49(1):46–53.

45. Shen L, Jhund PS, Petrie MC, et al. Declining risk of sudden death in heart failure. N Engl J Med 2017;377(1):41–51.

46. Bardy GH, Lee KL, Mark DB, et al. Amiodarone or an implantable cardioverter-defibrillator for congestive heart failure. N Engl J Med 2005;352(3):225–37.

47. Setoguchi S, Stevenson LW, Schneeweiss S. Repeated hospitalizations predict mortality in the community population with heart failure. Am Heart J 2007;154(2):260–6.

48. Kashani A, Barold SS. Significance of QRS complex duration in patients with heart failure. J Am Coll Cardiol 2005;46(12):2183–92.

49. Jarcho JA. Biventricular pacing. N Engl J Med 2006;355(3):288–94.

50. Levy WC, Mozaffarian D, Linker DT, et al. The Seattle Heart Failure Model: prediction of survival in heart failure. Circulation 2006;113(11):1424–33.

51. Allen LA, Stevenson LW, Grady KL, et al. Decision making in advanced heart failure: a scientific statement from the American Heart Association. Circulation 2012;125(15):1928–52.

52. Dunlay SM, Redfield MM, Jiang R, et al. Care in the last year of life for community patients with heart failure. Circ Heart Fail 2015;8(3):489–96.

53. Rogers JG, Patel CB, Mentz RJ, et al. Palliative care in heart failure: the PAL-HF randomized, controlled clinical trial. J Am Coll Cardiol 2017;70(3):331–41.

54. Mentz RJ, O'Connor CM, Granger BB, et al. Palliative care and hospital readmissions in patients with advanced heart failure: insights from the PAL-HF trial. Am Heart J 2018;204:202–4.

Contemporary Treatment of Heart Failure

Maya H. Barghash, MD*, Sean P. Pinney, MD

KEYWORDS

- Heart failure with reduced ejection fraction (HFrEF) • Pharmacotherapy in heart failure
- Device therapy in heart failure • Advanced heart failure • Stage D heart failure
- Mechanical circulatory support • Cardiac transplantation

KEY POINTS

- Heart failure is a complex clinical syndrome that commonly results from left ventricular myocardial dysfunction and leads to dyspnea, fatigue, and fluid retention.
- In addition to classifying heart failure by ejection fraction, it is imperative to characterize disease progression and symptom severity to guide therapy selection, obtain prognostic information, and determine optimal timing for referral for advanced therapies.
- Medical and device therapy should be optimized according to society guidelines for the management of heart failure with reduced ejection fraction.
- Identification of advanced or stage D heart failure is clinically important due to its progressive nature and high mortality. Referral to an advanced heart failure specialist is recommended in patients with 2 or more heart failure hospitalizations, limitations to neurohormonal antagonists, high diuretic requirement, a history of inotrope use, and poor functional capacity.
- There is a broad spectrum of clinical syndromes within New York Heart Association class IV or stage D heart failure and the INTERMACS classification is useful in describing patient profiles to guide both prognostication and timing for referral for advanced therapies.
- Advanced therapies, including left ventricular assist devices and cardiac transplantation, are indicated in select patients with stage D heart failure and improve mortality and quality of life.

INTRODUCTION

Heart failure (HF) is a clinical syndrome that results from any structural or functional impairment of ventricular filling or ejection of blood.[1] It can result from a variety of cardiac disorders affecting the endocardium, myocardium, pericardium, heart valves, or great vessels, with the most common cause being left ventricular (LV) myocardial dysfunction.[1] Dyspnea, fatigue, and fluid retention are the most common symptoms of HF and can lead to reduced exercise tolerance, pulmonary and splanchnic congestion, and edema.

Ejection fraction (EF) is an important component of HF classification, as it guides selection and response to therapy. Most clinical trials selected patients based on EF such that HF with reduced EF (HFrEF) represents patients with HF and an EF of $\leq 40\%$. HF with preserved EF (HFpEF) has been variably defined, but an EF $\geq 50\%$ has been proposed. Additional subclassifications include HFpEF-borderline (EF 41%–49%) and HFpEF-improved (>40%).[1]

Thus far, therapies to slow progression and improve survival have been demonstrated only in

Disclosure Statement: No financial disclosures.
Department of Medicine, Division of Cardiology, Zena and Michael A. Wiener Cardiovascular Institute, Mount Sinai Hospital, Icahn School of Medicine at Mount Sinai, One Gustave L. Levy Place, Box 1030, New York, NY 10029, USA
* Corresponding author.
E-mail address: maya.barghash@mountsinai.org

Card Electrophysiol Clin 11 (2019) 21–37
https://doi.org/10.1016/j.ccep.2018.11.005
1877-9182/19/© 2018 Elsevier Inc. All rights reserved.

patients with HFrEF, and this is the focus of the present review.

In addition to classifying HF by EF, it is imperative to characterize disease progression and symptom severity, both of which provide prognostic information and guide selection of therapy. The New York Heart Association (NYHA) classification quantifies the degree of functional limitation from HF and assigns patients to 1 of 4 functional classes.[2] The American College of Cardiology Foundation (ACCF)/American Heart Association (AHA) staging system of HF describes the development and progression of disease, from structural abnormalities in asymptomatic patients to symptomatic phases that can be altered my medical and device therapy[3] (Fig. 1).

This review focuses on the management of symptomatic HF, stages C and D. Stage D HF represents those with persistent and progressive signs and symptoms of HF despite medical and device therapy and represents a group of patients with high mortality, a subset of whom benefit from advanced therapies, including mechanical circulatory support and cardiac transplantation.[4]

PHARMACOTHERAPY FOR CHRONIC HEART FAILURE

Angiotensin-converting enzyme (ACE) inhibitors are recommended in all patients with HFrEF regardless of etiology or symptom severity (NYHA class I–IV) and have been shown to reduce the risk of death and hospitalization for HF. Although head-to-head comparisons of different ACE inhibitors have not been studied, available evidence suggests no differences between various ACE inhibitors in their effects on survival.[5–9] Trials evaluating the mortality benefit of ACE inhibitors did not dose adjust to therapeutic effect, but instead targeted a prespecified dose. Studies evaluating the efficacy of high versus low doses of ACE inhibitors found an impact on hospitalizations, but not mortality.[10] Angiotensin receptor blockers (ARBs) reduce morbidity and mortality in HFrEF and are recommended for patients with HFrEF who are intolerant of ACE inhibitors.[11–14] For both ACE inhibitors and ARBs, monitoring of blood pressure, renal function, and potassium should be done within 1 to 2 weeks of initiation and with subsequent dose adjustments.

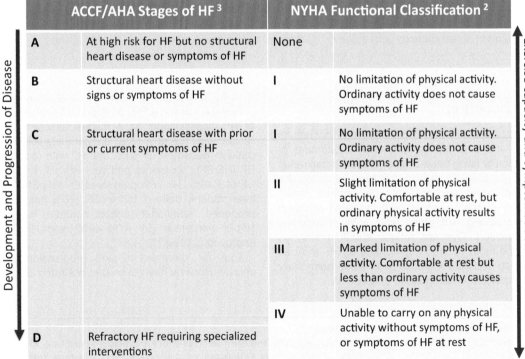

ACCF/AHA Stages of HF [3]		NYHA Functional Classification [2]	
A	At high risk for HF but no structural heart disease or symptoms of HF	None	
B	Structural heart disease without signs or symptoms of HF	I	No limitation of physical activity. Ordinary activity does not cause symptoms of HF
C	Structural heart disease with prior or current symptoms of HF	I	No limitation of physical activity. Ordinary activity does not cause symptoms of HF
		II	Slight limitation of physical activity. Comfortable at rest, but ordinary physical activity results in symptoms of HF
		III	Marked limitation of physical activity. Comfortable at rest but less than ordinary activity causes symptoms of HF
		IV	Unable to carry on any physical activity without symptoms of HF, or symptoms of HF at rest
D	Refractory HF requiring specialized interventions		

(left axis) Development and Progression of Disease

(right axis) Exercise capacity and symptomatic status of disease

Fig. 1. Comparison of ACCF/AHA Stages and NYHA Classes of HF. ACCF indicates American College of Cardiology Foundation; AHA indicated American Heart Association; HF, heart failure; NYHA, New York Heart Association. (*Adapted from* Yancy CW, Jessup M, Bozkurt B, et al. 2013 ACCF/AHA Guideline for the Management of Heart Failure. J Am Coll Cardiol. 2013; 62 (16):e147–239; with permission.)

The landmark trial of angiotensin receptor-neprilysin inhibitors found a cardiovascular mortality benefit over ACE inhibition.[15] Replacement with an ARB–neprilysin inhibitor (ARNi) sacubitril/valsartan is now recommended in patients with chronic NYHA class II or III HFrEF who are already on an ACE inhibitor or an ARB.[16] An ARNi is a combination of valsartan with sacubitril, an inhibitor of neprilysin. Neprilysin is a ubiquitous enzyme responsible for degradation of endogenous vasoactive peptides, including natriuretic peptides, bradykinin, adrenomedullin, angiotensin I and II, and endothelin-1, among others.[17] Sacubitril/valsartan is the first approved ARNi and was studied in a randomized trial evaluating stable symptomatic NYHA class II-III patients with HFrEF who were randomized to either sacubitril/valsartan or enalapril.[4] The ARNi significantly reduced the composite endpoint of cardiovascular death or HF hospitalization by 20% and the benefit was seen for both death and HF hospitalization. Side effects are similar to those seen with ACE inhibitors and include hypotension, renal insufficiency, and angioedema.

Specific beta-blockers are indicated in all patients with HFrEF with or without symptoms, reduce mortality and hospitalizations, and improve symptoms and quality of life on a background of ACE inhibition. Three beta-blockers have proven to be effective in reducing mortality in chronic HFrEF: bisoprolol,[18] sustained-release metoprolol (succinate),[19] both of which are beta 1 selective, and carvedilol,[20–23] which blocks beta-1, beta-2, and alpha receptors. Every effort should be made to titrate to the dose shown to be effective in clinical trials while monitoring closely for side effects of hypotension, bradycardia, fluid retention, and worsening HF.

Mineralocorticoid receptor antagonists (MRAs) are recommended in patients with symptomatic HFrEF (NYHA class II–IV) and have been shown to reduce mortality from both sudden death and HF.[24,25] MRA therapy should be avoided in those with significant renal insufficiency (creatinine [Cr] $\geq$2.5 in men, Cr $\geq$2.0 mg/dL in women, estimated glomerular filtration rate <30 mL/min per 1.73 m^2) or hyperkalemia (potassium >5.0 mEq/L). In addition to those with chronic HFrEF, MRAs are also indicated after myocardial infarction (MI) with LV dysfunction (EF $\leq$40%) in those with diabetes or symptomatic HF.[26]

The addition of hydralazine and isosorbide dinitrate to optimal therapy with ACE inhibitors and beta-blockers reduces mortality in NYHA class III-IV self-identified African American patients with HFrEF.[27,28] This vasodilator combination should not be used in place of ACE inhibitor treatment in ACE inhibitor–naïve patients, but can be considered in those who are intolerant of ACE inhibitors or ARBs[29–31] (**Fig. 2**).

Diuretics are recommended to improve symptoms in HFrEF in patients who have a prior history or present evidence of fluid retention.[32] Diuretics increase urinary sodium excretion, and improve symptoms and exercise tolerance in patients with HF.[33–35] The most commonly used are loop diuretics: furosemide, bumetanide, and torsemide. Sequential nephron blockade via diuretics that act on the proximal and distal collecting tubule, such as metolazone and thiazide diuretics, can be used to augment loop diuretics. Diuretic resistance can be observed in patients who are not adherent to prescribed sodium and fluid restriction, those taking nonsteroidal anti-inflammatory drugs, which counteract the effects of diuretics, or those with impaired renal function or perfusion.

Ivabridine is a sinoatrial node modulator that selectively inhibits the I_f current in the sinoatrial node leading to heart rate reduction. It has been shown to reduce HF hospitalizations in patients with HFrEF with NYHA class II to IV symptoms who are in sinus rhythm with a resting heart rate $\geq$70 beats per minute despite beta-blocker therapy.[36] Although the randomized trial found that ivabradine reduced the composite endpoint of cardiovascular death or HF hospitalization, this was driven by a reduction in hospitalizations. Only 25% of patients studied were on optimal doses of beta-blocker therapy, and it is important to maximize this before considering the addition of ivabradine.[16]

Digoxin has been shown to improve symptoms and quality of life and reduce HF hospitalizations in patients with HFrEF.[37–41] Lower plasma concentrations between 0.5 and 0.9 ng/mL have been effective in retrospective studies.

Systemic anticoagulation should be offered in patients with chronic HF and atrial fibrillation with an additional risk factor for stroke, such as history of hypertension, diabetes mellitus, prior stroke or transient ischemic attack, female gender, or age 75 and older.

Supplementation with omega-3 polyunsaturated fatty acids in symptomatic patients with HF has been shown to reduce cardiovascular mortality and can be used as adjunctive therapy.[42]

With regard to management of atrial and ventricular arrhythmias in patients with HF, amiodarone and dofetilide are the only antiarrhythmic agents that have neutral effects on mortality and are the preferred drugs for treating arrhythmias.[43,44]

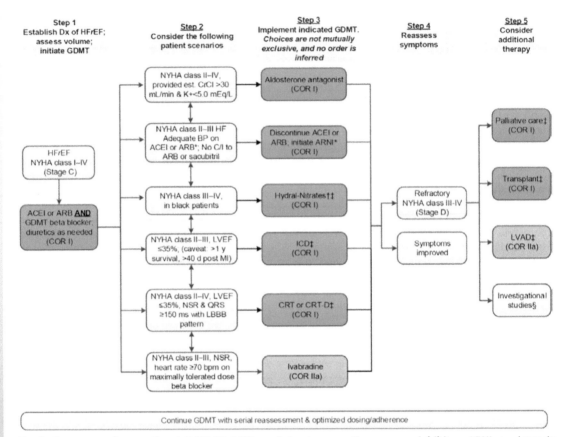

Fig. 2. Treatment of stage C and D HFrEF. ACEi, angiotensin-converting enzyme inhibitor; ARNI, angiotensin receptor-neprilysin inhibitor; BP, blood pressure; bpm, beats per minute; C/I, contraindication; COR, Class of Recommendation; CrCl, creatinine clearance; CRT-D, cardiac resynchronization therapy-device; Dx, diagnosis; GDMT, guideline-directed management and therapy; ISDN/HYD, isosorbide dinitrate hydral-nitrates; K+, potassium; NSR, normal sinus rhythm. (*From* Yancy CW, Jessup M, Bozkurt B, et al. 2017 ACC/AHA/HFSA focused update of the 2013 ACCF/AHA guideline for the management of heart failure: a report of the American College of Cardiology/American Heart Association ask Force on Clinical Practice Guidelines and the Heart Failure Society of America; J Am Coll Cardiol. 2017; 70(6): 776–803; with permission.)

DEVICE THERAPY FOR CHRONIC HEART FAILURE

Patients with HFrEF have an increased risk of sudden death due to ventricular arrhythmias, and neurohormonal antagonists have led to a substantial reduction in sudden death risk. Implantable cardioverter defibrillator (ICD) therapy has been shown to further reduce all-cause mortality in many randomized clinical trials. ICD therapy should be considered only after guideline-directed medical therapy (GDMT) has been optimized for 3 to 6 months in patients with expected survival of more than 1 year with good functional status.

ICD therapy is recommended for primary prevention of sudden cardiac death to reduce mortality in patients with HFrEF with an LVEF ≤35% with NYHA class II or III HF symptoms despite GDMT in nonischemic cardiomyopathy and ischemic cardiomyopathy at least 40 days after MI.[45,46] ICD therapy is also recommended in patients with HFrEF secondary to ischemic cardiomyopathy with an LVEF of 30% despite GDMT who are NYHA class I and at least 40 days post MI.[47–49]

Secondary prevention ICD therapy is indicated in patients who have survived a prior cardiac arrest or sustained ventricular tachycardia (VT) after reversible causes have been excluded, in patients with conditions associated with a high sudden death risk who experience unexplained syncope with or without evidence of sustained VT or ventricular fibrillation at electrophysiological study.[50–56]

Cardiac resynchronization therapy (CRT), or multisite ventricular pacing, can improve ventricular contractile function and reverse ventricular remodeling in patients with HFrEF with a prolonged QRS, typically 150 ms or greater with a left bundle branch (LBBB) pattern, and has been associated with reduced hospitalization and mortality. CRT is indicated in patients with HFrEF with an LVEF of 35% or less in sinus rhythm with an LBBB and a QRS duration of 150 ms or greater with NYHA class II to IV HF symptoms on GDMT.[57–61] CRT may be useful in patients with HFrEF in sinus rhythm with either a non-LBBB pattern and QRS of 150 ms or greater, an LBBB QRS duration of 120 to 149 ms, or if the underlying rhythm is atrial fibrillation and atrioventricular junctional ablation or pharmacologic rate control will achieve 100% ventricular pacing with CRT.[57–59,61–68]

CRT also can be considered in those with LVEF ≤35% undergoing a device implantation with a high anticipated requirement of right ventricular pacing (>40%),[64,69] or those patients with NYHA class I symptoms more than 40 days after MI with an LVEF of ≤30% in sinus rhythm with LBBB QRS ≥150 ms[60] (**Fig. 3**).

MECHANICAL SUPPORT

Stage D or advanced HF is characterized by progressive or persistent severe signs and symptoms of HF despite optimized medical, surgical, and device therapy.[4] Limited data suggest that stage D HF represents fewer than 1% of patients with HF.[70] Stage D HF carries a high mortality with medical therapy alone with survival of 11% to 25% with inotropic support at 1 year.[71,72] Aside from patients presenting with acute stage D HF and cardiogenic shock, recognition of stage D

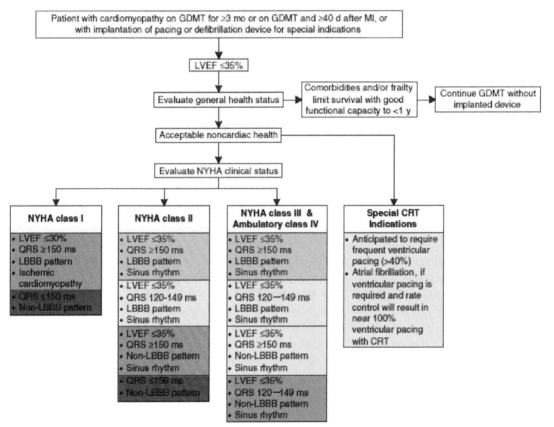

Fig. 3. Indications for CRT therapy in HFrEF. Colors correspond to the class of recommendations in the ACCF/AHA in **Fig. 1**. Benefit for NYHA class I and II patients has only been shown in CRT-D trials, and although patients may not experience immediate symptomatic benefit, late remodeling may be avoided along with long-term HF consequences. There are no trials that support CRT-pacing (without ICD) in NYHA class I and II patients. Thus, it is anticipated these patients would receive CRT-D unless clinical reasons or personal wishes make CRT-pacing more appropriate. In patients who are NYHA class III and ambulatory class IV, CRT-D may be chosen but clinical reasons and personal wishes may make CRT-pacing appropriate to improve symptoms and quality of life when an ICD is not expected to produce meaningful benefit in survival. (*From* Yancy CW, Jessup M, Bozkurt B, et al. 2013 ACCF/AHA Guideline for the Management of Heart Failure. J Am Coll Cardiol. 2013; 62 (16):e147–239; with permission.)

HF can be difficult because signs and symptoms wax and wane over time (**Fig. 4**).

Late recognition and referral of patients with stage D HF limits treatment options with advanced therapies because of resultant end-organ dysfunction, frailty, and poor nutritional and functional status, all of which can be prohibitive for advanced therapies consideration or lead to increased morbidity and mortality with advanced therapies.[4] The Interagency Registry for Mechanically Assisted Circulatory Support (INTERMACS) has defined patient profiles to facilitate risk stratification for advanced therapies[73] (**Fig. 5**) Patients in INTERMACS 1 through 3 are critical yet clearer to identify, as they require some level of inotropic and/or mechanical support. Patients in INTERMACS 4 to 7 profiles are harder to identify and many clinical clues and tools have been proposed to identify those who may benefit from an escalation to advanced therapies.[1,3,4,73,74] Signs of advanced HF include repeated HF hospitalizations, intolerance of neurohormonal antagonists due to hypotension or cardiorenal limitations, end-organ dysfunction, escalation of diuretics, refractory arrhythmias or frequent ICD shocks, and objective severe impairment of functional capacity (**Box 1**).

Intravenous inotropic agents are commonly given in the acute setting in patients with decompensated HFrEF with low cardiac index and clinical evidence of end-organ hypoperfusion. Despite improving hemodynamic compromise, positive inotropic agents have not demonstrated improved survival in patients with HF in either the hospital or outpatient setting. When patients fail to wean from intravenous inotropic support, this portends a poor prognosis and should signal a milestone for decision making and overall goals of care, whether advanced therapies or palliative care.[75–78]

In patients with INTERMACS profile 1 and 2 who present with critical cardiogenic shock or who are decompensating on a single inotrope, the primary goal of pharmacologic and mechanical circulatory support (MCS) is to provide short-term or long-term hemodynamic stabilization to augment cardiac output; maintain or restore end-organ perfusion; and reduce intracardiac filling pressures, ventricular volumes, wall stress, and myocardial oxygen consumption.[79] Appropriate

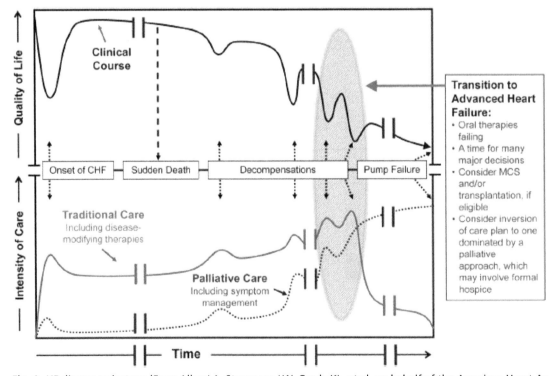

Fig. 4. HF disease trajectory. (*From* Allen LA, Stevenson LW, Grady KL, et al. on behalf of the American Heart Association Council on Quality of Care and Outcomes Research, Council on Cardiovascular Nursing, Council on Clinical Cardiology, Council on Cardiovascular Radiology and Intervention, and Council on Cardiovascular Surgery and Anesthesia. Decision making in advanced heart failure: a scientific statement from the American Heart Association. Circulation 2012;125; with permission.)

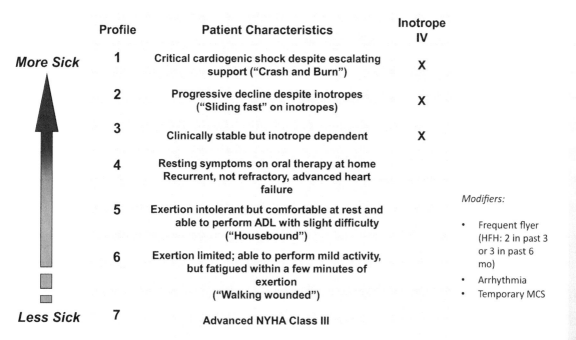

	Profile	Patient Characteristics	Inotrope IV
More Sick	1	Critical cardiogenic shock despite escalating support ("Crash and Burn")	X
	2	Progressive decline despite inotropes ("Sliding fast" on inotropes)	X
	3	Clinically stable but inotrope dependent	X
	4	Resting symptoms on oral therapy at home Recurrent, not refractory, advanced heart failure	
	5	Exertion intolerant but comfortable at rest and able to perform ADL with slight difficulty ("Housebound")	
	6	Exertion limited; able to perform mild activity, but fatigued within a few minutes of exertion ("Walking wounded")	
Less Sick	7	Advanced NYHA Class III	

Modifiers:

- Frequent flyer (HFH: 2 in past 3 or 3 in past 6 mo)
- Arrhythmia
- Temporary MCS

INTERMACS: **Inter**agency Registry of **M**echanically **A**ssisted **C**irculatory **S**upport

Fig. 5. INTERMACS classification. ADL, activities of daily living; HFH, heart failure hospitalizations; IV, intravenous. (*Adapted from* Stevenson LW, Pagani FD, Young JB, et al. INTERMACS profiles of advanced heart failure: the current picture. J Heart Lung Transplant 2009;28:535–41; with permission.)

device selection must be individualized according to the overall therapeutic goal, the anticipated duration and intensity of support required, and may be further influenced by anatomic considerations and the burden of comorbidities. Patients with INTERMACS profile 1 with critical cardiogenic shock are at particularly high risk for poor outcomes with durable MCS and may benefit from stabilization with temporary MCS[80] (**Fig. 6**).

For temporary MCS, intra-aortic balloon counterpulsation (IABP) is one of the most common and widely available temporary mechanical support options. Despite relatively modest augmentation of cardiac output (typically 0.5–1.0 L/min), the IABP can be useful in temporary hemodynamic stabilization of cardiogenic shock; however, randomized trials have not shown clear benefits over medical therapy with regard to 30-day survival.[81] The Impella (Abiomed, Danvers, MA) is a microaxial flow pump designed to propel blood directly from the LV to the aorta. The device is available in 3 versions that provide incremental flow augmentation over the IABP: Impella 2.5 (12F, 2.5 L/min flow), Impella CP (14F, 3.0–4.0 L/min flow), and Impella 5.0 (21F, 5.0 L/min flow). Despite increased hemodynamic support over IABP, it has been difficult to demonstrate incremental survival benefits of

Impella in patients with cardiogenic shock.[82,83] The TandemHeart (CardiacAssist, Pittsburgh, PA) is a left atrium to aorta assist device that uses a transseptal venous inflow cannula in the left atrium and a centrifugal pump to the femoral artery and can deliver 5.0 L/min of flow. Addition of an oxygenator to the circuit allows the device to support extracorporeal membrane oxygenation (ECMO), and it can also be configured using right atrial and pulmonary arterial cannulae to provide right ventricular or biventricular support. In small, randomized clinical trials, use of the TandemHeart has been associated with incremental improvement in cardiac index and mean arterial pressure and reduction in filling pressure compared with the IABP, but a higher risk of vascular trauma and limb ischemia due to the large-bore venous and arterial cannulae.[84]

Distinct from the previously described temporary support devices, central or peripheral venoarterial ECMO is a temporary MCS strategy that can provide biventricular mechanical support and oxygenation. Displacement of venous blood volume into the arterial system can increase LV afterload and further compromise left ventricular ejection in patients with HF and concomitant LV venting using inotropes, IABP, Impella, transseptal left atrial cannula, or surgical left atrial/LV cannula may be required. Anticoagulation is essential to prevent clotting within the circuit and complications include stroke, bleeding, and limb ischemia.[85] The choice between veno-arterial ECMO and temporary surgical left ventricular assist device (LVAD) as initial treatment for refractory cardiogenic shock depends on local expertise and the need for biventricular support and oxygenation.

For durable MCS in patients with advanced HF with INTERMACS profiles 1 to 5, LVADs have emerged as an increasingly important therapeutic option, particularly with the availability of continuous-flow pumps that have led to increased survival in advanced HF. LVADs are approved for extended-duration support as a bridge to recovery or explantation, transplantation, and destination therapy for patients who are not transplant candidates. Most devices in current use are axial flow (eg, Thoratec [Pleasanton, CA] Heartmate 2) or centrifugal flow (eg, HeartWare [Framingham, MA] HVAD, Thoratec Heartmate 3) pumps that provide continuous, nonpulsatile flow.[71,72,86–88] Clinical trial data have found that approximately 80% to 85% of LVAD-supported patients live 1 year, with an average survival of 3 years.[87–90] Improvement in event-free survival with lower rates of pump thrombosis has been seen with the centrifugal flow Heartmate 3 LVAD.[87,88] MCS should be considered in patients with HF with an estimated probability of 1-year survival of $\leq$85% with acceptable operative risk and with comorbid conditions that will not prohibit meaningful survival of more than 2 years with LVAD support[4] (**Fig. 7**).

Patients with biventricular failure may be successfully bridged to transplantation (BTT) with biventricular assist devices or a total artificial heart, but durable biventricular support is not currently available for destination therapy. Because of a mismatch between the burden of advanced HF and the availability of donor hearts, as well as generally poor long-term outcomes with medical therapy alone, LVAD is increasingly the preferred strategy for BTT in most patients who are good surgical candidates.

CARDIAC TRANSPLANTATION

Cardiac transplantation is considered the gold standard for the treatment of end-stage HF. Since the first successful cardiac transplantation in 1967, advances in immunosuppressive therapy have led to improved long-term survival of transplant recipients, with 1-year, 3-year, and 5-year posttransplant survival rates of 87.8%, 78.5%, and 71.7% in adults, respectively, and a median survival of 10.7 years[91,92] (**Fig. 8**). Similarly, cardiac transplantation has been shown to improve functional status, with most recipients reporting normal functional capacity and improved health-related quality of life.[91,93,94] The greatest survival benefit is seen in those patients who are at highest risk of death from advanced HF.[95] Cardiopulmonary exercise testing helps refine candidate

Intermacs Continuous Flow LVAD/BiVAD Implants: 2013 – 2016, n = 10,726

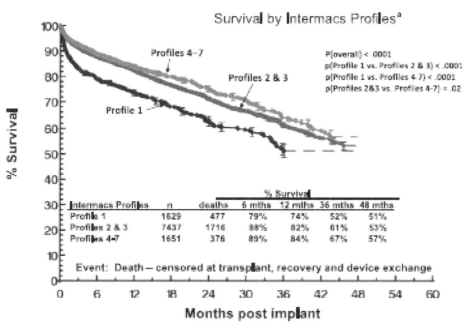

Survival by Intermacs Profiles[a]

P(overall) < .0001
p(Profile 1 vs. Profiles 2 & 3) < .0001
p(Profile 1 vs. Profiles 4-7) < .0001
p(Profiles 2&3 vs. Profiles 4-7) = .02

Intermacs Profiles	n	deaths	6 mths	12 mths	36 mths	48 mths
Profile 1	1629	477	79%	74%	52%	51%
Profiles 2 & 3	7437	1716	88%	82%	61%	53%
Profiles 4-7	1651	376	89%	84%	67%	57%

Event: Death — censored at transplant, recovery and device exchange

Fig. 6. Kaplan-Meier survival curves stratified by INTERMACS profile at the time of implant. [a] Nine patients with unspecified patient profile at time of implant. (*Data from* Kirklin JK, Pagani FD, Kormos RL, et al. Eighth annual INTERMACS report: special focus on framing the impact of adverse events. 2017 INTERMACS report. J Heart Lung Transplant 2017;36:1080–86.)

Intermacs Continuous Flow LVAD/BiVAD Implants: 2008 – 2016, n = 17633

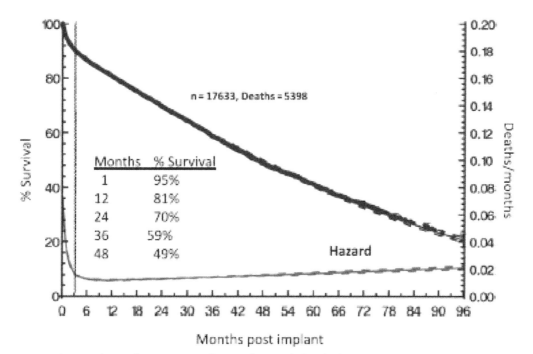

n = 17633, Deaths = 5398

Months	% Survival
1	95%
12	81%
24	70%
36	59%
48	49%

Hazard

Fig. 7. Parametric survival curve for continuous-flow implants including both LVADs and BiVADs. BiVAD, biventricular assist device. (*Data from* Kirklin JK, Pagani FD, Kormos RL, et al. Eighth annual INTERMACS report: special focus on framing the impact of adverse events. 2017 INTERMACS Report. J Heart Lung Transplant 2017;36:1080–86.)

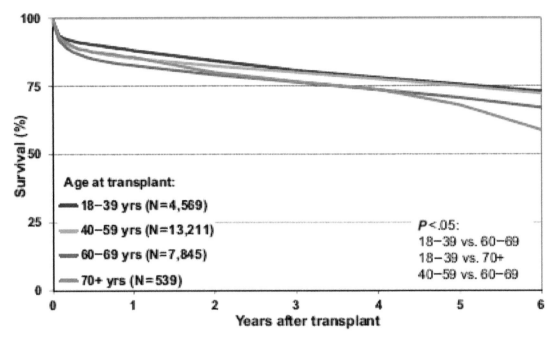

Fig. 8. Adult heart transplant survival: Kaplan-Meier survival by recipient age group January 2009 to June 2015. (*Data from* Lund LH, Khush KK, Cherikh WS, et al. International Society for Heart and Lung Transplantation. The Registry of the International Society for heart and lung transplantation: thirty-fourth adult heart transplantation report-2017; focus theme: allograft ischemic time. J Heart Lung Transplant 2017;36(10):1037–46.)

selection.[96–100] Selected patients with stage D HF and poor prognosis should be referred to a cardiac transplantation center for evaluation and transplant consideration.

Cardiac transplantation is a limited resource because of the shortage of available donor organs and so not only is patient selection crucial, but bridging strategies with MCS in transplant-eligible patients with stage D HF is increasing. Appropriate patients to consider listing for heart transplantation are those with a peak Vo_2 on cardiopulmonary exercise testing of less than 10 mL/kg per minute or less than 50% of predicted.[92] Candidacy is also based on other clinical parameters for patients with a peak Vo_2 of 10 to 14 mL/kg per minute as discussed in the previous MCS evaluation. Appropriate patient selection for MCS and transplantation requires patient evaluation based on severity of HF as well as operative risk, comorbid conditions, psychosocial stability, and ability to adhere to self-care after MCS and transplantation. The decision to select a patient for MCS or transplantation is complex and best made by an experienced and multidisciplinary team[101] (**Fig. 9**).

BEHAVIORAL MODIFICATION

Education for the patient and family, particularly during transitional points of care; that is, between hospital discharge and the outpatient setting, is an essential component of HF self-care.[1] A 1-hour nurse educator–delivered teaching session at the time of hospital discharge for HF can increase HF self-care and medication adherence, and subsequently reduce the risk of rehospitalization.[102] Further, open communication between clinicians and nurses, medication reconciliation, carefully planned transitions between care settings, and consistent documentation are patient safety initiatives that should be in place for all patients with HF.[1] Multidisciplinary approaches to care can reduce rehospitalization rates for HF, and scheduling an early follow-up visit within 7 to 14 days and early telephone follow-up within 3 days of hospital discharge are reasonable initiatives.[1,103,104] Programs involving specialized follow-up by a multidisciplinary team decrease all-cause hospitalizations and mortality, but this is not the case for programs focusing only on HF self-care.[105–109]

Dietary sodium restriction is commonly recommended to patients with HF and is endorsed by many guidelines.[1,110–112] The data on which this recommendation is drawn are not robust, with some observational data finding an association among dietary sodium intake, fluid retention, and risk for hospitalization,[113,114] and other data with signals to worsening neurohormonal profile with sodium restriction in HF.[115–117]

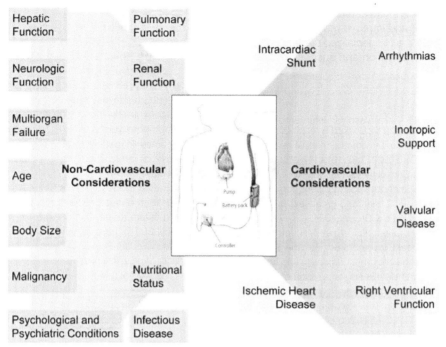

Hepatic Function

Pulmonary Function

Intracardiac Shunt

Arrhythmias

Neurologic Function

Renal Function

Multiorgan Failure

Inotropic Support

Age   **Non-Cardiovascular Considerations**

Cardiovascular Considerations

Valvular Disease

Body Size

Malignancy

Nutritional Status

Ischemic Heart Disease

Right Ventricular Function

Psychological and Psychiatric Conditions

Infectious Disease

Fig. 9. Evaluating candidates for durable support. (*From* Wilson SR, Mudge GH, Stewart GC, et al. Evaluation for a ventricular assist device: selecting the candidate. Circulation 2009;119:2225–32; with permission.)

Recommendations for fluid restriction in HF are largely driven by clinical experience. Sodium and fluid balance recommendations are best implemented in the context of weight-monitoring and symptom-monitoring programs. Limiting fluid intake to approximately 2 L per day is usually adequate for most hospitalized patients who are not diuretic resistant or significantly hyponatremic. In one study, patients on a similar sodium and diuretic regimen showed higher readmission rates with higher fluid intake, suggesting that fluid intake affects HF outcomes.[113]

A U-shaped distribution curve has been suggested in which mortality is greatest in cachectic patients with HF; lower in normal, overweight, and mildly obese patients; and higher again in more severely obese patients.[118] Exercise training in patients with HF is safe, and meta-analyses have demonstrated that cardiac rehabilitation reduces mortality and hospitalizations, and improves functional capacity, exercise duration, and health-related quality of life.[119,120]

Supportive cardiology and palliative care for HF are integral to help address symptoms, psychosocial stressors, caregiver support, frailty, depression, quality of life, and support for complex decision making in advanced HF surrounding goals of care and advanced HF therapies.[121,122]

SUMMARY

HF is a complex clinical syndrome caused by a variety of disorders that lead to impairment of ventricular filling and ejection of blood. The most common cause of HF arises from LV myocardial dysfunction, which in turn has many etiologies. The clinical syndrome is characterized by dyspnea, fatigue, and fluid retention, and can be seen with preserved or reduced EF. The major advances in medical, surgical, and device therapy have been demonstrated in HFrEF and have led to remarkable improvements in survival and quality of life. Medical and device therapy should be optimized according to society guidelines for the management of HFrEF.

In addition to classifying HF by EF, it is imperative to characterize disease progression and symptom severity using the ACCF/AHA stages of HF and the NYHA functional classification to guide therapy selection, obtain prognostic information, and determine optimal timing for referral for advanced therapies. Identification of advanced or stage D HF is clinically important because of its progressive nature and high mortality. In addition to clinical clues that help identify stage D HF, there is a broad spectrum of clinical profiles put forth by INTERMACS that are useful in guiding prognostication and referral for advanced therapies. Advanced therapies with LVAD and transplantation are indicated in select patients with stage D HF and improve mortality and quality of life. Early referral to specialized centers is imperative for patient selection and success with these therapies.

REFERENCES

1. Yancy CW, Jessup M, Bozkurt B, et al. 2013 ACCF/AHA guideline for the management of heart failure. J Am Coll Cardiol 2013;62(16):e147–239.
2. The Criteria Committee of the New York Heart Association. Nomenclature and criteria for diagnosis of diseases of the heart and great vessels. 9th edition. Boston: Little & Brown; 1994.
3. Hunt SA, Abraham WT, Chin MH, et al. 2009 focused update incorporated into the ACC/AHA 2005 guidelines for the diagnosis and management of heart failure in adults: a report of the American College of Cardiology Foundation/ American Heart Association Task Force on Practice Guidelines. J Am Coll Cardiol 2009;53:e1–90.
4. Fang JC, Ewald GA, Allen LA, et al. Advanced (stage D) heart failure: a statement from the Heart Failure Society of America Guidelines Committee. J Card Fail 2015;21(6):519–34.
5. Pfeffer MA, Braunwald E, Moye LA, et al. Effect of captopril on mortality and morbidity in patients with left ventricular dysfunction after myocardial infarction: results of the survival and ventricular enlargement trial: the SAVE Investigators. N Engl J Med 1992;327:669–77.
6. The CONSENSUS Trial Study Group. Effects of enalapril on mortality in severe congestive heart failure: results of the Cooperative North Scandinavian Enalapril Survival Study (CONSENSUS). N Engl J Med 1987;316:1429–35.
7. The SOLVD Investigators. Effect of enalapril on survival in patients with reduced left ventricular ejection fractions and congestive heart failure. N Engl J Med 1991;325:293–302.
8. The SOLVD Investigators. Effect of enalapril on mortality and the development of heart failure in asymptomatic patients with reduced left ventricular ejection fractions. N Engl J Med 1992;327: 685–91.
9. Garg R, Yusuf S. Overview of randomized trials of angiotensin-converting enzyme inhibitors on mortality and morbidity in patients with heart failure: Collaborative Group on ACE Inhibitors Trials. JAMA 1995;273:1450–6.
10. Packer M, Poole-Wilson PA, Armstrong PW, et al, ATLAS Study Group. Comparative effects of low and high doses of the angiotensin-converting enzyme inhibitor, lisinopril, on morbidity and mortality in chronic heart failure. Circulation 1999;100: 2312–8.
11. Cohn JN, Tognoni G. A randomized trial of the angiotensin-receptor blocker valsartan in chronic heart failure. N Engl J Med 2001;345:1667–75.
12. Pfeffer MA, Swedberg K, Granger CB, et al. Effects of candesartan on mortality and morbidity in patients with chronic heart failure: the CHARM-Overall programme. Lancet 2003;362:759–66.
13. Konstam MA, Neaton JD, Dickstein K, et al. Effects of high-dose versus low-dose losartan on clinical outcomes in patients with heart failure (HEAAL study): a randomised, double-blind trial. Lancet 2009;374:1840–8.
14. Pitt B, Segal R, Martinez EA, et al. Randomised trial of losartan versus captopril in patients over 65 with heart failure (Evaluation of Losartan in the Elderly Study, ELITE). Lancet 1997;349:747–52.
15. McMurray JJV, Packer M, Desai AS, et al. Angiotensin-neprilysin inhibition versus enalapril in heart failure. N Engl J Med 2014;371(11):993–1004.
16. Yancy CW, Jessup M, Bozkurt B, et al. 2017 ACC/AHA/HFSA focused updated of the 2013 ACCF/AHA guideline for the management of heart failure: a report of the American College of Cardiology/ American Heart Association task force on clinical practice guidelines and the Heart Failure Society of America. Circulation 2017;136:e137–61.
17. Barghash MH, Desai AS. First-in-class composite angiotensin receptor-neprilysin inhibitors in practice. Clin Pharmacol Ther 2017;102(2):265–8.
18. CBIS II Authors. The cardiac insufficiency bisoprolol study II (CIBISII): a randomised trial. Lancet 1999;353:9–13.
19. Effect of metoprolol CR/XL in chronic heart failure: metoprolol CR/XL randomised intervention trial in congestive heart failure (MERIT-HF). Lancet 1999; 353:2001–7.
20. Packer M, Bristow MR, Cohn JN, et al. The effect of carvedilol on morbidity and mortality in patients with chronic heart failure: U.S. Carvedilol Heart Failure Study Group. N Engl J Med 1996;334: 1349–55.
21. Colucci WS, Packer M, Bristow MR, et al. Carvedilol inhibits clinical progression in patients with mild symptoms of heart failure: US Carvedilol Heart Failure Study Group. Circulation 1996;94: 2800–6.
22. Packer M, Coats AJ, Fowler MB, et al. Effect of carvedilol on survival in severe chronic heart failure. N Engl J Med 2001;344:1651–8.
23. Australia/New Zealand Heart Failure Research Collaborative Group. Randomised, placebo-controlled trial of carvedilol in patients with congestive heart failure due to ischaemic heart disease. Lancet 1997;349:375–80.
24. Pitt B, Zannad F, Remme WJ, et al, Randomized Aldactone Evaluation Study Investigators. The effect of spironolactone on morbidity and mortality in

patients with severe heart failure. N Engl J Med 1999;341:709–17.

25. Zannad F, McMurray JJ, Krum H, et al. Eplerenone in patients with systolic heart failure and mild symptoms. N Engl J Med 2011;364:11–21.

26. Pitt B, Remme W, Zannad F, et al. Eplerenone, a selective aldosterone blocker, in patients with left ventricular dysfunction after myocardial infarction. N Engl J Med 2003;348:1309–21.

27. Carson P, Ziesche S, Johnson G, et al, Vasodilator-Heart Failure Trial Study Group. Racial differences in response to therapy for heart failure: analysis of the vasodilator-heart failure trials. J Card Fail 1999;5:178–87.

28. Taylor AL, Ziesche S, Yancy C, et al. Combination of isosorbide dinitrate and hydralazine in blacks with heart failure. N Engl J Med 2004;351:2049–57.

29. Cohn JN, Johnson G, Ziesche S, et al. A comparison of enalapril with hydralazine-isosorbide dinitrate in the treatment of chronic congestive heart failure. N Engl J Med 1991;325:303–10.

30. Fonarow GC, Chelimsky-Fallick C, Stevenson LW, et al. Effect of direct vasodilation with hydralazine versus angiotensin-converting enzyme inhibition with captopril on mortality in advanced heart failure: the Hy-C trial. J Am Coll Cardiol 1992;19:842–50.

31. Cohn JN, Archibald DG, Ziesche S, et al. Effect of vasodilator therapy on mortality in chronic congestive heart failure: results of a Veterans Administration Cooperative Study. N Engl J Med 1986;314:1547–52.

32. Patterson JH, Adams KF Jr, Applefeld MM, et al. Oral torsemide in patients with chronic congestive heart failure: effects on body weight, edema, and electrolyte excretion: Torsemide Investigators Group. Pharmacotherapy 1994;14:514–21.

33. Cody RJ, Kubo SH, Pickworth KK. Diuretic treatment for the sodium retention of congestive heart failure. Arch Intern Med 1994;154:1905–14.

34. Wilson JR, Reichek N, Dunkman WB, et al. Effect of diuresis on the performance of the failing ventricle in man. Am J Med 1981;70:234–9.

35. Richardson A, Bayliss J, Scriven AJ, et al. Double-blind comparison of captopril alone against furosemide plus amiloride in mild heart failure. Lancet 1987;2:709–11.

36. Swedberg K, Komajda M, Bohm M, et al. Ivabridine and outcomes in chronic heart failure (SHIFT): a randomised placebo-controlled study. Lancet 2010;376:875–85.

37. The Digitalis Investigation Group. The effect of digoxin on mortality and morbidity in patients with heart failure. N Engl J Med 1997;336:525–33.

38. The Captopril-Digoxin Multicenter Research Group. Comparative effects of therapy with captopril and digoxin in patients with mild to moderate heart failure. JAMA 1988;259:539–44.

39. Dobbs SM, Kenyon WI, Dobbs RJ. Maintenance digoxin after an episode of heart failure: placebo-controlled trial in outpatients. Br Med J 1977;1:749–52.

40. Lee DC, Johnson RA, Bingham JB, et al. Heart failure in outpatients: a randomized trial of digoxin versus placebo. N Engl J Med 1982;306:699–705.

41. Guyatt GH, Sullivan MK, Fallen EL, et al. A controlled trial of digoxin in congestive heart failure. Am J Cardiol 1988;61:371–5.

42. Tavazzi L, Maggioni AP, Marchioli R, et al. Effect of n-3 polyunsaturated fatty acids in patients with chronic heart failure (the GISSI-HF trial): a randomized, double-blind, placebo-controlled trial. Lancet 2008;372:1223–30.

43. Singh SN, Fletcher RD, Fisher SG, et al. Amiodarone in patients with congestive heart failure and asymptomatic ventricular arrhythmia: survival trial of antiarrhythmic therapy in congestive heart failure. N Engl J Med 1995;333:77–82.

44. Torp-Pederson C, Moller M, Bloch-Thomsen PE, et al. Dofetilide in patients with congestive heart failure and left ventricular dysfunction: Danish Investigations of Arrhythmia and Mortality on Dofetilide Study Group. N Engl J Med 1999;341:857–65.

45. Moss AJ, Zareba W, Hall WJ, et al. Prophylactic implantation of a defibrillator in patients with myocardial infarction and reduced ejection fraction. N Engl J Med 2002;346:877–83.

46. Bardy GH, Lee KL, Mark DB, et al. Amiodarone or an implantable cardioverter-defibrillator for congestive heart failure. N Engl J Med 2005;352:225–37.

47. Moss AJ, Hall WJ, Cannon DS, et al. Improved survival with an implanted defibrillator in patients with coronary disease at high risk for ventricular arrhythmia: Multicenter Automatic Defibrillator Implantation Trial Investigators. N Engl J Med 1996;335:1933–40.

48. Buxton AE, Lee KL, Fisher JD, et al. A randomized study of the prevention of sudden death in patients with coronary artery disease: Multicenter Unsustained Tachycardia Trial Investigators. N Engl J Med 1999;341:1882–90.

49. Hohnloser SH, Kuck KH, Dorian P, et al. Prophylactic use of an implantable cardioverter-defibrillator after acute myocardial infarction. N Engl J Med 2004;351:2481–8.

50. Zipes DP, Camm AJ, Borggrefe M, et al. ACC/AHA/ESC 2006 guidelines for management of patients with ventricular arrhythmias and the prevention of sudden cardiac death: a report of the American College of Cardiology/American Heart Association Task Force and the European Society of Cardiology

Committee for Practice Guidelines (Writing Committee to develop guidelines for management of patients with ventricular arrhythmias and the prevention of sudden cardiac death). J Am Coll Cardiol 2006;48:e247–346.

51. The Antiarrhythmics versus Implantable Defibrillators (AVID) Investigators. A comparison of antiarrhythmic-drug therapy with implantable defibrillators in patients resuscitated from near-fatal ventricular arrhythmias. N Engl J Med 1997;337:1576–83.

52. Wever EF, Hauer RN, van Capelle FL, et al. Randomized study of implantable defibrillator as first-choice therapy versus conventional strategy in postinfarct sudden death survivors. Circulation 1995;91:2195–203.

53. Siebels J, Kuck KH. Implantable cardioverter defibrillator compared with antiarrhythmic drug treatment in cardiac arrest survivors (the Cardiac Arrest Study Hamburg). Am Heart J 1994;127:1139–44.

54. Connolly SJ, Gent M, Roberts RS, et al. Canadian implantable defibrillator study (CIDS): a randomized trial of the implantable cardioverter defibrillator against amiodarone. Circulation 2000;101:1297–302.

55. Kuck KH, Cappato R, Siebels J, et al. Randomized comparison of antiarrhythmic drug therapy with implantable defibrillators in patients resuscitated from cardiac arrest: the Cardiac Arrest Study Hamburg (CASH), 2000 (CASH). Circulation 2000;102:748–54.

56. Connolly SJ, Hallstrom AP, Cappato R, et al. Meta-analysis of the implantable cardioverter defibrillator secondary prevention trials. AVID, CASH and CIDS studies. Antiarrhythmics vs implantable defibrillatorstudy, 2000 study. Cardiac Arrest Study Hamburg. Canadian Implantable Defibrillator Study. Eur Heart J 2000;21:2071–8.

57. Cleland JG, Daubert JC, Erdmann E, et al. The effect of cardiac resynchronization on morbidity and mortality in heart failure. N Engl J Med 2005;352:1539–49.

58. Bristow MR, Saxon LA, Boehmer J, et al. Cardiac resynchronization therapy with or without an implantable defibrillator in advanced chronic heart failure. N Engl J Med 2004;350:2140–50.

59. Abraham WT, Fisher WG, Smith AL, et al. Cardiac resynchronization in chronic heart failure. N Engl J Med 2002;356:1845–53.

60. Moss AJ, Hall WJ, Cannom DS, et al. Cardiac-resynchronization therapy for the prevention of heart-failure events. N Engl J Med 2009;361:1329–38.

61. Tang AS, Wells GA, Talajic M, et al. Cardiac resynchronization therapy for mild-to-moderate heart failure. N Engl J Med 2010;363:2385–95.

62. Linde C, Abraham WT, Gold MR, et al. Randomized trial of cardiac resynchronization in mildly symptomatic heart failure patients and in asymptomatic patients with left ventricular dysfunction and previous heart failure symptoms. J Am Coll Cardiol 2008;52:1834–43.

63. Brignole M, Gammage M, Puggioni E, et al. Comparative assessment of right, left, and biventricular pacing in patients with permanent atrial fibrillation. Eur Heart J 2011;32:2420–9.

64. Brignole M, Botto G, Mont L, et al. Cardiac resynchronization therapy in patients undergoing atrioventricular junction ablation for permanent atrial fibrillation: a randomized trial. Eur Heart J 2011;32:2420–9.

65. Doshi RN, Daoud EG, Fellows C, et al. Left ventricular-based cardiac stimulation post AV nodal ablation evaluation (the PAVE study). J Cardiovasc Electrophysiol 2005;16:1160–5.

66. Gasparini M, Auricchio A, Regoli F, et al. Four-year efficacy of cardiac resynchronization therapy on exercise tolerance and disease progression: the importance of performing atrioventricular junction ablation in patients with atrial fibrillation. J Am Coll Cardiol 2006;248:734–43.

67. Wilton SB, Leung AA, Ghali WA, et al. Outcomes of cardiac resynchronization therapy in patients with versus those without atrial fibrillation: a systematic review and meta-analysis. Heart Rhythm 2011;8:1088–94.

68. Upadhyay GA, Chouhry NK, Auricchio A, et al. Cardiac resynchronization in patients with atrial fibrillation: a meta-analysis of prospective cohort studies. J AM Coll Cardiol 2008;52:1239–46.

69. Wilkoff BL, Cook JR, Epstein AE, et al. Dual-chamber pacing or ventricular backup pacing in patients with an implantable defibrillator: the Dual Chamber and VVI Implantable Defibrillator (DAVID) Trial. JAMA 2002;288:115–23.

70. Ammar KA, Jacobsen SJ, Mahoney DW, et al. Prevalence and prognostic significance of heart failure stages: application of the American College of Cardiology/American Heart Association heart failure staging criteria in the community. Circulation 2007;115:1563–70.

71. Rose EA, Gelijns AC, Moskowitz AJ, et al. Long-term use of a left ventricular assist device for end-stage heart failure. N Engl J Med 2001;345:1435–43.

72. Rogers JG, Butler J, Lansman SL, et al. Chronic mechanical circulatory support for inotrope-dependent heart failure patients who are not transplant candidates: results of the INTREPID trial. J Am Coll Cardiol 2007;50:741–7.

73. Stevenson LW, Pagani FD, Young JB, et al. INTERMACS profiles of advanced heart failure: the current picture. J Heart Lung Transplant 2009;28:535–41.

74. Metra M, Pinikowski P, Dickstein K, et al. Advanced chronic heart failure: a position statement from the study group on advanced heart failure of the heart failure association of the European Society of Cardiology. Eur J Heart Fail 2007;9:684–94.

75. Allen LA, Stevenson LW, Grady KL, et al, on behalf of the American Heart Association Council on Quality of Care and Outcomes Research, Council on Cardiovascular Nursing, Council on Clinical Cardiology, Council on Cardiovascular Radiology and Intervention, and Council on Cardiovascular Surgery and Anesthesia. Decision making in advanced heart failure: a scientific statement from the American Heart Association. Circulation 2012; 125:1928–52.

76. Abraham WT, Adams KF, Fonarow GC, et al. In-hospital mortality in patients with acute decompensated heart failure requiring intravenous vasoactive medications: an analysis from the Acute Decompensated Heart Failure National Registry (ADHERE). J Am Coll Cardiol 2005;46: 57–64.

77. Cuffe MS, Califf RM, Adams KF Jr, et al. Short-term intravenous milrinone for acute exacerbation of chronic heart failure: a randomized controlled trial. JAMA 2002;287:1541–7.

78. Elkayam U, Tasissa G, Binanay C, et al. Use and impact of inotropes and vasodilator therapy in hospitalized patients with severe heart failure. Am Heart J 2007;153:98–104.

79. Rihal CS, Naidu SS, Givertz MM, et al. 2015 SCAI/ ACC/HFSA/STS clinical expert consensus statement on the use of percutaneous mechanical circulatory support devices in cardiovascular care: endorsed by the American Heart Association, the Cardiological Society of India, and Sociedad Latino Americana de Cardiologia Intervencion; Affirmation of Value by the Canadian Association of Interventional Cardiology-Association Canadienne de Cardiologie d'intervention. J Am Coll Cardiol 2015;65:e7–26.

80. Holman WL, Pae WE, Teuteberg JJ, et al. INTERMACS: interval analysis of registry data. J Am Coll Surg 2009;2008:755–61.

81. Thiele H, Zeymer U, Neumann FJ, et al, for Investigators I-SIT. Intraaortic balloon support for myocardial infarction with cardiogenic shock. N Engl J Med 2012;367:1287–96.

82. Seyfarth M, Sibbing D, Bauer I, et al. A randomized clinical trial to evaluate the safety and efficacy of a percutaneous left ventricular assist device versus intra-aortic balloon pumping for treatment of cardiogenic shock caused by myocardial infarction. J Am Coll Cardiol 2008;52: 1584–8.

83. Cheng JM, den Uil CA, Hoeks SE, et al. Percutaneous left ventricular assist devices vs. intra-aortic balloon pump counterpulsation for treatment of cardiogenic shock: a meta-analysis of controlled trials. Eur Heart J 2009;30:2102–8.

84. Thiele H, Sick P, Boudriot E, et al. Randomized comparison of intra-aortic balloon support with a percutaneous left ventricular assist device in patients with revascularized acute myocardial infarction complicated by cardiogenic shock. Eur Heart J 2005;26:1276–83.

85. Kapur NK, Esposito M. Hemodynamic support with percutaneous devices in patients with heart failure. Heart Fail Clin 2015;11(2):215–30.

86. Slaughter MS, Rogers JG, Milano CA, et al, for the HeartMate II Investigators. Advanced heart failure treated with continuous-flow left ventricular assist devices. N Engl J Med 2009;361(23): 2241–51.

87. Mehra MR, Naka Y, Uriel N, et al, for the MOMENTUM 3 Investigators. A fully magnetically levitated circulatory pump for advanced heart failure. N Engl J Med 2017;376:440–50.

88. Mehra MR, Goldstein DJ, Uriel N, et al, for the MOMENTUM 3 Investigators. Two-year outcomes with a magnetically levitated cardiac pump in heart failure. N Engl J Med 2018;378:1386–95.

89. Starling RC, Naka Y, Boyle AJ, et al. Results of the post-U.S. Food and Drug Administration – approval study with a continuous flow ventricular assist device as bridge to heart transplantation: a prospective study using the INTERMACS (Interagency Registry for Mechanically Assisted Circulatory Support). J Am Coll Cardiol 2011;57: 1890–8.

90. Kirklin JK, Pagani FD, Kormos RL, et al. Eighth annual INTERMACS report: special focus on framing the impact of adverse events. 2017 INTERMACS Report. J Heart Lung Transplant 2017;36: 1080–6.

91. Stehlik J, Edwards LB, Kucheryavaya AY, et al. The registry of the International Society for Heart and Lung Transplantation: twenty-eighth adult heart transplant report–2011. J Heart Lung Transplant 2011;30:1078–94.

92. Lund LH, Khush KK, Cherikh WS, et al, International Society for Heart and Lung Transplantation. The registry of the International Society for Heart and Lung Transplantation: thirty-fourth adult heart transplantation report-2017; focus theme: allograft ischemic time. J Heart Lung Transplant 2017; 36(10):1037–46.

93. Grady KL, Naftel DC, Kobashigawa J, et al. Patterns and predictors of quality of life at 5 to 10 years after heart transplantation. J Heart Lung Transplant 2007;26:535–43.

94. Kobashigawa JA, Leaf DA, Lee N, et al. A controlled trial of exercise rehabilitation after heart transplantation. N Engl J Med 1999;340: 272–7.

95. Deng MC, De Meester JM, Smits JM, et al. Effect of receiving a heart transplant: analysis of a national cohort entered on to a waiting list, stratified by heart failure severity: Comparative Outcome and Clinical Profiles in Transplantation (COCPIT) Study Group. BMJ 2000;321:540–5.

96. Mancini DM, Eisen H, Kussmaul W, et al. Value of peak exercise oxygen consumption for optimal timing of cardiac transplantation in ambulatory patients with heart failure. Circulation 1991;83: 778–86.

97. Lund LH, Aaronson KD, Mancini DM. Predicting survival in ambulatory patients with severe heart failure on beta-blocker therapy. Am J Cardiol 2003;92:1350–4.

98. Goda A, Lund LH, Mancini D. The Heart Failure Survival Score outperforms the peak oxygen consumption for heart transplantation selection in the era of device therapy. J Heart Lung Transplant 2011;30:315–25.

99. Butler J, Khadim G, Paul KM, et al. Selection of patients for heart transplantation in the current era of heart failure therapy. J Am Coll Cardiol 2004;43: 787–93.

100. Ferreira AM, Tabet JY, Frankenstein L, et al. Ventilatory efficiency and the selection of patients for heart transplantation. Circ Heart Fail 2010;3: 378–86.

101. Wilson SR, Mudge GH, Stewart GC, et al. Evaluation for a ventricular assist device: selecting the appropriate candidate. Circulation 2009;119: 2225–32.

102. Koelling TM, Johnson ML, Cody RJ, et al. Discharge education improves clinical outcomes in patients with chronic heart failure. Circulation 2005;111:179–85.

103. Krumholz HM, Chen YT, Wang Y, et al. Predictors of readmission among elderly survivors of admission with heart failure. Am Heart J 2000;139: 72–7.

104. Hernandez AF, Greiner MA, Fonarow GC, et al. Relationship between early physician follow-up and 30-day readmission among Medicare beneficiaries hospitalized for heart failure. JAMA 2010; 303:1716–22.

105. McAlister FA, Stewart S, Ferrua S, et al. Multidisciplinary strategies for the management of heart failure patients at high risk for admission: a systematic review of randomized trials. J Am Coll Cardiol 2004;44:810–9.

106. Fonarow GC, Abraham WT, Albert NM, et al. Influence of a performance-improvement initiative on quality of care for patients hospitalized with heart failure: results of the Organized Program to Initiate Lifesaving Treatment in Hospitalized Patients with Heart Failure (OPTIMIZE-HF). Arch Intern Med 2007;167:1493–502.

107. Rich MW, Beckham V, Wittenberg C, et al. A multidisciplinary intervention to prevent the readmission of elderly patients with congestive heart failure. N Engl J Med 1995;333:1190–5.

108. McAlister FA, Lawson FM, Teo KK, et al. A systematic review of randomized trials of disease management programs in heart failure. Am J Med 2001;110:378–84.

109. Grady KL, Dracup K, Kennedy G, et al. Team management of patients with heart failure: a statement for healthcare professionals from the Cardiovascular Nursing Council of the American Heart Association. Circulation 2000;102: 2443–56.

110. Lindenfeld J, Albert NM, Boehmer JP, et al. HFSA 2010 comprehensive heart failure practice guideline. J Card Fail 2010;16:e1–194.

111. Dickstein K, Cohen-Solal A, Filippatos G, et al. ESC guidelines for the diagnosis and treatment of acute and chronic heart failure 2008: the task force for the diagnosis and treatment of acute and chronic heart failure 2008 of the European Society of Cardiology: developed in collaboration with the Heart Failure Association of the ESC (HFA) and endorsed by the European Society of Intensive Care Medicine (ESICM). Eur Heart J 2008;29:2388–442.

112. Malcom J, Arnold O, Howlett JG, et al. Canadian Cardiovascular Society Consensus Conference guidelines on heart failure–2008 update: best practices for the transition of care of heart failure patients, and the recognition, investigation and treatment of cardiomyopathies. Can J Cardiol 2008;24:21–40.

113. Lennie TA, Song EK, Wu JR, et al. Three gram sodium intake is associated with longer event-free survival only in patients with advanced heart failure. J Card Fail 2011;17:325–30.

114. Arcand J, Ivanov J, Sasson A, et al. A high-sodium diet is associated with acute decompensated heart failure in ambulatory heart failure patients: a prospective follow-up study. Am J Clin Nutr 2011;93: 332–7.

115. Damgaard M, Norsk P, Gustafsson F, et al. Hemodynamic and neuroendocrine responses to changes in sodium intake in compensated heart failure. Am J Physiol Regul Integr Comp Physiol 2006;290:R1294–301.

116. Volpe M, Magri P, Rao MA, et al. Intrarenal determinants of sodium retention in mild heart failure: effects of angiotensin-converting enzyme inhibition. Hypertension 1997;30:168–76.

117. Paterna S, Gaspare P, Fasullo S, et al. Normal-sodium diet compared with low-sodium diet in compensated congestive heart failure: is sodium an old enemy or a new friend? Clin Sci (Lond) 2008;114:221–30.

118. Habbu A, Lakkis NM, Dokainish H. The obesity paradox: fact or fiction? Am J Cardiol 2006;98: 944–8.

119. O'Connor CM, Whellan DJ, Lee KL, et al. Efficacy and safety of exercise training in patients with chronic heart failure: HF-ACTION randomized controlled trial. JAMA 2009;301: 1439–50.

120. Piepoli MF, Davos C, Francis DP, et al. Exercise training meta-analysis of trials in patients with chronic heart failure (ExTraMATCH). BMJ 2004;328:189.

121. Adler ED, Goldfinger JZ, Kalman J, et al. Palliative care in the treatment of advanced heart failure. Circulation 2009;120:2597–606.

122. Goodlin SJ. Palliative care in congestive heart failure. J Am Coll Cardiol 2009;54:386–96.

CRT Role in HF Management and Implant Techniques

Why Dyssynchrony Matters in Heart Failure?

Bhupendar Tayal, MD, PhD[a], Peter Sogaard, MD, DMSc[a],*, Niels Risum, MD, PhD[b]

KEYWORDS

- Dyssynchrony • Cardiac resynchronization therapy • Heart failure

KEY POINTS

- Cardiac resynchronization therapy (CRT) is an electrical therapy to resolve an electrical problem. Any method to predict CRT response must specifically reflect the electrical substrate.
- Time-to-peak dyssynchrony is too unspecific for prediction of response because dyssynchrony by this approach may reflect the presence of scar or fibrosis even in the absence of a conduction delay.
- New methods are based on the actual physiology of activation delay–induced heart failure (HF) and are superior to time-to-peak methods in predicting CRT response.
- Time-to-peak dyssynchrony may still be used for prognosis in HF patients without signs of delayed ventricular activation and for monitoring CRT response.

INTRODUCTION

The term, *dyssynchrony*, refers to discoordination in contraction of myocardial wall segments. Myocardial dyssynchrony has been described in a series of different pathologies, such as ischemic heart disease,[1,2] hypertrophic cardiomyopathy,[3] pulmonary hypertension,[4] congenital heart defects,[5,6] arrhythmogenic right ventricular cardiomyopathy,[7] hypertension,[8] and metabolic syndrome.[9] Heart failure (HF) is a clinical syndrome that can be caused by a range of different structural and functional abnormalities. Although electrical and mechanical dyssynchrony is frequently reported in patients with HF,[10–12] mechanical dyssynchrony can be observed in HF patients despite the absence of electrical dyssynchrony.[12]

Mechanical dyssynchrony gained significance with the introduction of cardiac resynchronization therapy (CRT) device for the treatment of patients with HF. In the setting of CRT, however, it is important to differentiate between various types of dyssynchrony, that is, specific patterns of dyssynchrony must be identified that are amenable to resynchronization. In other words, follow the physiology of activation delay–induced HF. This review discusses the evolving concept of dyssynchrony and how it can be applied in patients with HF who are considered for device therapy.

SELECTION CRITERIA FOR CARDIAC RESYNCHRONIZATION THERAPY

Thus far, the mainstay for patient selection for CRT implantation has been the presence of electrical dyssynchrony. Initially, a QRS widening to a duration to greater than or equal to 120 ms was one of the selection criteria. Despite overall improvement in morbidity and mortality, a significant percentage of patients (30%–40%) showed inadequate response.[13] The effect has primarily been

Disclosure: P. Sogaard: Consultant, Biotronik; Advisory board, Astra Zeneca; Research grants; Biotronik and GE Healthcare. N. Risum and B. Tayal: None.
[a] Department of Cardiology, Aalborg University Hospital, Hobrovej 18-22, Aalborg 9100, Denmark;
[b] Department of Cardiology, Rigshospitalet, Copenhagen University Hospital, Blegdamsvej 9, Copenhagen 2100, Denmark
* Corresponding author.
E-mail address: p.soegaard@rn.dk

cardiacEP.theclinics.com

observed in patients with left bundle branch block (LBBB) and wide QRS (≥150 ms).[14,15] Therefore, the current guidelines recommend presence of LBBB with wide QRS (≥150 ms) as class IA indication for CRT implantation.[16,17]

NOT ALL PATIENTS WITH LEFT BUNDLE BRANCH BLOCK BY ECG ARE THE SAME

A significant number of HF patients have LBBB,[18] but not all of them are LBBB myopathy. Surface ECGs may sometimes be unreliable in diagnosing true LBBB with an activation delay, as demonstrated by invasive electrophysiologic studies.[19,20] Approximately one-third of patients are misdiagnosed as LBBB just by the present ECG criteria and have more than 1 septal breakthrough site indicating a lack of true activation delay.[19,21] A stricter definition to diagnose LBBB by ECG has been proposed by Straus and colleagues,[22] with 2 specific changes to distinguish it from interventricular conduction delays: (1) longer QRS duration—greater than or equal to 130 ms in women and greater than or equal to 140 ms in men and (2) mid-QRS notching in 2 contiguous leads. This definition of LBBB has shown additional value in identifying CRT responders beyond the current criteria for CRT.[23]

LEFT BUNDLE BRANCH BLOCK AND ACTIVATION DELAY DYSSYNCHRONY

Presence of LBBB causes early activation of the septum and a delayed activation of the LV free wall because the free wall is activated by the myocardial fiber-to-myocardial fiber conduction rather than by the Purkinje system due to block of the left bundle.[24] This inefficient contraction pattern leads to a series of changes, including reduction of the septal workload along with its hypoperfusion, increased workload of the free wall, asymmetric hypertrophy of the LV free wall, and LV remodeling and development of cardiomyopathy.[25] Pacing by CRT with a right ventricular septal lead and LV lead restores a simultaneous activation of the LV, attenuating the activation delay.[26] Identification of a mechanical delay as a consequence of abnormal electrical activation is important because this serves as a substrate for optimal response to CRT. The substrate for optimal CRT response is the activation delay and the challenge is to identify this by echocardiography.

ACTIVATION DELAY BY ECHOCARDIOGRAPHY

A few methods are discussed that have shown convincing results with the potential of clinical use.

Typical Left Bundle Branch Block Contraction Pattern

Risum and colleagues[23] used 2-D speckle tracking echocardiography to define a typical contraction pattern in patients with LBBB, thereby identifying true LBBB activation delay–induced HF. Three characteristics features were described: (1) early septal contraction within the 70% of the aortic valve closure (AVC) from the start of QRS, (2) prestretch of the lateral wall, and (3) delayed contraction of the lateral wall after the AVC (**Fig. 1**).[27] AVC time was determined from the pulsed Doppler left ventricular (LV) outflow curve. It should be examined in both apical 4-chamber and long-axis views. In a study including only patients with LBBB, Risum and colleagues[23] demonstrated that approximately one-third of patients with LBBB by ECG did not show LBBB contraction but had other structural or mechanical characteristics to explain the LBBB-like changes in the ECG, such as scar or hypertrophy. Identification of this contraction pattern is even superior to some of the stricter ECG criteria proposed for defining LBBB because strain pattern also provides information on myocardial performance, which cannot be gathered by ECG. The investigators further demonstrated in a prospective study with 4 years' follow-up that the absence of a typical LBBB contraction pattern prior to the implantation of CRT was associated with a 3-fold increase in mortality risk in comparison to those with a typical contraction pattern.[27] These findings were found independent of QRS width. This is important because the current guidelines are still unclear regarding the group of patients with intermediate QRS width (QRS 120–149 ms). Besides being a relatively simple method, another advantage of this method is the low interobserver variability, which is one of the most important criticisms of dyssynchrony methods.

The concept of identifying an activation delay by studying the myocardial mechanical patterns also may be applied to patients with right ventricular pacing (RVP) and HF. Upgrade to CRT in RVP patients is performed based on the discretion of the treating physician because the guidelines are ambiguous. RVP and development of HF are not always related. Like LBBB patients, the question is whether these patients have a mechanical problem due to the pacing-induced activation delay or simply a problem due to a sick myocardium with fibrosis or scarring. Tayal and colleagues[28] applied the strain pattern in patients with RVP and HF and found that presence of this contraction pattern prior to upgrade to CRT was associated with outcome comparable to that in patients with LBBB and wide QRS (≥150 ms).

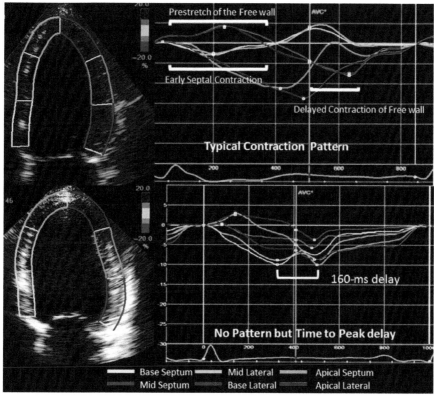

Fig. 1. Typical contraction pattern. Two examples of contraction pattern are shown from patients having LBBB. The upper panel figure shows the typical contraction pattern with early septal contraction and prestretch of the free wall followed by the delayed contraction of the free wall. In the lower panel, this contraction pattern is not observed but there is significant delay by time-to-peak method between the septum and LV free wall.

Apical Rocking and Septal Flash

Looking for apical rocking and septal flash is based on the concept of identifying activation-contraction physiology compatible with a typical LBBB activation pattern.[29] Apical rocking is the horizontal movement of the LV apex, first toward right due to free wall stretch and later toward left due to free wall contraction caused by the time-delay in septal to lateral activation (**Fig. 2**). Septal flash is the representation of the early septal activation during isovolumic contraction time, which is suppressed by the counteracting later activated lateral walls. In a retrospective series of 1060 patients with various QRS morphology, the investigators observed that presence of this apical rocking and septal flash was associated with an approximately 60% reduction in mortality with a median follow-up period of 46 months. Among patients who had septal flash and apical rocking at baseline, 92% of them had correction of this contraction pattern post–device therapy. The 8% of patients who did not resynchronize post-CRT had severe cardiomyopathy with very low ejection fraction along with dilatation of ventricle. It was

shown recently that to achieve better mechanical resynchronization, timely device implantation is important before it is too late and the ventricle becomes severely dilated.[30] Delaying device implantation strategy to optimize HF medication increases the risk of LV dilatation, because the recommended HF medications may not necessarily help patients with LBBB myopathy.[31]

Cross-correlation Analysis

Cross-correlation analysis (CCA) of the tissue Doppler imaging (TDI) acceleration curves is another method that can identify activation delay–induced HF.[32,33] CCA uses complex waveforms analysis and is performed on a software publicly available. Tissue velocity data from opposing wall are imported from the color-coded TDI images of apical views. By applying automated algorithm, these velocity data are first converted to acceleration curves and they are then moved against each other in both directions frame-by-frame to identify the time delay that provides the best correlation between the contraction of the opposing walls (**Figs. 3** and **4**). Basically, by

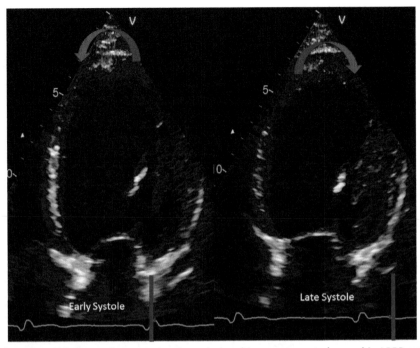

Fig. 2. Apical rocking. This figure demonstrates the apical rocking movement observed in LBBB patients with a significant activation delay–induced HF. The apex of the LV moves horizontally, first toward the right ventricle in the early systole (*right* panel) and later toward the free wall in the late systole (*left* panel). This is due to the early activation of the septum and delayed activation of the LV free wall.

this method, the time delay is derived between the opposing myocardial walls, which would produce a coordinated LV contraction. A time delay of greater than or equal to 35 ms prior to CRT is considered significant dyssynchrony by CCA. Risum and colleagues[33] studied 131 patients and found that presence of significant activation delay by CCA was associated with reduced all-cause death at the end of 4 years after CRT implantation in comparison to those without significant activation delay by CCA (14% vs 40%). Furthermore, lack of dyssynchrony by CCA in patients with intermediate QRS duration (120–149 ms) had a 4-fold increased risk of outcome events. This method has considerably less intraobserver and interobserver variability because it is performed on software rather than manually.

ACTIVATION DELAY VERSUS TIME-TO-PEAK DYSSYNCHRONY

Nearly all the early methods of dyssynchrony assessment were based on the time-to-peak concept, where dyssynchrony is determined by differences in time-to-peak movements of the opposing wall segments. The major pitfall in using a time-to-peak method is conceptual. Whether time-to-peak dyssynchrony is measured using TDI velocities, displacement, deformation, or any

other movement, not all dyssynchrony by this approach necessarily reflects an activation delay. Large time-to-peak differences can be seen due to scar, fibrosis, heterogeneities in a failing heart, and even changes in loading conditions (see **Fig. 3**).[34–36] Such associations between varying degrees of contractility and conduction delay have been elegantly demonstrated by Lumens and colleagues[37] using computer modeling and real-life patients examples.

Although a significant activation delay usually leads to a large time-to-peak difference dyssynchrony, the latter may be too unspecific in identifying the underlying electrical substrate.[26] This has been clearly demonstrated by the failure of the Echocardiography Guided Cardiac Resynchronization Therapy (EchoCRT) trial.[38] In EchoCRT trial, 809 patients with HF with narrow QRS (<130 ms) and presence of mechanical dyssynchrony were randomized to CRT-on and CRT-off in 1:1 ratio. Mechanical dyssynchrony was measured by applying longitudinal TDI time-to-peak and radial strain time-to-peak delay. Patients with CRT-on had a worse prognosis and specifically increased mortality was observed in younger patients who were randomized to CRT-on. Recently, a substudy of EchoCRT demonstrated that approximately 50% of the patients with dyssynchrony by time-to-peak methods had no

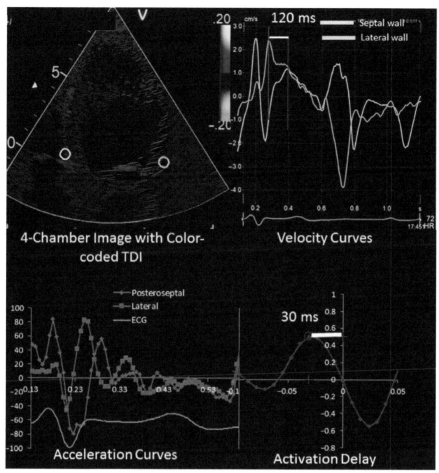

Fig. 3. No activation delay by CCA. This is an example of no activation delay by CCA but dyssynchrony by time-to-peak method. In the upper right panel, TDI velocity curves are shown. A significant dyssynchrony by time-to-peak is observed with an opposing wall delay of 120 ms (≥65 ms) between the timing of peak tissue velocities of the septum and the lateral wall. The lower left panel shows the acceleration curve derived from the tissue velocity data and lower right panel shows the activation delay between these 2 walls. There is an activation delay of 30 ms, which suggest that there is no dyssynchrony by CCA.

activation delay dyssynchrony by CCA. In addition, this study demonstrated that patients with lack of dyssynchrony by CCA who were randomized to CRT-on at baseline had the worst outcome.[39] Thus, the role of time-to-peak dyssynchrony is limited in selection of patients for CRT. Another important concern associated with estimation of time-to-peak dyssynchrony is its poor reproducibility.[40]

Several single-center studies have demonstrated independent of each other that presence of dyssynchrony by time-to-peak parameters—both radial strain delay and TDI dyssynchrony—are associated with improved outcome and volumetric response after CRT.[41–43] In comparison to these time-to-peak parameters, however, methods more specifically identifying activation delay have been associated with significantly

greater improvement in outcome after CRT (**Table 1**). This further supports the concept of following the physiology of activation delay–induced HF when assessing candidates for CRT implantation.

TIME-TO-PEAK DYSSYNCHRONY AS A PROGNOSTIC MARKER

Although time-to-peak dyssynchrony has proved inferior in selection of patients for CRT in comparison to other methods, prognostic information can be derived from such parameters. Several studies have shown that persistence or onset of new mechanical dyssynchrony is related to adverse cardiac events, in particular ventricular arrhythmias in patients with CRT.[39,44–47] Applying different approaches of measurement of

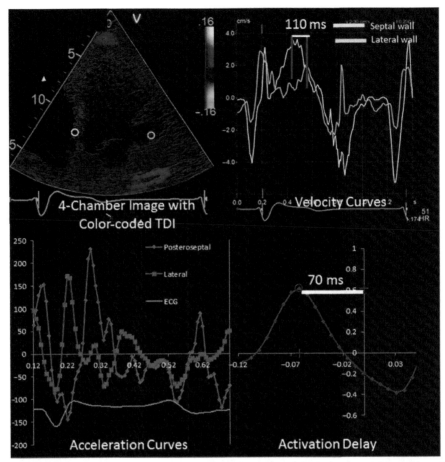

Fig. 4. Activation delay by CCA. This is another example of activation delay by CCA and dyssynchrony by time-to-peak. In the upper right panel, a significant dyssynchrony by time-to-peak method is observed with an opposing wall delay of 110 ms between the timing of peak tissue velocities of the septum and the lateral wall. The lower left panel shows the acceleration curve derived from the tissue velocity data and lower right panel shows the activation delay between these 2 walls. In this example, it can be observed that at an activation delay of 70 ms, there is a significant change in the correlation between the opposing wall movement (from −0.2 to +0.6).

mechanical dyssynchrony, these studies have shown similar results. Any conventional method of time-to-peak or even CCA could be applied to measure this dyssynchrony prior to and after CRT implantation. Although most studies have measured follow-up dyssynchrony at 6-months, it can be measured before discharge of the patient after device implantation. In patients with persistence or worsening of dyssynchrony, a close follow-up strategy and eventually changing LV lead position or turning CRT off could be considered if dyssynchrony persists.

Furthermore, time-to-peak dyssynchrony can be applied in identification of HF patients at high risk of sudden cardiac death. This could be helpful in identification of patients who would benefit from the implantation of a defibrillator device in some specific patient groups like the nonischemic cardiomyopathy where the evidence is scarce.[48] In

experimental animal models, it is demonstrated that dyssynchronous heart causes protein dysregulation increasing the susceptibility to arrhythmias.[49] In a prospective study of 104 patients, Bader and colleagues[50] showed that at 1 -year follow-up HF patients with dyssynchrony had more than a 3-fold increased risk of adverse cardiac events in comparison to those without dyssynchrony. Haugaa and colleagues[51] calculated mechanical dispersion applying standard deviation of time-to-peak of the segmental longitudinal strain in dilated cardiomyopathy and found that increased mechanical dispersion was associated with a higher risk for ventricular arrhythmias.

FUTURE IMPLICATIONS

The current international guidelines recommend CRT implantation in patients with LBBB and wide

Table 1
Comparing studies with and without methods of mechanical

Studies	Patient Inclusion Criteria	Dyssynchrony Method Applied	Event Rate
Recent CRT trials			
MADIT-CRT[53]	NYHA class I–II, LVEF<35%, QRS ≥120 ms	None	25%–30% at the end of 2.3 y
RAFT[54]	NYHA class II–III, LVEF<35%, QRS ≥120 ms	None	30%–40% at the end of 6 y
Time-to-peak dyssynchrony as an additional criterion			
Gorcsan et al,[43] 2010	NYHA class II–IV, LVEF<35%, QRS ≥120 ms	Radial strain delay (≥130 ms)	25%-30% at the end of 4 y
Gorcsan et al,[43] 2010	NYHA class II–IV, LVEF<35%, QRS ≥120 ms	Opposing wall delay by TDI (≥65 ms)	25%–30% at end of 4 y
Gorcsan et al,[43] 2010	NYHA class II–IV, LVEF<35%, QRS ≥120 ms	Yu index (≥32 ms)	25%–30% at end of 4 y
Activation delay as an additional criterion			
Risum et al,[27] 2015	NYHA class II–IV, LVEF<35%, QRS ≥120 ms, and LBBB morphology	Contraction pattern	10%–12% at the end of 4 y
Stankovic et al,[29] 2016	NYHA class II–IV, LVEF<35%, QRS ≥120 ms	Apical rocking and septal flash	25% at the end of nearly 12 y
Risum et al,[33] 2013	NYHA class II–IV, LVEF<35%, QRS ≥120 ms	CCA	10%–15% at the end of 4.5 y

Abbreviations: NYHA, New York Heart Association; MADIT-CRT, multicenter automatic defibrillator implantation trial with cardiac resynchronization therapy; RAFT, *resynchronization/defibrillation for ambulatory heart failure trial*.

QRS (≥150 ms), although it is not recommended in patients with narrow QRS (<130 ms). Dyssynchrony assessment can be helpful in selection of patients where the guidelines are unclear, such as patients with LBBB and intermediate QRS duration, patients with RVP, and patients with non-LBBB and wide QRS. Moreover, dyssynchrony can be applied for risk assessment at follow-up after device implantation particularly in nonresponders. Patients with persistent or new onset of dyssynchrony after device implanted should be reviewed for LV lead position or even device removal if necessary. Wireless LV endocardial CRT system can be considered in some nonresponders where LV free wall cannot be targeted due to anatomic limitations of the cardiac veins.[52]

SUMMARY

Assessment of mechanical dyssynchrony by specific echo techniques provides prognostic information in activation delay–induced HF both before and after implantation.

REFERENCES

1. Huang WS, Huang CH, Lee CL, et al. Relation of early post-stress left ventricular dyssynchrony and the extent of angiographic coronary artery disease. J Nucl Cardiol 2014;21(6):1048–56.
2. Mollema SA, Liem SS, Suffoletto MS, et al. Left ventricular dyssynchrony acutely after myocardial infarction predicts left ventricular remodeling. J Am Coll Cardiol 2007;50(16): 1532–40.
3. Nagakura T, Takeuchi M, Yoshitani H, et al. Hypertrophic cardiomyopathy is associated with more severe left ventricular dyssynchrony than is hypertensive left ventricular hypertrophy. Echocardiography 2007;24(7):677–84.
4. Lopez-Candales A, Dohi K, Rajagopalan N, et al. Right ventricular dyssynchrony in patients with pulmonary

hypertension is associated with disease severity and functional class. Cardiovasc Ultrasound 2005;3:23.

5. Zhong SW, Zhang YQ, Chen LJ, et al. Ventricular twisting and dyssynchrony in children with single left ventricle using three-dimensional speckle tracking imaging after the fontan operation. Echocardiography 2016;33(4):606–17.

6. Friedberg MK, Silverman NH, Dubin AM, et al. Right ventricular mechanical dyssynchrony in children with hypoplastic left heart syndrome. J Am Soc Echocardiogr 2007;20(9):1073–9.

7. Prati G, Vitrella G, Allocca G, et al. Right ventricular strain and dyssynchrony assessment in arrhythmogenic right ventricular cardiomyopathy: cardiac magnetic resonance feature-tracking study. Circ Cardiovasc Imaging 2015;8(11):e003647.

8. Kwon BJ, Lee SH, Park CS, et al. Left ventricular diastolic dyssynchrony in patients with treatment-naive hypertension and the effects of antihypertensive therapy. J Hypertens 2015;33(2):354–65.

9. Crendal E, Walther G, Dutheil F, et al. Left ventricular myocardial dyssynchrony is already present in nondiabetic patients with metabolic syndrome. Can J Cardiol 2014;30(3):320–4.

10. Iuliano S, Fisher SG, Karasik PE, et al. Department of veterans affairs survival trial of antiarrhythmic therapy in congestive heart F. QRS duration and mortality in patients with congestive heart failure. Am Heart J 2002;143(6):1085–91.

11. Bleeker GB, Schalij MJ, Molhoek SG, et al. Relationship between QRS duration and left ventricular dyssynchrony in patients with end-stage heart failure. J Cardiovasc Electrophysiol 2004; 15(5):544–9.

12. Ghio S, Constantin C, Klersy C, et al. Interventricular and intraventricular dyssynchrony are common in heart failure patients, regardless of QRS duration. Eur Heart J 2004;25(7):571–8.

13. Ypenburg C, Westenberg JJ, Bleeker GB, et al. Noninvasive imaging in cardiac resynchronization therapy–part 1: selection of patients. Pacing Clin Electrophysiol 2008;31(11):1475–99.

14. Sipahi I, Carrigan TP, Rowland DY, et al. Impact of QRS duration on clinical event reduction with cardiac resynchronization therapy: meta-analysis of randomized controlled trials. Arch Intern Med 2011;171(16):1454–62.

15. Sipahi I, Chou JC, Hyden M, et al. Effect of QRS morphology on clinical event reduction with cardiac resynchronization therapy: meta-analysis of randomized controlled trials. Am Heart J 2012; 163(2):260–7.e263.

16. Tracy CM, Epstein AE, Darbar D, et al. 2012 ACCF/AHA/HRS focused update of the 2008 guidelines for device-based therapy of cardiac rhythm abnormalities: a report of the American College of Cardiology Foundation/American Heart Association Task Force on Practice Guidelines. J Am Coll Cardiol 2012; 60(14):1297–313.

17. Brignole M, Auricchio A, Baron-Esquivias G, et al. 2013 ESC guidelines on cardiac pacing and cardiac resynchronization therapy: the Task Force on cardiac pacing and resynchronization therapy of the European Society of Cardiology (ESC). Developed in collaboration with the European Heart Rhythm Association (EHRA). Eur Heart J 2013;34(29):2281–329.

18. Baldasseroni S, Opasich C, Gorini M, et al. Left bundle-branch block is associated with increased 1-year sudden and total mortality rate in 5517 outpatients with congestive heart failure: a report from the Italian network on congestive heart failure. Am Heart J 2002;143(3):398–405.

19. Vassallo JA, Cassidy DM, Marchlinski FE, et al. Endocardial activation of left bundle branch block. Circulation 1984;69(5):914–23.

20. Auricchio A, Fantoni C, Regoli F, et al. Characterization of left ventricular activation in patients with heart failure and left bundle-branch block. Circulation 2004;109(9):1133–9.

21. Grant RP, Dodge HT. Mechanisms of QRS complex prolongation in man; left ventricular conduction disturbances. Am J Med 1956;20(6):834–52.

22. Strauss DG, Selvester RH, Wagner GS. Defining left bundle branch block in the era of cardiac resynchronization therapy. Am J Cardiol 2011;107(6):927–34.

23. Risum N, Strauss D, Sogaard P, et al. Left bundle-branch block: the relationship between electrocardiogram electrical activation and echocardiography mechanical contraction. Am Heart J 2013;166(2): 340–8.

24. Prinzen FW, Hunter WC, Wyman BT, et al. Mapping of regional myocardial strain and work during ventricular pacing: experimental study using magnetic resonance imaging tagging. J Am Coll Cardiol 1999;33(6):1735–42.

25. Vernooy K, Verbeek XA, Peschar M, et al. Left bundle branch block induces ventricular remodelling and functional septal hypoperfusion. Eur Heart J 2005;26(1):91–8.

26. Risum N, Jons C, Olsen NT, et al. Simple regional strain pattern analysis to predict response to cardiac resynchronization therapy: rationale, initial results, and advantages. Am Heart J 2012;163(4):697–704.

27. Risum N, Tayal B, Hansen TF, et al. Identification of typical left bundle branch block contraction by strain echocardiography is additive to electrocardiography in prediction of long-term outcome after cardiac resynchronization therapy. J Am Coll Cardiol 2015;66(6):631–41.

28. Tayal B, Gorcsan J 3rd, Delgado-Montero A, et al. Comparative long-term outcomes after cardiac resynchronization therapy in right ventricular paced patients versus native wide left bundle branch block patients. Heart Rhythm 2016;13(2):511–8.

29. Stankovic I, Prinz C, Ciarka A, et al. Relationship of visually assessed apical rocking and septal flash to response and long-term survival following cardiac resynchronization therapy (PREDICT-CRT). Eur Heart J Cardiovasc Imaging 2016;17(3):262–9.

30. Tayal B, Sogaard P, Delgado-Montero A, et al. Interaction of left ventricular remodeling and regional dyssynchrony on long-term prognosis after cardiac resynchronization therapy. J Am Soc Echocardiogr 2017;30(3):244–50.

31. Sze E, Samad Z, Dunning A, et al. Impaired recovery of left ventricular function in patients with cardiomyopathy and left bundle branch block. J Am Coll Cardiol 2018;71(3):306–17.

32. Olsen NT, Mogelvang R, Jons C, et al. Predicting response to cardiac resynchronization therapy with cross-correlation analysis of myocardial systolic acceleration: a new approach to echocardiographic dyssynchrony evaluation. J Am Soc Echocardiogr 2009;22(6):657–64.

33. Risum N, Williams ES, Khouri MG, et al. Mechanical dyssynchrony evaluated by tissue Doppler cross-correlation analysis is associated with long-term survival in patients after cardiac resynchronization therapy. Eur Heart J 2013;34(1):48–56.

34. Tigen K, Karaahmet T, Kirma C, et al. Diffuse late gadolinium enhancement by cardiovascular magnetic resonance predicts significant intraventricular systolic dyssynchrony in patients with nonischemic dilated cardiomyopathy. J Am Soc Echocardiogr 2010;23(4):416–22.

35. Lin LY, Wu CK, Juang JM, et al. Myocardial regional interstitial fibrosis is associated with left intraventricular dyssynchrony in patients with heart failure: a cardiovascular magnetic resonance study. Sci Rep 2016;6:20711.

36. Lafitte S, Bordachar P, Lafitte M, et al. Dynamic ventricular dyssynchrony: an exercise-echocardiography study. J Am Coll Cardiol 2006;47(11):2253–9.

37. Lumens J, Tayal B, Walmsley J, et al. Differentiating electromechanical from non-electrical substrates of mechanical discoordination to identify responders to cardiac resynchronization therapy. Circ Cardiovasc Imaging 2015;8(9):e003744.

38. Ruschitzka F, Abraham WT, Singh JP, et al. Cardiac-resynchronization therapy in heart failure with a narrow QRS complex. N Engl J Med 2013;369(15):1395–405.

39. Tayal B, Gorcsan J 3rd, Bax JJ, et al. Cardiac resynchronization therapy in patients with heart failure and narrow QRS complexes. J Am Coll Cardiol 2018;71(12):1325–33.

40. Chung ES, Leon AR, Tavazzi L, et al. Results of the predictors of response to CRT (PROSPECT) trial. Circulation 2008;117(20):2608–16.

41. Bax JJ, Bleeker GB, Marwick TH, et al. Left ventricular dyssynchrony predicts response and prognosis after cardiac resynchronization therapy. J Am Coll Cardiol 2004;44(9):1834–40.

42. Yu CM, Zhang Q, Fung JW, et al. A novel tool to assess systolic asynchrony and identify responders of cardiac resynchronization therapy by tissue synchronization imaging. J Am Coll Cardiol 2005;45(5):677–84.

43. Gorcsan J 3rd, Oyenuga O, Habib PJ, et al. Relationship of echocardiographic dyssynchrony to long-term survival after cardiac resynchronization therapy. Circulation 2010;122(19):1910–8.

44. Tayal B, Gorcsan J 3rd, Delgado-Montero A, et al. Mechanical dyssynchrony by tissue Doppler cross-correlation is associated with risk for complex ventricular arrhythmias after cardiac resynchronization therapy. J Am Soc Echocardiogr 2015;28(12):1474–81.

45. Haugaa KH, Marek JJ, Ahmed M, et al. Mechanical dyssynchrony after cardiac resynchronization therapy for severely symptomatic heart failure is associated with risk for ventricular arrhythmias. J Am Soc Echocardiogr 2014;27(8):872–9.

46. Gorcsan J 3rd, Sogaard P, Bax JJ, et al. Association of persistent or worsened echocardiographic dyssynchrony with unfavourable clinical outcomes in heart failure patients with narrow QRS width: a subgroup analysis of the EchoCRT trial. Eur Heart J 2016;37(1):49–59.

47. Kutyifa V, Pouleur AC, Knappe D, et al. Dyssynchrony and the risk of ventricular arrhythmias. JACC Cardiovasc Imaging 2013;6(4):432–44.

48. Kober L, Thune JJ, Nielsen JC, et al. Defibrillator implantation in patients with nonischemic systolic heart failure. N Engl J Med 2016;375(13):1221–30.

49. Spragg DD, Leclercq C, Loghmani M, et al. Regional alterations in protein expression in the dyssynchronous failing heart. Circulation 2003;108(8):929–32.

50. Bader H, Garrigue S, Lafitte S, et al. Intra-left ventricular electromechanical asynchrony. A new independent predictor of severe cardiac events in heart failure patients. J Am Coll Cardiol 2004;43(2):248–56.

51. Haugaa KH, Goebel B, Dahlslett T, et al. Risk assessment of ventricular arrhythmias in patients with nonischemic dilated cardiomyopathy by strain echocardiography. J Am Soc Echocardiogr 2012;25(6):667–73.

52. Reddy VY, Miller MA, Neuzil P, et al. Cardiac resynchronization therapy with wireless left ventricular endocardial pacing: the SELECT-LV study. J Am Coll Cardiol 2017;69(17):2119–29.

53. Moss AJ, Hall WJ, Cannom DS, et al. Cardiac-resynchronization therapy for the prevention of heart-failure events. N Engl J Med 2009;361(14):1329–38.

54. Tang AS, Wells GA, Talajic M, et al. Cardiac-resynchronization therapy for mild-to-moderate heart failure. N Engl J Med 2010;363(25):2385–95.

Cardiac Magnetic Resonance as a Tool to Assess Dyssynchrony

Edmond Obeng-Gyimah, MD, Saman Nazarian, MD, PhD*

KEYWORDS

- Mechanical dyssynchrony • Myocardial tagging • Displacement encoding with stimulated echoes
- Tissue velocity mapping • Cardiac resynchronization therapy

KEY POINTS

- There is a high rate of nonresponse to cardiac resynchronization therapy (CRT).
- To optimize the benefit to risk/cost ratio, objective methods for improved patient selection beyond electrocardiographic evidence of dyssynchrony are necessary.
- Mechanical dyssynchrony is an important target of CRT and appears to predict CRT response.
- Cardiac MRI provides high-resolution strain images to assess dyssynchrony with reduced interobserver variability.
- Cardiac MRI also provides scar distribution with added predictive value to dyssynchrony assessment.

INTRODUCTION

Current guidelines support (class I) cardiac resynchronization therapy (CRT) for patients in sinus rhythm; presenting with left ventricular (LV) dysfunction with ejection fraction less than 35% on optimally tolerated medical therapy; left bundle branch block (LBBB) with QRS duration greater than 150 ms; and New York Heart Association class II, III, or ambulatory class IV symptoms.[1] CRT is also reasonable (class IIa) in patients with LBBB and QRS duration of 120 to 149 ms.[1] CRT improves cardiovascular outcomes by treating mechanical dyssynchrony,[2] and prolonged QRS duration (electrical dyssynchrony) has been used as a surrogate of mechanical dyssynchrony since the inception of the technology. Although CRT is effective at improving cardiac indices and

symptoms for most patients, up to 40% who meet guideline criteria do not respond to therapy.[3–5] Many studies have proposed patient selection algorithms to improve CRT response with several concentrating on measurement of dyssynchrony. Some studies suggest that electrical dyssynchrony, as determined by QRS prolongation, may not always correlate with mechanical dyssynchrony.[6,7] Recently, Sillanmäki and colleagues[6] analyzed single-photon emission computed tomography (SPECT) and myocardial perfusion imaging (MPI) data in a cohort of 43 patients with LBBB based on the strict Strauss criteria.[8] Comparison of electrocardiographic (ECG), vector ECG, and SPECT/MPI data showed that only 60% of the patients with electrical dyssynchrony also had mechanical dyssynchrony. Also, in some cases, QRS duration may better predict interventricular dyssynchrony

Disclosures: Dr S. Nazarian is a consultant for Siemens, Biosense Webster, and CardioSolv. Dr S. Nazarian also serves as principal investigator for research funding from Biosense Webster, Imricor, and Siemens. The University of Pennsylvania Conflict of Interest Committee manages all commercial arrangements.
Department of Medicine, Cardiovascular Division, Clinical Cardiac Electrophysiology Section, Perelman School of Medicine at the University of Pennsylvania, Philadelphia, PA, USA
* Corresponding author. Section of Cardiac Electrophysiology, University of Pennsylvania, Perelman School of Medicine, 3400 Spruce Street/Founders 9, Philadelphia, PA 19104.
E-mail address: saman.nazarian@uphs.upenn.edu

rather than intraventricular dyssynchrony, the latter of which has been shown to be the main target for CRT response.[9,10]

Several tools and methods are available to measure mechanical dyssynchrony. Because of its relatively low cost and wide availability, echocardiography is the most commonly used methodology. The PROSPECT trial[11] analyzed several objective echo measurements for dyssynchrony including M-mode and Tissue Doppler imaging (TDI), which did not appear to predict response to CRT. The investigators posited the negative results as due to high M-mode and TDI interobserver and intraobserver variability, thus reducing power to detect differences. Subsequently the STAR[12] and TARGET[13] trials showed speckle tracking echocardiography strain measurement as a reliable indicator of CRT response.

Advanced imaging modalities, including cardiac MRI and computed tomography (CT),[14] have also been used for dyssynchrony assessment for CRT response prediction. Compared with echocardiography, these modalities provide high spatial resolution imaging capable of providing complementary venous anatomic and scar characterization. In this article, a brief technical overview of MRI sequences and analytical techniques for dyssynchrony evaluation and the evidence for its utility in evaluating CRT response are presented. The advantages and limitations of MRI as a tool for measuring dyssynchrony compared with other modalities are also examined.`

MEASUREMENT OF DYSSYNCHRONY WITH CARDIAC MRI

Three main methods are used with MRI to measure LV dyssynchrony by assessing strain. These include myocardial tagging, phase-contrast tissue velocity mapping, and displacement encoding with stimulated echoes (DENSE). Zerhouni and colleagues[15] first described myocardial tagging with MRI in the late 1980s as a novel method for strain assessment.[10,16] With this method, radiofrequency pulses (ie, tags) are placed parallel to the imaging plane at end diastole (at earliest detection of R wave on ECG). A series of tags are used to produce a gridlike pattern on imaging. The tags, which have altered the myocardial signal signature at specific sites, deform with myocardial motion during systole. Deformation in various directions (longitudinal, circumferential, or radial) can then be quantified with special processing programs to yield specific strain and strain rate values. Semi-automated or automated algorithms, such as HARP (Harmonic Phase), can be used for strain analysis. Cardiovascular magnetic resonance

(CMR) myocardial tagging is similar to speckle tracking used in echocardiography, especially in its ability to measure circumferential strain. However, CMR has improved spatial resolution and reproducibility.[10,14] However, myocardial tagging results in relatively large grids, with limited spatial resolution compared with other techniques described as follows.[17,18]

MRI Tissue Velocity Mapping is similar to TDI as used in echocardiography, and a good correlation between the two has been established by multiple studies.[10,19–21] However, MRI is able to provide multiplanar 3-dimensional velocities and is not limited by acoustic windows of the chest.[16] The idea is that a proton spin inside a magnetic field gathers a phase shift relative to nonmobile spins and that the phase shift is proportional to velocity. On imaging, stationary tissue appears gray, and moving tissues are black or light depending on the direction of movement. Velocity information can then be processed to calculate deformation and strain with high spatial resolution. Important limitations, however, include long acquisition and breathhold times and relatively low temporal resolution.[19,21] In addition, velocity error measurements can compound during strain calculation.

DENSE is a more advanced MRI technique used to calculate strain and to assess dyssynchrony. The concept is similar to tissue velocity mapping except that displacement, instead of velocity, is encoded.[16,17] Another important difference is that DENSE measures strain directly and offers improved temporal resolution while maintaining high spatial resolution.[17] This methodology combines the advantages of tissue velocity mapping and myocardial tagging.[22]

Assessing dyssynchrony may be important before CRT implantation. Scar and coronary venous anatomy information may also inform patient selection as well as better strategies for LV lead positioning. Patients with scar burden greater than 15% as determined by late gadolinium-enhanced (LGE) MRI appear to have poor prognosis after CRT.[23,24] Cardiac MRI remains the gold standard for scar assessment and coupled with strain analysis, could be the ideal imaging tool before CRT implantation. Future strategies to liberalize the ability to position the LV lead outside the venous distribution will amplify the utility of LGE and dyssynchrony assessment for optimization of CRT outcomes.

DOES DYSSYNCHRONY ASSESSMENT WITH CARDIAC MRI PREDICT CARDIAC RESYNCHRONIZATION THERAPY RESPONSE?

The nonresponse rate with CRT remains suboptimal at 30%. Importantly, some patients have worsening outcomes after CRT implantation. Many risk assessment strategies, including biomarkers and echocardiographic parameters besides ejection fraction, have been used to predict response. Mixed results have been noted from echocardiographic studies, with the PROSPECT[11] trial failing to find any predictors, whereas TARGET[13] and STAR[12] trials noted that speckle tracking strain analysis predicted response. The techniques for assessing dyssynchrony with MRI still remain in their infancy mostly for research purposes, and large, prospective, multicenter trials have not been undertaken to evaluate their performance. However, increasing data from small studies show ample promise. In 2008, Bilchick and colleagues[23] used a previously validated index of circumferential strain, the circumferential uniformity ratio (CURE),[7] with 0 representing pure dyssynchrony and 1 perfect synchrony. The investigators noted that the CURE index was associated with CRT response with 90% accuracy. Specificity was 71% but improved to 86% when delayed enhancement imaging was added.

Subsequently in 2013, another study by Cochet and colleagues[25] evaluated MRI dyssynchrony to predict reverse remodeling following CRT implantation in 60 patients meeting guideline criteria for CRT implantation. Dyssynchrony, based on radial displacement and delayed enhancement data were acquired. Reverse remodeling was defined as a decrease in LV end systolic volume (LVESV) by ≥15%, by 6 months after device implantation. The investigators noted that intraventricular dyssynchrony independently predicted reverse remodeling with sensitivity and specificity of 67% and 75%, respectively. In addition, scar by delayed enhancement was an independent predictor of response, and specifically, worsened outcome was reported when LV pacing was directly on the scar. Mechanical dyssynchrony performed better than QRS duration as predictor of response.

Another elegant study by Bilchick and colleagues[26] in 2014 added to the utility of MRI as a credible tool to evaluate dyssynchrony and to predict CRT response. In this study, MRI was obtained in 75 patients before CRT system implantation. Strain values based on CURE on cine DENSE images were computed for these patients. Scar data were also obtained with delayed enhancement imaging. In addition, mechanical stretch at the site of LV lead placement and delayed electrical activation as determined by Q-LV were measured. Following a median of 2.6 years, all 4 parameters predicted CRT response among 40 patients (53%) who had improved LV indices. Notably, a CURE index value >0.70 was associated with 12-fold increase in the risk of death.

SUMMARY

Many patients respond to CRT, and benefit from improvement in heart failure symptoms and reduced mortality. On the other hand, a significant proportion of patients do not respond, and are exposed to higher risk of infection, potential proarrhythmia, and higher medical costs. Therefore, improved methods for patient selection, beyond ECG evidence of dyssynchrony, are necessary. Cardiac MRI is a promising tool for the evaluation of mechanical dyssynchrony to predict CRT response. Various methods are available to measure dyssynchrony with MRI. The myocardial tagging technique is the most commonly used, but the recently developed cine DENSE methodology provides accurate assessment of myocardial displacement and circumferential strain with higher resolution. Specific strain measurements also have been evaluated, with circumferential strain shown to be more reproducible and predictive compared with longitudinal strain.[27] Cardiac CT also can provide strain and limited scar assessment, as well coronary venous anatomy information for pre-CRT implantation planning. However, functional CT images are associated with additional radiation exposure and there is scant evidence for evaluating dyssynchrony compared with echocardiography and MRI. Echocardiographic parameters are promising, especially in light of the TARGET and STAR trials. However, image quality is affected by thoracic acoustic windows and there is relatively high interobserver variability. The utility of MRI lies not only in its ability to provide high spatial resolution strain images, but also as a gold standard for scar assessment.[26] In addition, although of lower spatial resolution than CT, MRI can provide coronary venous anatomic images to help with preimplantation planning. Some limitations are notable. Variations in strain values exist using different software manufacturers and standardization is paramount.[28,29] In addition, large, multicenter trials will be needed before wide adoption. Also, significant artifacts can be present on MRI of patients with preexisting devices. For most patients who are undergoing new CRT implantation, the presented evidence suggests consideration of cardiac MRI for dyssynchrony and scar assessment as part of preimplant evaluation.

REFERENCES

1. Epstein AE, DiMarco JP, Ellenbogen KA, et al. 2012 ACCF/AHA/HRS focused update incorporated into the ACCF/AHA/HRS 2008 guidelines for device-based therapy of cardiac rhythm abnormalities: a

report of the American College of Cardiology Foundation/American Heart Association Task Force on Practice Guidelines and the Heart Rhythm Society. J Am Coll Cardiol 2013;61(3):e6–75.

2. Fudim M, Borges-Neto S. A troubled marriage: when electrical and mechanical dyssynchrony don't go along. J Nucl Cardiol 2018. https://doi.org/10.1007/s12350-018-1227-6.

3. Auger DA, Bilchick KC, Gonzalez JA, et al. Imaging left-ventricular mechanical activation in heart failure patients using cine DENSE MRI: validation and implications for cardiac resynchronization therapy. J Magn Reson Imaging 2017;46(3):887–96.

4. Behar JM, Mountney P, Toth D, et al. Real-time X-MRI-guided left ventricular lead implantation for targeted delivery of cardiac resynchronization therapy. JACC Clin Electrophysiol 2017;3(8):803–14.

5. Bakos Z, Markstad H, Ostenfeld E, et al. Combined preoperative information using a bullseye plot from speckle tracking echocardiography, cardiac CT scan, and MRI scan: targeted left ventricular lead implantation in patients receiving cardiac resynchronization therapy. Eur Heart J Cardiovasc Imaging 2014;15(5):523–31.

6. Sillanmäki S, Lipponen JA, Tarvainen MP, et al. Relationships between electrical and mechanical dyssynchrony in patients with left bundle branch block and healthy controls. J Nucl Cardiol 2018. https://doi.org/10.1007/s12350-018-1204-0.

7. Leclercq C, Faris O, Tunin R, et al. Systolic improvement and mechanical resynchronization does not require electrical synchrony in the dilated failing heart with left bundle-branch block. Circulation 2002;106(14):1760–3.

8. Strauss DG, Selvester RH, Wagner GS. Defining left bundle branch block in the era of cardiac resynchronization therapy. Am J Cardiol 2011;107(6):927–34.

9. Bax JJ, Abraham T, Barold SS, et al. Cardiac resynchronization therapy: Part 1–issues before device implantation. J Am Coll Cardiol 2005;46(12):2153–67.

10. Aggarwal NR, Martinez MW, Gersh BJ, et al. Role of cardiac MRI and nuclear imaging in cardiac resynchronization therapy. Nat Rev Cardiol 2009;6(12):759–70.

11. Chung ES, Leon AR, Tavazzi L, et al. Results of the predictors of response to CRT (PROSPECT) trial. Circulation 2008;117(20):2608–16.

12. Tanaka H, Nesser HJ, Buck T, et al. Dyssynchrony by speckle-tracking echocardiography and response to cardiac resynchronization therapy: results of the Speckle Tracking and Resynchronization (STAR) study. Eur Heart J 2010;31(14):1690–700.

13. Khan FZ, Virdee MS, Palmer CR, et al. Targeted left ventricular lead placement to guide cardiac resynchronization therapy: the TARGET study: a randomized, controlled trial. J Am Coll Cardiol 2012;59(17):1509–18.

14. Tee M, Noble JA, Bluemke DA. Imaging techniques for cardiac strain and deformation: comparison of echocardiography, cardiac magnetic resonance and cardiac computed tomography. Expert Rev Cardiovasc Ther 2013;11(2):221–31.

15. Zerhouni EA, Parish DM, Rogers WJ, et al. Human heart: tagging with MR imaging–a method for noninvasive assessment of myocardial motion. Radiology 1988;169(1):59–63.

16. Ibrahim el SH. Myocardial tagging by cardiovascular magnetic resonance: evolution of techniques–pulse sequences, analysis algorithms, and applications. J Cardiovasc Magn Reson 2011;13:36.

17. Aletras AH, Ding S, Balaban RS, et al. DENSE: displacement encoding with stimulated echoes in cardiac functional MRI. J Magn Reson 1999;137(1):247–52.

18. Spottiswoode BS, Zhong X, Hess AT, et al. Tracking myocardial motion from cine DENSE images using spatiotemporal phase unwrapping and temporal fitting. IEEE Trans Med Imaging 2007;26(1):15–30.

19. Delfino JG, Fornwalt BK, Oshinski JN, et al. Role of MRI in patient selection for CRT. Echocardiography 2008;25(10):1176–85.

20. Westenberg JJ, Lamb HJ, van der Geest RJ, et al. Assessment of left ventricular dyssynchrony in patients with conduction delay and idiopathic dilated cardiomyopathy: head-to-head comparison between tissue Doppler imaging and velocity-encoded magnetic resonance imaging. J Am Coll Cardiol 2006;47(10):2042–8.

21. McVeigh ER. MRI of myocardial function: motion tracking techniques. Magn Reson Imaging 1996;14(2):137–50.

22. Budge LP, Helms AS, Salerno M, et al. MR cine DENSE dyssynchrony parameters for the evaluation of heart failure: comparison with myocardial tissue tagging. JACC Cardiovasc Imaging 2012;5(8):789–97.

23. Bilchick KC, Dimaano V, Wu KC, et al. Cardiac magnetic resonance assessment of dyssynchrony and myocardial scar predicts function class improvement following cardiac resynchronization therapy. JACC Cardiovasc Imaging 2008;1(5):561–8.

24. White JA, Yee R, Yuan X, et al. Delayed enhancement magnetic resonance imaging predicts response to cardiac resynchronization therapy in patients with intraventricular dyssynchrony. J Am Coll Cardiol 2006;48(10):1953–60.

25. Cochet H, Denis A, Ploux S, et al. Pre- and intra-procedural predictors of reverse remodeling after cardiac resynchronization therapy: an MRI study. J Cardiovasc Electrophysiol 2013;24(6):682–91.

26. Bilchick KC, Kuruvilla S, Hamirani YS, et al. Impact of mechanical activation, scar, and electrical timing on cardiac resynchronization therapy response and clinical outcomes. J Am Coll Cardiol 2014;63(16):1657–66.

27. Helm RH, Leclercq C, Faris OP, et al. Cardiac dyssynchrony analysis using circumferential versus longitudinal strain: implications for assessing cardiac resynchronization. Circulation 2005;111(21): 2760–7.

28. Cao JJ, Ngai N, Duncanson L, et al. A comparison of both DENSE and feature tracking techniques with tagging for the cardiovascular magnetic resonance assessment of myocardial strain. J Cardiovasc Magn Reson 2018;20(1):26.

29. Jeung MY, Germain P, Croisille P, et al. Myocardial tagging with MR imaging: overview of normal and pathologic findings. Radiographics 2012;32(5): 1381–98.

Updated Clinical Evidence for Effective Cardiac Resynchronization Therapy in Congestive Heart Failure and Timing of Implant

Natalia Hernandez, MD, David T. Huang, MD*

KEYWORDS

- Heart failure • Left bundle branch block • Right bundle branch block
- Cardiac resynchronization therapy • Cardiac remodeling

KEY POINTS

- Cardiac resynchronization therapy leads to morbidity and mortality benefit in select patients with heart failure.
- A combination of severely symptomatic heart failure with severe left ventricular dysfunction, left bundle branch block, widened QRS duration, and sinus rhythm have been demonstrated to have the most consistent data leading to improvement with cardiac resynchronization therapy.
- Patients with early or mild heart failure symptoms, as well as non–left bundle branch block or atrial fibrillation may derive benefit from cardiac resynchronization therapy as well, although evidence is not as robust.

INTRODUCTION

Over the past 20 plus years, cardiac resynchronization therapy with defibrillation (CRT-D) or without defibrillation (CRT-P) has become a well-recognized therapeutic modality for patients with congestive heart failure (CHF). The remarkable database of knowledge has been compiled over time, from the simple first pilot study of 20 patients in 1996 to complex trials involving thousands of patients, and it continues to evolve as investigations continue the search to address further outstanding inquiries. Today, data are now available to properly identify patients with specific heart failure who are expected to respond and derive morbidity as well as mortality benefit from CRT. On the other hand, we have also learned that not every patient with dyssynchrony will improve with this therapy. It is therefore imperative to understand the predictors of response to CRT, factors such as widened QRS duration, morphology of bundle branch block, and underlying rhythm as well as timing to implement therapy with respect to degrees of heart failure symptoms and left ventricular (LV) dysfunction. Patient characteristics associated with less favorable CRT outcomes are recognized as well,

Conflicts of interest: N. Hernandez: none. D.T. Huang, Research grant support from Biosense Webster, Medtronic, Boston Scientific and Abbott; Fellowship grant support from Medtronic, Boston Scientific, Abbott and Biotronik.
Department of Cardiology, University of Rochester Medical Center, 601 Elmwood Avenue, Rochester, NY 14642, USA
* Corresponding author. University of Rochester Medical Center, 601 Elmwood Avenue Box 679, Rochester, NY 14642.
E-mail address: David_Huang@urmc.rochester.edu

Card Electrophysiol Clin 11 (2019) 55–65
https://doi.org/10.1016/j.ccep.2018.11.008
1877-9182/19/© 2018 Elsevier Inc. All rights reserved.

including non–left bundle branch block (LBBB) conduction abnormalities, atrial fibrillation, and less symptomatic heart failure. Despite all the data and understanding, challenges to overcome non- or underresponse to CRT remain.

PERSPECTIVE AND IMPLICATION FROM HISTORIC CLINICAL TRIALS

The pathway leading to pacing as therapy for patients with CHF started shortly after the invention of artificial pacemakers, when they were thought to provide symptomatic relief to patients with heart failure even with single right ventricular (RV) pacing through restoration of adequate heart rate. Further investigations demonstrated the importance of atrioventricular synchrony, given potential issues with pacing only the ventricle, such as pacemaker syndrome.[1] In early 1990s, synchronized atrioventricular pacing was demonstrated to improve signs and symptoms of heart failure in patients with cardiomyopathy.[2,3] Around the same time period, Bakker and colleagues[4] first examined the effect of pacing both the RV and LV by using y-adaptors for the ventricular pacing port and conventional dual chamber pacemakers in 12 patients with CHF. They reported improved LV function and clinical HF symptoms. Shortly after, Cazeau and colleagues[5] reported their results of biventricular pacing improving CHF clinical outcomes in a series of 20-patient cohort. Thus, biventricular pacing, termed as "cardiac resynchronization therapy," became recognized as a potentially effective nonpharmacologic treatment for patients with CHF and aberrancy on surface electrocardiogram (ECG). Starting with the MUSTIC and MIRACLE trials in 1998, multiple randomized trials aimed to further assess the efficacy of CRT in heart failure were undertaken. As a direct result of these trials, CRT was approved by Food and Drug Administration for patients with heart failure with prominent symptoms in 2001.

CARDIAC RESYNCHRONIZATION THERAPY IN ADVANCED CONGESTIVE HEART FAILURE

MUSTIC, the first randomized controlled trial that demonstrated clinical benefit from CRT in heart failure, was published in 2001.[6] Of the major CRT trials, this study had the smallest number of participants with the shortest follow-up time of 3 months. The study included 131 participants with QRS duration of 150 msec or more, New York Heart Association (NYHA) class III for at least 1 month while receiving optimal pharmacologic treatment. This was a crossover study, and the enrolled patients were randomized first to either

12 weeks of medical therapy with CRT or medical therapy alone. Of note, beta-blockers were not considered to be part of the standard therapy for heart failure during the enrollment period in the MUSTIC trial. Thus, CRT was compared with medical therapy which included primarily of angiotensin-converting enzyme inhibitors and diuretics. Compared with medical therapy alone, CRT therapy with medical therapy resulted in a 62% distance increase in the 6- minute walk test, the study primary end point, as well as a 67% decrease in the incidence of heart failure hospitalizations and a 32% improvement in quality of life scores, both as part of the secondary end points.

MIRACLE was the first double-blind randomized controlled trial with 2 arms of CRT-P with medical therapy versus medical therapy alone.[7] Enrollment began around the same time as MUSTIC, recruiting 453 patients with a mean follow-up of 6 months. MIRACLE and subsequent studies included patients with narrower QRS durations as compared with MUSTIC, $\geq$130 msec (some of the later trials included patients with QRS of $\geq$120 msec). The enrolled population was characterized by advanced symptomatic heart failure, with NYHA functional class III and IV. Medical therapy used as control included the full spectrum of heart failure medications, adhering to the practice guidelines of the time, including beta-blockers. The study demonstrated positive effects of CRT in qualified patients based on improvement in 3 primary end points: 6-minute walking test, quality of life, and NYHA functional class. Published in 2003, MIRACLE implantable cardioverter defibrillator (ICD) was conducted by the same group of investigators to assess CRT combined with defibrillator in patients with advanced heart failure (NYHA class III and IV) and high risk for life-threatening ventricular arrhythmias.[8] This trial compared CRT-D plus medical therapy to optimal medical therapy alone. Number of participants enrolled reached 369. After a 6-month follow-up period, the results with CRT-D demonstrated greater symptomatic improvement with reduced NYHA class, increased exercise tolerance, and improved quality of life but no significant differences in left ventricular ejection fraction (LVEF) or mortality. Also published in 2003, CONTAK CD was the first trial to compare CRT-D with ICD against a background of "optimized" medical therapy (OMT), although beta-blockers were not strictly included.[9] The trial enrolled 501 participants with moderately to severely symptomatic heart failure. The results demonstrated CRT was associated with a 15% improvement in composite end point of all-cause mortality, heart failure hospitalization, and ventricular tachycardia/ventricular fibrillation events in all enrolled patients. The study specifically noted a 22% improvement in the subgroup with higher degree of symptomatic heart failure.

To date, the COMPANION trial remains one of the largest CRT trials with 1520 participants enrolled. Reported in 2004, COMPANION studied the effectiveness of both CRT-P and CRT-D in the same trial in patients with CHF with NYHA class III and IV symptoms.[10] The results demonstrated mortality benefit in the group treated with CRT with and without defibrillation plus medical therapy as compared with the medical therapy alone after about 1 year of follow-up. A combination of all-cause mortality and hospitalization from any cause was prespecified as the primary end point. The results demonstrated a 20% reduction in the composite primary end point afforded by CRT regardless of defibrillation status. Secondary analysis revealed a significant 36% reduction in all-cause mortality for the CRT-D group and a less robust decrease for the CRT-P group. Breaking the secondary end points down further, reduction of cardiovascular and heart events or death was evident in both groups with the following decrease: CRT-P/CRT-D groups by 25%/28% and 34%/40%, respectively. Along with some of the other previous studies, COMPANION paved the way for treating patients with heart failure with CRT without defibrillation.

CARDIAC RESYNCHRONIZATION THERAPY IN MILD CONGESTIVE HEART FAILURE

The REVERSE trial, published in 2008, was the first CRT study to include patients with less symptomatic heart failure, NYHA class I and II, and expanded the inclusion of LVEF to less than or equal to 40%,[11] The trial enrolled 684 patients randomized to CRT-P or CRT-D with OMT versus OMT alone. Patients were followed for 12 months and the impact of CRT was assessed based on composite CHF clinical response as well as cardiac remodeling effects as assessed by LV end-systolic volume index and other measures of LV remodeling. The trial demonstrated an effective reverse cardiac remodeling with the CRT treatment group demonstrating a greater improvement in LV volume, -18.4 ± 29.5 mL/m^2 versus -1.3 ± 23.4 mL/m^2 in the control group. Concurrently, there was noted a 56% relative risk reduction in time to the first hospitalization for heart failure with CRT. Of note, the data showed CRT was not associated with improved symptomatic status, physical performance, or quality of life in this mildly symptomatic cohort. No mortality benefit was seen in CRT group, which may have been the result of a relatively low event rate in healthier and younger patients with heart failure. Arguably, a longer

intervention period might have demonstrated a potential survival benefit with CRT.

Another landmark trial, MADIT CRT, was published in 2009 and left its mark by demonstrating that CRT when offered to patients earlier in heart failure course with mild symptoms, could result in lower mortality, morbidity, and slow the progression of the disease.[12] For the first time in CRT trials, the control group in MADIT CRT included not just guideline-directed medical therapy but also an ICD as prescribed by the device guidelines at the time. Total study population consisted of 1820 asymptomatic patients with ischemic cardiomyopathy, NYHA class I, or mildly symptomatic with either ischemic or nonischemic cardiomyopathy, NYHA class II, and a stricter LVEF range of less than or equal to 30%. Enrolled patients were randomized to receive either CRT-D and OMT or ICD with OMT. The average follow-up was 2.4 years. The results showed that CRT was associated a significant 34% reduction in the prespecified composite primary end point of all-cause mortality or nonfatal heart failure event. The figure was driven primarily by a 41% reduction in heart failure events. This result extended to NYHA class II, but not to NYHA class I participants, and was not affected by the cause of heart failure. Favorable cardiac adaptation was observed with an increase of LVEF by 11% in CRT group, as compared with 3% increase in the control group. The remodeling benefit could be observed within the first few months after CRT implantation.

Investigators of the RAFT trial also evaluated the additive impact of CRT on morbidity and mortality against that of a control group with defibrillation therapy.[13] RAFT enrolled 1798 patients with mildly to moderately symptomatic heart failure (about 80% of participants were assessed as NYHA class II, the rest NYHA class III) and LVEF of less than or equal to 30%, with a relatively long follow-up among trials of 40 months. Intervention arm included OMT combined with CRT-D system. Of particular note, patients with controlled rhythms other than sinus, such as atrial fibrillation, flutter, and atrial pacing, were included as well in RAFT. The results, as reported in 2010, demonstrated that CRT led to a 25% relative reduction in the primary end point, consisting of all-cause mortality and CHF hospitalization. The results were driven predominantly by positive results in patients with LBBB, wider QRS duration (>150 msec), and LVEF less than 20%. A significant relative risk reduction associated with CRT-D was also shown in secondary end points, with a 25% reduction of all-cause mortality and a 24% of cardiovascular death. Incidentally, the 32% reduction of heart failure hospitalizations was offset by a 39% higher number of device-related hospitalizations in CRT-D group.

A substudy of MADIT CRT, published in 2011 by Zareba and colleagues,[14] specifically focused on determination of influence of QRS morphology on benefit provided by CRT, including morbidity, mortality, and cardiac remodeling. Data were analyzed based on the 1817 enrollees of the original trial, with the same study arms of CRT-D versus ICD alone and symptomatic distribution (NYHA class I or II). Benefit associated with CRT-D was realized in patients with LBBB with a 53% relative risk reduction for primary end point of all-cause mortality or heart failure event. Patients with non-LBBB conduction patterns did not derive any benefit from CRT in the subgroup analyses. These patients with non-LBBB were further stratified to groups with intraventricular conduction delay (IVCD) and right bundle branch block (RBBB) and CRT in those with IVCD was observed to be associated with a trend for higher mortality. A greater improvement in reverse cardiac remodeling was observed in patients with LBBB, whereas patients with non-LBBB demonstrated only modest change. The investigators noted that the benefit associated with CRT primary end point were driven mainly by clinical improvement noted in patients with LBBB, mildly symptomatic (NYHA class II), ischemic or nonischemic heart failure, QRS duration of greater than 150 msec. Patient with non-LBBB conduction defect and asymptomatic ischemic heart failure with LBBB, NYHA class I, did not derive any significant benefit.

CARDIAC RESYNCHRONIZATION THERAPY—LONG-TERM EFFECTS

With every trial assessing new therapy, the outcome is assessed during a predetermined and limited period. Question always remains about whether patients will continue to receive benefit beyond the reported monitoring time frame. In 2005, the CARE-HF trial confirmed that positive effects of CRT on mortality and morbidity persist during a relatively longer follow-up period of 36 months.[15] With 813 patients, about half of the participants in COMPANION by number, 2 arms were evaluated: CRT with OMT or OMT alone, without prespecified differentiation of defibrillation status in the CRT group. Markers of mechanical dyssynchrony were used as an inclusion criterion in addition to electrical dyssynchrony evidenced by the widened QRS duration. The results demonstrated CRT, at 2 years, was associated with a 33% reduction in all-cause mortality, most of which (83%) resulted from cardiovascular causes, representing mortality rate of 18% in the CRT group versus 25.1% noted in medical therapy group. Composite secondary end point, consisting of all-cause mortality and hospitalization for worsening heart failure, was lower in the CRT group by 46% compared with OMT. In addition, CRT recipients demonstrated greater improvement in symptomatic status and quality of life.

The long-term outcome of the MADIT CRT trial was published by Goldenberg and colleagues[16] in 2014, and the long-term impact of CRT was evaluated by means of intention-to-treat analysis in patients who participated in the original study, over a median follow-up of 5.6 years in addition to the 2.4-year follow-up during the primary trial. The report followed patients in 2 phases, with 1691 patients who made up all the surviving patients from the original MADIT CRT trial in phase I and 854 patients who enrolled in the posttrial registry in phase II. The results confirmed the observed benefits of CRT for the enrolled patient persisted over the long-term posttrial follow-up. Because of the large discrepancies noted, the investigators reported the results designated by the baseline ECG bundle branch aberrancy patterns. A highly significant 50% relative risk reduction for the primary end point, which included all-cause mortality or heart failure event, was observed in patients with LBBB with CRT therapy as compared with ICD alone. Multivariate regression analysis showed a 41% reduction in the long-term risk of death and a 62% reduction in nonfatal heart failure events with CRT-D versus ICD. The Kaplan-Meier curves of freedom from death and nonfatal heart failure events for patients with LBBB between CRT-D group versus ICD group diverged early at 1 year following randomization and remained well separated through 7 years of follow-up, suggesting early and sustained benefits observed. For patients with non-LBBB conduction defects, clinical benefits were not seen at 2.4 years and could not be demonstrated at long-term follow-up.

CARDIAC RESYNCHRONIZATION THERAPY IN PACING

Because of the observed association between high amount of single RV pacing and progressive LV systolic dysfunction, the role of CRT was also investigated in patients who require high amounts of ventricular pacing in the BLOCK HF trial.[17] The study enrolled selected patients with indications for pacing with atrioventricular block, NYHA class I, II, or III heart failure, and a higher LVEF of less than or equal to 50%. All patients underwent either a CRT-P or CRT-D and were randomly assigned to standard RV pacing or biventricular pacing by electronic programming. The prespecified primary outcome was defined as the death from any cause, any heart failure that required intravenous therapy, or a greater than or equal to 15% increase in the LV end-systolic volume index. After an averaged follow-up of 37 months, 190 of 342 patients (55.6%) in the single RV pacing group, as compared with 160 of 349 (45.8%) in the biventricular pacing group, reached primary outcome. The results in patients who received a defibrillator (CRT-D) did not differ from those with a pacemaker (CRT-P). Following this trial, the standard-of-care for patients with ventricular dysfunction at any symptomatic stage who require pacing or have a need for high degrees of ventricular pacing due to high-degree atrioventricular block is to implant a CRT device.

CARDIAC RESYNCHRONIZATION THERAPY AND DYSSYNCHRONY IN CLINICAL TRIALS

Patients with heart failure are subject to cardiac electrical dyssynchrony as well as mechanical dyssynchrony. Since 1991, when a widened QRS duration was shown to be correlated with compromised cardiac function,[18] it remains to date the gold-standard indicator for electrical ventricular dyssynchrony and a main qualifying criteria for CRT. An overwhelming majority of classic CRT trials used electrical dyssynchrony assessed by QRS width as a part of inclusion criteria. CARE HF and ECHO CRT are the only large trials to date that used mechanical dyssynchrony seen on echocardiography as an inclusion criterion in addition to ECG data.

There are data that mechanical dyssynchrony demonstrated through cardiac imaging may also be a strong predictor for response to CRT.[19] Investigators of the EchoCRT trial attempted to answer the question whether mechanical dyssynchrony as detected by transthoracic echocardiography in the setting of a normal QRS duration on ECG in patients with CHF could be a useful criterion for CRT.[20] The study enrolled 809 participants with moderate to severe heart failure symptoms (NYHA III and IV), LVEF less than 35%, and narrow QRS duration ($\leq$130 msec), who had evidence of mechanical LV dyssynchrony on echocardiography and met indications for ICD. All patients underwent device implantation with a biventricular pacing defibrillator system, with the CRT therapy randomly assigned to be turned on or off. The defined primary end point consisted of all-cause mortality or heart failure hospitalization. The study was terminated prematurely after a mean follow-up period of 19.4 months due to a lack of effectiveness of

CRT in the studied population. In the group randomized to CRT, 116 out of 404 patients reached primary efficacy outcome as compared with 102 of the 405 patients in the control group. However, there was a concerning trend observed for increased death in the CRT group of 45 versus 26 in the control group. The EchoCRT stands as a notable negative trial for CRT and has essentially halted any further studies evaluating the role of CRT in patients with heart failure with a narrow QRS duration ($\leq$130 msec).

CARDIAC RESYNCHRONIZATION THERAPY IN WOMEN

Consistently through CRT trials, women represented a minority of participants with an overall representation of less than 35% of total number of patients enrolled. Earlier studies, MUSTIC, MIRACLE, and COMPANION, included the largest women proportion (32%) of all participants. A total of 453 women partook in MADIT-CRT, the largest absolute number in these CRT trials. The reported results of MUSTIC, MIRACLE, and COMPANION were not clear in terms of benefit distribution between men and women. Report from COMPANION demonstrated benefit in mortality from any causes and heart failure events in male enrollees, but no benefit for women. CARE HF, a later study, reported that men and women have similar benefits from CRT. Results of the REVERSE trial showed no significant clinical difference between genders in terms of morbidity and mortality, but demonstrated a more prominent positive effect on cardiac remodeling in women with a more notable improvement in LV end-systolic volume index with CRT. MADIT-CRT and its substudies demonstrated that women with heart failure develop LBBB more frequently and gain the more clinical benefit from CRT regardless of QRS duration. RAFT, described more prominent benefits in both morbidity and mortality in women. The overall available data on the impact of CRT in women is suggest a positive response especially in the later trials perhaps even stronger than men, possibly due to a combination with updated medical therapy. **Table 1** lists all of the major trials examining the response to CRT reported by gender subgroups of women as compared with men.

CARDIAC RESYNCHRONIZATION THERAPY AND ATRIAL FIBRILLATION

Most of the completed CRT trials excluded patients with rhythms other than sinus, and only 2

Table 1
List of major trials examining the response to CRT reported by gender subgroups of women and as compared with men

Trial	Women %/Number	Result in Women Compared to Men		
		All-Cause Mortality	HF Hospitalization	Cardiac Remodeling
MUSTIC	32/32	—	—	—
MIRACLE	32/142	—	—	—
MIRACLE ICD	23/86	—	—	—
COMPANION	32/388	Benefit in men, but no benefit in women	Benefit in men, no benefit in women	-
CONTAK CD	16/80	—	—	—
CARE HF	27/216	Benefit similar to men	Benefit similar to men	
REVERSE	21/131	No benefit in heart failure clinical composite response in both men and women		More benefit
MADIT CRT	25/453	More benefit	More benefit	—
RAFT	17/308	More benefit	More benefit	—
MADIT-CRT QRS morphology	22/394	More benefit in LBBB	More benefit in LBBB	—
MADIT-CRT long term	23/203	More benefit	More benefit	—

trials, CONTAK CD and RAFT, enrolled participants with atrial arrhythmias. Results of the larger among the 2, RAFT trial revealed the benefit afforded by CRT and OMT, in mildly to moderately symptomatic heart failure that could be extrapolated on patients with sinus or atrial paced rhythm. However, in patients with permanent atrial fibrillation or flutter, even with adequate rate control, no significant clinical improvement was recognized with CRT over ICD and OMT.[12] MADIT-CRT included a small subset of patients with history of paroxysmal atrial fibrillation before enrollment in the trial[12] and noted less significant CRT-D impact compared with patient without a history of atrial arrhythmia.

CRT was compared with non-CRT device in regard to impact of LVEF and physical performance in patients with atrial fibrillation undergoing atrioventricular junction (AVJ) ablation in the PAVE trial that included 184 patients, with normal or mildly reduced LVEF and mild to moderate symptoms.[21] CRT was associated with significant improvement of the end point parameters, with a more pronounced benefit when baseline LVEF was at least moderately reduced at 45% or less. CERTIFY, the largest dedicated trial to assess effect of CRT in patients with atrial fibrillation, was conducted as a prospective observational study and published in 2013.[22] Results demonstrated that outcomes

for patients with atrial fibrillation after AVJ ablation were comparable to ones for patients with sinus rhythm. The study enlisted 7384 patients with severely reduced LVEF, moderate to severe symptoms (NYHA III and IV), and widened QRS duration of greater than 120 msec, who received CRT (D or P). The outcomes for 443 participants with AVJ ablation and 895 patients with rate-control strategy were compared against 6046 CRT recipients in sinus rhythm after a median follow-up of 37 months. For the patients with atrial fibrillation who underwent AVJ ablation, a 52% reduction in all-cause mortality was demonstrated compared with those managed medically, irrespective of other variables. Reverse cardiac remodeling after AVJ ablation for AF was comparable to the patients in sinus rhythm and was better than the patients in medically managed AF arm. Alarmingly, rate-controlled atrial fibrillation group not only failed to demonstrate any benefit from CRT but was also characterized by increased mortality, both total and cardiac, when compared with sinus rhythm and AVJ ablation groups. Further details on the discussion of the role of AVJ ablation and CRT in these patients will be presented in Jonathan S. Steinberg's article, "Role of Atrioventricular Junctional Ablation and Cardiac Resynchronization Therapy in Patients With Chronic Atrial Fibrillation," in this issue.

CARDIAC RESYNCHRONIZATION THERAPY IN NON-LBBB ABERRANCY

Although the beneficial impact of CRT in heart failure with LBBB has been strongly supported by the available date, the effects in patients with other infranodal or interventricular conduction abnormalities has been controversial and in many cases suboptimal.[23] Data in such patients are often less robust due to lower numbers in the major trials and results are derived often through subgroup analyses. Zareba and colleagues[14] reported on a MADIT CRT substudy focused on outcomes of CRT-D in patients with asymptomatic or mildly symptomatic CHF based on baseline QRS morphology. This report involved the largest number of 228 patients with RBBB (13% of the 1817 total patients enrolled in MADIT CRT) and 308 patients with IVCD (17%). Their analyses demonstrated no benefit realized with CRT by the entire group with non-LBBB conduction abnormalities in the primary end point of heart failure progression and secondary end points of ventricular tachyarrhythmia event rates. These results were confirmed even after stratification based on age, symptoms, QRS duration, and echocardiographic findings. In fact, the report noted CRT in patients with IVCD was associated with a trend for increased mortality. RAFT and COMPANION trials enrolled smaller numbers of patients with non-LBBB and reported neutral CRT impact for this group. **Table 2** presents a compiled data on the major CRT trials, which included patients with non-LBBB aberrancy, QRS duration, and the reported results with CRT.

Several potential factors have been hypothesized to be responsible for bundle branch block pattern type discrepancies observed in response to CRT. Hara and colleagues[24] postulated that patients with a combination of RBBB plus mechanical dyssynchrony identify a subgroup of patient who may benefit from long-term CRT. They prospectively analyzed a cohort of 278 consecutive patients with advanced symptomatic heart failure, all of whom were screened for presence of ventricular mechanical dyssynchrony and/or radial strain using echocardiography. Based on the results, patients with LBBB had a higher prevalence of mechanical dyssynchrony and more favorable response to CRT as evidenced by decreased mortality and need for advanced heart failure therapies. Patients with non-LBBB ECG patterns with dyssynchrony had similar clinical outcomes as compared with patients with LBBB and those with non-LBBB and lack of detected mechanical dyssynchrony experienced less favorable clinical outcomes.

Others have noted that not every RBBB pattern seen on ECG represents the same conduction defect and some can also exhibit concurrent left-sided conduction disturbance or may have other intraventricular conduction delays leading to "atypical RBBB" patterns. A post hoc breakdown of clinical benefits associated with CRT for patients RBBB with left anterior fascicular block (LAFB) were compared with patients with RBBB and no left fascicular blocks serving as controls among MADIT-CRT participants was presented by Tompkins and colleagues.[25] They noted more significant reductions in LV and LA volumes at 1 year in patients with RBBB with no left fascicular blocks versus those with RBBB plus LAFB as well as the control group. However, this did not translate into any detectable clinical difference in the long-term (3 years) all-cause mortality or heart failure hospitalizations.

Pastore and colleagues[26] categorized patients with RBBB even further, describing those with ECG patterns displaying RBBB in the precordial leads and a less prominent S-wave in the lateral limb leads as "atypical RBBB." In their retrospective analysis, atypical RBBB pattern was found to be associated with longer measured onset of QRS to the left ventricular activation times (as measured by the implanted LV lead, Q-LV times) than patients with typical RBBB pattern, although both groups were shorter than the patients with LBBB. During a 2-year follow-up in these 66 CRT recipients with RBBB, 35 of the patients with atypical RBBB realized a significantly better clinical response to CRT based on measured LV function, NYHA CHF classification, heart failure–related hospitalizations or deaths.[27] A potential relationship between very wide QRS (>180 msec), BBB, and CRT-D versus ICD effect was studied by Sundaram and colleagues[28] on 24,960 CRT-D recipients from Medicare registry. Their results suggest that CRT in patients with non-LBBB with QRS duration greater than 180 msec is associated with reduced mortality and heart failure hospitalizations and no benefit with CRT seen in patients with QRS duration 150 to 179 msec. Of note, the observed benefit in the non-LBBB with QRS duration greater than 180 msec patient group is less than that in patients with LBBB.

To address these differences in a prospective fashion, ENHANCE CRT investigated whether positioning the LV lead in CRT at the site of latest activation based on Q-LV time compared with a standard anatomic approach would have an impact on outcomes. The primary results were presented in 2018.[29] The investigators randomized 248 patients with non-LBBB, mean LVEF of 26%, predominantly NYHA class III to targeted or

Table 2
List of major CRT trials, which included non-LBBB aberrancy patients, QRS duration, selected clinical characteristics, and results

Trial	Study Groups	Non-LBBB %/Number	RBBB %/Number	IVCD %/Number	NYHA Class	QRS, msec	Results
COMPANION	CRT-D or CRT-P vs OMT	—	11/161	—	III-IV	>120	Insignificant morbidity and mortality benefit
RAFT	CRT-D vs ICD	20/368	9/161	11/207	II-III	>120	No benefit in non-LBBB
MADIT CRT	CRT-D vs ICD	29/536	12/228	17/308	I-II	>130	No benefit in non-LBBB Increased mortality in IVCD
Tompkins et al (MADIT-CRT)	RBBB + LAFB, RBBB w/o LAFB vs RBBB	—	100/219 LAFB 80 Non LAFB 52	—	I-II	>130	Morbidity and mortality benefit for RBBB with non-LAFB, no benefit for RBBB + LAFB
Pastore et al	Typical vs atypical RBBB	—	66/35 atypical	—	—	—	Significantly higher CRT response in atypical RBBB
Sundaram et al	CRT-D vs ICD	18/4394	—	—	II-IV	>150	Mortality and morbidity benefit for QRS>180 msec, no benefit for QRS 150–179 msec
ENCHANCE CRT	Targeted vs anatomic LV lead placement	100/248	150	98	III-IV	>120	Improvement of composite clinical score and reverse cardiac remodeling in all non-LBBB patients, no difference in outcomes with targeted LV lead positioning

anatomic LV lead placement approach. ECG characteristics included sinus rhythm only, widened QRS duration of 120 msec or greater, and QRS morphology as RBBB in 60.5% participants and IVCD in 39.5%. The primary end point was assessed by a blinded investigator after a 12-month follow-up and composed of a composite score that included cardiovascular deaths, heart failure events, NYHA functional class, and patient assessment. The results of the trial turned out to be neutral, with no significant differences in the outcomes between 2 arms of LV implant strategy and the subgroups based on RBBB, IVCD, gender, or LVEF. There was, however, a notable improvement in composite score (67.2% in targeted and 72.8% in anatomic group), LVEF (5.8% and 5.5%), and quality of life as compared with baseline clinical status at study entry. ENHANCE CRT did not include a concurrent control group. Compared with MADIT-CRT, this study included more symptomatic patient group and did not suggest any evidence for increase mortality with CRT, although the follow-up period is shorter. Of note, ENHANCE CRT is, at this time, nonpeer reviewed and the final publication is anticipated.

The medical community has accepted and adapted the results of EchoCRT in not prescribing CRT to patients with narrow QRS duration and ventricular dyssynchrony assessed by echocardiogram due to adverse results noted. Questions about CRT in patients with non-LBBB remain; future trials are needed to acquire even more definitive data and to address more explicit queries. Dissimilar to LBBB, it is clear that patients with non-LBBB dyssynchrony is a heterogenous group with respect to CRT and reasonably should not be viewed collectively nor prescribed the same specific treatment to the entire cohort. Moreover, strategies of delivering CRT may be influenced by these data and future clinical outcomes. Implanting the left ventricular lead in the posterolateral or lateral nonapical sites may be corporately beneficial for patients with LBBB; other locations around the LV or even in the RV will need to be explored and addressed.

Known data, and the associated warning, for some of these patients of CRT resulting in possible adverse outcomes should not be overlooked when clinical decisions are being made in the treatment of these patients with CRT. Future studies, in the authors' view, will need to define aberrancy ECG patterns more specifically and, for at least some of these patients, be accompanied by more advanced imaging to investigate the inter- and intraventricular dyssynchrony more precisely. Realizing that subdividing the patient cohorts even further will expectedly result in difficult

recruitment issues, the multiple and diverse variates involved in investigating CRT in the non-LBBB group is certainly going to be more challenging. This is already reflected in the current lack of universally accepted resolve for this group despite the many trials on CRT that have already been conducted.

CARDIAC RESYNCHRONIZATION THERAPY PRACTICE GUIDELINES

The accruement of data and knowledge regarding CRT has been reflected in the professional society Practice Guidelines, which have evolved over time. CRT was first listed in the 2002 version of the Cardiac Device Guidelines and recommended for advanced symptomatic heart failure with severely reduced LVEF, regardless of the cause, plus a widened QRS duration of 130 msec or more without further conduction disturbance distinction, as a Class IIa recommendation.[30] In the 2008 Guidelines, CRT was upgraded to Class I recommendation for advanced symptomatic heart failure with wide QRS; whereas categories of atrial fibrillation, high RV pacing requirement, and mild to moderate symptoms were included as CRT qualifiers as Class II recommendations if additional criteria were met.[31] The most recently updated Guidelines from 2012 expanded further the indications for CRT with specification of recommendations based on bundle branch block patterns, QRS duration, atrial fibrillation, and, for the first time, addressing patients with asymptomatic heart failure as CRT candidates.[32] Patients with NYHA Class II – ambulatory Class IV CHF symptoms and LBBB with QRS of greater than or equal to 150 msec in sinus rhythm are considered the most appropriate candidates for CRT, assigned as Class I recommendation. Patients with LBBB and aforementioned characteristics, but with narrower QRS of greater than or equal to 120 msec, can be considered as reasonable CRT candidates (Class II recommendations). Asymptomatic (NYHA CHF Class I) status was supported by less data and is specified in patients with ischemic heart disease with LVEF less than or equal to 30%. It is worthy to point out that the expansion of CRT to patients with early and mildly symptomatic CHF is now supported with more robust data. Patients with non-LBBB with severely symptomatic heart failure with advanced LV dysfunction can be considered for CRT as well, given QRS is wide enough (at least 120 msec for class IIb and 150 msec for class IIa). Patients with asymptomatic heart failure, non-LBBB ECG pattern, and narrower QRS should not receive CRT.

SUMMARY

With the knowledge of the relationship between ventricular dysfunction and conduction aberrancy, CRT has been adapted and has become an important treatment modality for patients with heart failure. The clinician's responsibility in appropriately prescribing CRT with updated selection criteria therefore needs to be emphasized. Even with the abundance of data compiled over the last 20 years, the understanding of CRT is still not yet comprehensive. Definite progress has been made in identifying appropriate patients for this therapy, but there are still subgroups of patients in whom further research is needed to better understand the details of resynchronizing the aberrant ventricular conduction and to more precisely preselect the responders.

It is evident that patients with severe LV dysfunction, specifically ejection fraction less than or equal to 35%, are consistently identified as one of the qualifying parameters for response to CRT. Earlier trials assessed predominantly patients with advanced heart failure symptoms, and the trials individually and collectively demonstrated convincing outcomes. From the mid 2000s, patients with milder symptoms were also recruited and found to benefit from CRT. These results allowed the incorporation of a wider symptomatic spectrum of patients with heart failure with dyssynchrony to be considered for CRT. It is reasonable to surmise that CRT may be an effective treatment to prevent progression of CHF status in patients with more preserved LV function and early symptomatic classes. Trials with this intention have been designed, but to date, not yet carried out.

Despite all the advancements in the field, there remain substantial subsets of patients who fail to respond to CRT satisfactorily. Further enhancement of CRT response may take place in multiple directions, including more advanced understanding of cardiac dyssynchrony and modalities for its assessment, evaluation of cardiac substrate to avoid suboptimal LV lead positions, multisite pacing, and continuous reassessment of CRT response. CRT as a therapy will certainly continue to evolve and will expand its role in improving patients with heart failure and dyssynchrony.

REFERENCES

1. Samet P, Bernstein WH, Medow A, et al. Effect of alterations in ventricular rate on cardiac output in complete heart block. Am J Cardiol 1964;14:477–82.
2. Hochleitner M, Hörtnagl H, Ng CK, et al. Usefulness of physiologic dual-chamber pacing in drug-resistant idiopathic dilated cardiomyopathy. Am J Cardiol 1990;66:198–202.
3. Brecker SJ, Xiao HB, Sparrow J, et al. Effects of dual-chamber pacing with short atrioventricular delay in dilated cardiomyopathy. Lancet 1992;340: 1308–12.
4. Bakker PF, Meijburg HW, de Vries JW, et al. Biventricular pacing in end-stage heart failure improves functional capacity and left ventricular function. J Interv Card Electrophysiol 2000;4:395–404.
5. Cazeau S, Ritter P, Lazarus A, et al. Multisite pacing for end-stage heart failure: early experience. Pacing Clin Electrophysiol 1996;19:1748–57.
6. Cazeau S, Leclercq C, Lavergne T, et al, for the Multisite Stimulation in Cardiomyopathies (MUSTIC) Study Investigators. Effects of multisite biventricular pacing in patients with heart failure and intraventricular conduction delay. N Engl J Med 2001;344: 873–80.
7. Abraham WT, Fisher WG, Smith AL, et al. Cardiac resynchronization in chronic heart failure. N Engl J Med 2002;346:1845–53.
8. Young JB, Abraham WT, Smith AL, et al. Combined cardiac resynchronization and implantable cardioversion defibrillation in advanced chronic heart failure: the MIRACLE ICD Trial. J Am Med Assoc 2003;289:2685–94.
9. Higgins SL, Hummel JD, Niazi IK, et al. Cardiac resynchronization therapy for the treatment of heart failure in patients with intraventricular conduction delay and malignant ventricular tachyarrhythmias. J Am Coll Cardiol 2003;42:1454–9.
10. Bristow MR, Saxon LA, Boehmer J, et al. Cardiac-resynchronization therapy with or without an implantable defibrillator in advanced chronic heart failure. N Engl J Med 2004;350:2140–50.
11. Linde C, Abraham WT, Gold MR, et al, for the REVERSE (REsynchronization reVErses Remodeling in Systolic left vEntricular dysfunction) Study Group. Randomized trial of cardiac resynchronization in mildly symptomatic heart failure patients and in asymptomatic patients with left ventricular dysfunction and previous heart failure symptoms. J Am Coll Cardiol 2008;52:1834–43.
12. Moss AJ, Hall WJ, Cannom DS, et al. Cardiac-resynchronization therapy for the prevention of heart-failure events. N Engl J Med 2009;361:1329–38.
13. Tang AS, Wells GA, Talajic M, et al. Cardiac-resynchronization therapy for mild-to-moderate heart failure. N Engl J Med 2010;363:2385–95.
14. Zareba W, Klein H, Cygankiewicz I, et al. Effectiveness of cardiac resynchronization therapy by QRS morphology in the multicenter automatic defibrillator implantation trial-cardiac resynchronization therapy (MADIT-CRT). Circulation 2011;123:1061–72.
15. Cleland JG, Daubert JC, Erdmann E, et al. The effect of cardiac resynchronization on morbidity and

mortality in heart failure. N Engl J Med 2005;352:1539–49.

16. Goldenberg I, Kutyifa V, Klein HU, et al. Survival with cardiac-resynchronization therapy in mild heart failure. N Engl J Med 2014;370:1694–701.

17. Curtis AB, Worley SJ, Adamson PB, et al, for the Biventricular versus Right Ventricular Pacing in heart Failure Patients with Atrioventricular Block (BLOCK HD) Trial Investigators. Biventricular pacing for atrioventricular block and systolic dysfunction. N Engl J Med 2013;368:1585–93.

18. Xiao HB, Lee CH, Gibson DG. Effect of left bundle branch block on diastolic function in dilated cardiomyopathy. Br Heart J 1991;66(6):443–7.

19. Bax JJ, Gorcsan J 3rd. Echocardiography and noninvasive imaging in cardiac resynchronization therapy: results of the PROSPECT (Predictors of Response to Cardiac Resynchronization Therapy) study in perspective. J Am Coll Cardiol 2009;53:1933–43.

20. Ruschitzka F, Abraham WT, Singh JP, et al. Cardiac-resynchronization therapy in heart failure with a narrow QRS complex. N Engl J Med 2013;369:1395–405.

21. Doshi RN, Daoud EG, Fellows C, et al, PAVE Study Group. Left ventricular-based cardiac stimulation post AV nodal ablation evaluation (the PAVE study). J Cardiovasc Electrophysiol 2005;16:1160–5.

22. Gasparini M, Leclercq C, Lunati M, et al. Cardiac resynchronization therapy in patients with atrial fibrillation: the CERTIFY study (cardiac resynchronization therapy in atrial fibrillation patients multinational registry). JACC Heart Fail 2013;1:500–7.

23. Nery PB, Ha AC, Keren A, et al. Cardiac resynchronization therapy in patients with left ventricular systolic dysfunction and right bundle branch block: a systematic review. Heart Rhythm 2011;8:1083–7.

24. Hara H, Oyenuga OA, Tanaka H, et al. The relationship of QRS morphology and mechanical dyssynchrony to long-term outcome following cardiac resynchronization therapy. Eur Heart J 2012;33:2680–91.

25. Tompkins C, Kutyifa V, McNitt S, et al. Effect on cardiac function of cardiac resynchronization therapy in patients with right bundle branch block (from the Multicenter Automatic Defibrillator Implantation Trial with Cardiac Resynchronization Therapy [MADIT-CRT] trial). Am J Cardiol 2013;112:525–9.

26. Pastore G, Maines M, Marcantoni L, et al. ECG parameters predict left ventricular conduction delay in patients with left ventricular dysfunction. Heart Rhythm 2016;13:2289–96.

27. Pastore G, Morani G, Maines M, et al. Patients with right bundle branch block and concomitant delayed left ventricular activation respond to cardiac resynchronization therapy. Europace 2017. https://doi.org/10.1093/europace/eux362.

28. Sundaram V, Sahadevan J, Waldo AL, et al. Implantable cardioverter-defibrillators with versus without resynchronization therapy in patients with a QRS duration >180 ms. J Am Coll Cardiol 2017;69:2026–36.

29. Singh JP, Berger RD, Doshi RN et al. Targeted left ventricular lead implantation in non-left bundle branch block patients: primary results of ENHANCE CRT pilot study. Boston: Heart Rhythm Society Scientific Sessions. Presented May 10, 2018. [abstract B-LBCT01-03].

30. Gregoratos G, Abrams J, Epstein AE, et al. ACC/AHA/NASPE 2002 guideline update for implantation of cardiac pacemakers and antiarrhythmia devices–summary article: a report of the American College of Cardiology/American heart association task force on practice guidelines (ACC/AHA/NASPE Committee to update the 1998 pacemaker guidelines). J Am Coll Cardiol 2002;40:1703–19.

31. Epstein AE, DiMarco JP, Ellenbogen KA, et al, American College of Cardiology/American Heart Association Task Force on Practice Guidelines (Writing Committee to Revise the ACC/AHA/NASPE 2002 Guideline Update for Implantation of Cardiac Pacemakers and Antiarrhythmia Devices); American Association for Thoracic Surgery; Society of Thoracic Surgeons. ACC/AHA/HRS 2008 guidelines for device-based therapy of cardiac rhythm abnormalities: a report of the American College of Cardiology/American heart association task force on practice guidelines (Writing Committee to Revise the ACC/AHA/NASPE 2002 guideline update for implantation of cardiac pacemakers and antiarrhythmia devices): developed in collaboration with the American association for Thoracic Surgery and society of Thoracic Surgeons. Circulation 2008;117:e350–408.

32. Tracy CM, Epstein AE, Darbar D, et al. 2012 ACCF/AHA/HRS focused update incorporated into the ACCF/AHA/HRS 2008 guidelines for device-based therapy of cardiac rhythm abnormalities: a report of the American College of Cardiology Foundation/American heart association task force on practice guidelines and the heart rhythm society. Circulation 2013;127:e283–352.

How to Implant Cardiac Resynchronization Therapy in a Busy Clinical Practice

Daniel J. Friedman, MD, Kevin P. Jackson, MD*

KEYWORDS

- Cardiac resynchronization therapy • Biventricular pacemaker • Venography • Coronary sinus
- Venoplasty

KEY POINTS

- Compared with peripheral venography, high-quality local venography provides more detailed information about subclavian stenosis and occlusion.
- High-quality occlusive CS venography is essential for identifying the optimal target vessel and for efficient and effective lead delivery.
- Adoption of an interventional approach to CS cannulation and lead delivery with a telescoping guide system can result in improvements in procedure efficiency and efficacy.
- Competency in subclavian venoplasty and snaring techniques are essential to maintain efficiency and effectiveness during difficult cases.

INTRODUCTION

Over the past 20 years, implantation and management of cardiac resynchronization therapy (CRT) devices has evolved considerably. However, despite improvements in devices, leads, implant tools, and programming options, the comprehensive care of CRT patients remains challenging and time consuming for the electrophysiologist. Efficient and effective CRT implantation is imperative to reduce the procedural risk for patients, improve post-procedure recovery, and facilitate long-term improvement. Furthermore, because of procedure length and complexity, CRT implantation can expose the electrophysiologist to the cumulative effects of radiation exposure and the weight of protective lead. This article reviews several strategies used in our practice to improve efficiency, safety, and effectiveness of CRT implantation.

PREPROCEDURE

Efficient CRT implantation is greatly facilitated by preprocedure planning. Although several studies have suggested that specialized preprocedure imaging with strain echocardiography[1,2] or cardiac MRI[3] may have the potential to improve left ventricular (LV) lead targeting, a detailed understanding of a transthoracic echocardiogram, electrocardiogram, the results of the most recent coronary angiogram, and a high-quality occlusive

---

Disclosure Statement: Dr D.J. Friedman has received educational grants from Boston Scientific, Medtronic, and Abbot; and research grants from Biosense Webster, Boston Scientific, and the National Cardiovascular Data Registry. Dr K.P. Jackson has received research grants from Medtronic; and serves as a consultant for Medtronic, Merit Medical, and Bristol Myers Squib.
Electrophysiology Section, Duke University Hospital, 2301 Erwin Road, Duke North 7451F, Durham, NC 27710, USA
* Corresponding author.
E-mail address: k.j@duke.edu

Card Electrophysiol Clin 11 (2019) 67–74
https://doi.org/10.1016/j.ccep.2018.11.009

coronary sinus (CS) venogram may provide much of the same information. For example, it has been demonstrated that areas of ventricular infarct are typically drained by diminutive CS tributaries.[4] If a patient were to have a diminutive CS branch draining a thinned, severely hypokinetic LV segment, it is unlikely that this small branch would represent an appropriate target. In addition, the use of these specialized imaging studies typically incurs additional cost and time on the patient's behalf. Of note, a recent study assessing the utility of preprocedure computed tomography venogram before CRT implant did not demonstrate that a preprocedure understanding of CS anatomy shorted procedure duration or improved outcomes.[5]

Patients requiring upgrade from an existing transvenous device to a CRT device can represent a particular challenge because of venous stenosis or occlusion. Although patient counseling and preprocedure planning may be augmented by a preoperative understanding of the peripheral venous anatomy, we do not routinely obtain preprocedure venous imaging (except when existing hardware will be extracted) because peripheral venograms systematically overestimate the severity of subclavian stenosis.[6]

INTRAPROCEDURAL
Peripheral and Central Venography

CRT implant strategy focuses on optimizing LV lead implantation while minimizing risks associated with prolonged procedure and fluoroscopy times and is facilitated by the use of contrast injection through specially shaped catheters for CS access and lead delivery. To avoid the risks associated with contrast administration, adequate prehydration can safely obviate restricting contrast use to the absolute minimum. An example prehydration regimen includes bolus hydration with isotonic fluid (normal saline) at an infusion rate of 3 mL/kg starting 1 hour before the procedure followed by 1 mL/kg during and 6 hours after the procedure. This approach has been highly effective at preventing contrast-induced nephropathy but can at times require post-procedure diuretics. There is no acutely observed increased risk of renal failure with this approach.[7]

Performing an upper extremity venogram for all CRT implants expedites fluoroscopically guided axillary vein access over the first rib. Use of the axillary vein is associated with lower risk of pneumothorax[8] and long-term lead failure.[9] For de novo device implantations, the venogram is performed after creating the device pocket simultaneous with the first venipuncture. In this way, the vein is filled with contrast making it easily visible

and engorged, improving first pass success, thereby improving efficiency and reducing complications.

For patients with existing leads undergoing upgrade to a CRT system, the venogram is typically obtained before obtaining venous access to help plan the procedure. When the peripheral venogram suggests a possible occlusion, a more lateral access (usually over the second rib) may be preferred because it allows for the insertion of a 5F catheter short sheath proximal to the occlusion. Through this sheath, a local venogram is performed, often revealing a small tract around the existing leads (**Fig. 1**); sometimes the local venogram demonstrates that the vein is moderately stenosed but actually not occluded. When the local venogram confirms an occlusion, more lateral axillary vein access is valuable because it provides a "running start" for wire and catheter manipulation.

Venoplasty

Although primary venous obstruction with de novo device implantation is rare, the incidence of partial or complete obstruction from preexisting leads or prior instrumentation is fairly common. In approximately 25% of patients with an existing cardiovascular implantable electronic device, there is venous obstruction to some degree, with severe or complete obstruction in up to 10% of patients. Vessel stenosis usually occurs peripherally in the subclavian vein; however, central obstruction or obstruction at multiple locations is not uncommon. Factors associated with a higher chance of stenosis include greater total lead diameter, time since implant, and the presence of multiple leads.[10]

When the local venogram demonstrates a stenotic but not occluded vessel, the operator often chooses between successive dilatation of the vein with progressively larger dilators or venoplasty. In the case of CRT upgrade or implantation of multiple leads, venoplasty is preferred because it results in a larger vein lumen allowing for improved sheath maneuverability. The skill set required to perform successful venoplasty involves basic interventional knowledge and technical skills that are not standardly acquired during formal cardiac electrophysiology training. Therefore, it is advisable to include an interventional cardiologist or interventional radiologist with the introduction of this procedure. Once the implanting physician becomes comfortable with the tools and techniques, venoplasty can generally be safely and successfully performed without assistance, thereby improving procedural efficiency.

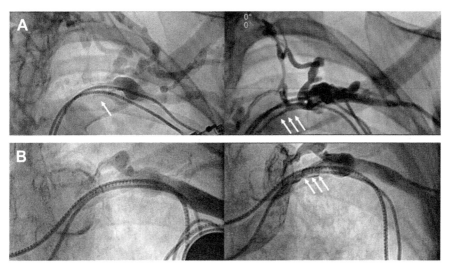

Fig. 1. A comparison of peripheral (*left*) and local (*right*) venograms from patients with prior implantable devices undergoing upgrade to CRT devices. (*A*) A faint beak (*single arrow*) is noted on the peripheral venogram but only extensive collaterals are definitively visualized; with the local venogram, a tract is noted (*triple arrows*). (*B*) No definite beak is observed; with the local venogram, a small tract is noted just inferior to the leads (*triple arrows*). In both cases, these tracts were traversed and successful subclavian venoplasty was performed.

Successful venoplasty relies on a high-quality local venography with complete vessel opacification (via manual injection through a 5F catheter short sheath; **Fig. 2**A). Appropriate wire selection for traversing the stenosis depends largely on the severity of the stenosis. When a tract is visualized alongside the existing leads, probing with an angled hydrophilic 0.035-inch guidewire usually suffices. A wire torque device is helpful in allowing fine manipulation of the wire tip. Once the lesion is crossed, the floppy guidewire needs to be exchanged for a stiffer 0.035-inch wire (Amplatz Extra-Stiff, Cook Medical, Bloomington, IN) for venoplasty. This is done by advancing a long, hydrophilic exchange catheter over the hydrophilic wire, allowing for wire exchange while preserving

access across the occlusion (**Fig. 2**B). Once the lesion is crossed, the operator must confirm that the wire or catheter has reentered the true lumen of the vein before proceeding with balloon venoplasty. This is done by advancing the wire into the inferior vena cava or the pulmonary artery, or by injecting a small amount of contrast through the hollow lumen of the exchange catheter.

For long or total occlusions, a hybrid 0.035-inch wire with a floppy hydrophilic leading segment followed by a stiff proximal segment (Glidewire Advantage, Terumo Medical Corp, Somerset, NJ) allows fine manipulation through the occlusion with excellent support for venoplasty thereby avoiding the need for a wire exchange. With this wire, it is imperative that the location of the distal

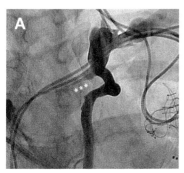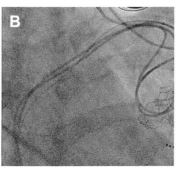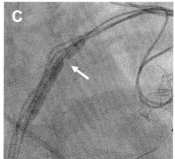

Fig. 2. Subclavian venoplasty. (*A*) Local venogram demonstrating a small beak (*asterisks*). (*B*) The channel was successfully traversed with an angled tip hydrophilic 0.035-inch wire; over this wire is an exchange catheter, which is used to exchange the floppy hydrophilic wire for a stiff 0.035-inch wire. (*C*) Balloon inflation with a 6 × 40 non-compliant balloon (white arrow indicates resolving waist during balloon inflation).

wire tip is confirmed to be intraluminal by advancing below the diaphragm or into the pulmonary artery. On occasion, a narrow or total occlusion cannot be crossed by a 0.035-inch wire or peripheral angioplasty balloon. In this situation, a smaller 0.014- or 0.018-inch hydrophilic wire is used and a coronary balloon (typically 2- to 3-mm diameter) is used to "predilate" the lesion.

Once the occlusion is crossed and a stiff 0.035-inch wire is confirmed to be distal to the lesion and intraluminal, a 6 mm × 40 mm noncompliant peripheral angioplasty balloon is advanced just beyond the most distal aspect of the stenosis (relative to the pocket) and inflated to rated burst pressure or until the lesion waste is eliminated (**Fig. 2**C). A 9-mm diameter balloon is preferred when more than one lead is being implanted. Inflations are made progressively more proximal until all stenoses are opened. If a stenosis is present near the venotomy site, then the final inflation is often performed with the proximal aspect of the balloon visible from within the pocket. **Table 1** includes a list of tools commonly used for venoplasty.

Although small venous dissections and contrast extravasations are common (40%),[6] these occurrences are typically of no clinical consequent;

venoplasty is considered safe so long as the guidewire is confirmed intraluminal before ballooning. It is important to consider that vessel patency after venoplasty is temporary (minutes to hours) and therefore ballooning may need to be repeated in the setting of prolonged cases. Vessel stenting is not required and should be avoided because entrapment of the existing leads. For a more detailed overview of subclavian venoplasty, readers are referred to a recent comprehensive review on the topic.[11]

Coronary Sinus Cannulation

Failure to cannulate the coronary sinus is a common reason for failed LV lead implantation. Traditionally, CS intubation is performed by advancing a 0.035-inch hydrophilic wire to the region of the CS ostium via a preformed guide catheter and probing to locate the CS ostium. Without the ability to directly visualize the CS however, the operator must guess at its presumptive location (thus termed the "poke and pray" method). Procedural efficiency is greatly improved using an "interventional" approach with a telescoping guide system connected to a contrast injection system, which allows for direct CS visualization and intubation

Table 1
Interventional CRT toolkit

Tool	Example
Venoplasty	
0.035-inch hydrophilic angled guidewire	Angled Glidewire (Terumo Medical)
0.035-inch wire with an angled hydrophilic leading tip with a stiff proximal end	Glidewire Advantage (Terumo Medical)
Stiff 0.035-inch wire	Amplatz Extra Stiff (Cook Medical)
Wire torque device	0.010–0.038-inch wire Torque Device (Terumo Medical)
4F hydrophilic crossing catheter	Cook CXI Support Catheter 0.035-inch (Cook Medical)
Peripheral angioplasty balloon (6-mm for single lead, 9-mm balloon if multiple leads)	6 mm × 40 mm, 70-cm shaft, noncompliant Mustang balloon (Boston Scientific)
Left ventricular lead delivery	
9F catheter CS sheath with braided core	Worley Advanced CSG Braided Core series, 40-cm, standard curve (Merit Medical)
Lead delivery sheath with target vein selector	Worley Advanced Lateral Vein Introducer (Merit Medical)
0.014-inch unipolar pacing and recording wire	Visionwire (Biotronik)
Contrast injection system	Worley Advanced Contrast Administration Kit (Merit Medical)
Snaring	
10-mm 4F catheter Goose neck snare	4F catheter, 10-mm loop, 65-cm One Snare (Merit Medical)

with or without the use of a hydrophilic wire. This system, which includes a large 9F catheter outer sheath and an inner, braided guide designed to be torqued directly into the CS, is connected to a Y-adaptor, allowing for concurrent contrast injection in the presence of a 0.035-inch wire. With this system, the braided inner guide is initially advanced to the tricuspid annulus or right ventricle, confirmed with a small puff of contrast. Counterclockwise torque is applied as the inner guide is drawn back and directed toward the inferior septum. A small drop is usually seen on fluoroscopy once the tip of the inner guide falls over the tricuspid annulus, and contrast injection identifies the CS ostium. At this point, depending on operator preference and anatomy, the hydrophilic wire is advanced to the distal CS and used to advance the inner guide and CS sheath into the CS, or the system is advanced into the CS without the use of a wire.

Occasionally a prominent Thebesian valve or tortuous proximal segment may prevent the large 9F catheter CS access sheath from advancing. In this situation, it is often possible to advance a 5F catheter straight, hydrophilic inner guide catheter over the hydrophilic wire to create a "rail" over which the CS sheath is advanced. If the hydrophilic catheter is successfully advanced but there is still resistance to advancement of the larger sheath, a rigid 0.035-inch wire is exchanged through the small sheath to provide additional support (**Fig. 3**). An alternative approach involves using an occlusive balloon as an "anchor." With this technique, a 0.035-inch wire is manipulated to the distal CS or anterior interventricular vein and a small, compliant peripheral or coronary angioplasty balloon advanced over the wire.[12] With balloon inflation, traction is applied to the balloon

thereby straightening the tortuous segment and allowing CS sheath advancement.

Coronary Sinus Venography

Optimal vein selection and lead implantation is greatly facilitated by high-quality occlusive venography. Venograms are typically performed in the anteroposterior and left anterior oblique projections. Although it is often possible to identify a target branch with a single view, venography in two views can improve understanding of the take-off and course of all possible target branches. This information is essential when identifying a target branch, identifying a "plan B" branch, determining how long to attempt a first-choice branch versus when to move on, and how to best select inner guide catheters for CS branch cannulation and subsequent lead delivery. Although performing venography in two views does require additional time and contrast, it can yield crucial information that often saves time and contrast in the long run.

Target Branch Cannulation and Lead Delivery

Similar to CS intubation, access to the target branch within the CS and subsequent advancement of the LV lead is traditionally performed using an "over-the-wire" technique. Without direct visualization of the CS tributaries during wire probing, the operator is left to guess at the target branch location. Additionally, if the 0.014-inch wire alone is used to guide the LV lead to the target location, there is often inadequate support through tortuous or narrow segments. Reliance on a 0.014-inch wire alone for LV lead placement, therefore, is often suboptimal and adds unnecessary time to the procedure.

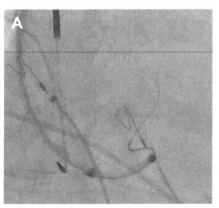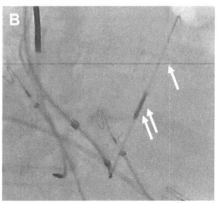

Fig. 3. Use of a 5F straight, hydrophilic catheter to support sheath advancement beyond a tortuous proximal CS segment. (*A*) Extreme angulation of the CS ostium with wire support alone. (*B*) A "rail" system to support sheath advancement, including a stiff 0.035-inch wire (*single arrow*) and a 5F hydrophilic catheter (*double arrow*).

An "interventional" technique of using inner catheters with contrast injection can greatly expedite and improve LV lead placement. This technique involves cannulation of the target branch with a two-component, telescoping catheter system consisting of a 5F catheter target vein selector connected to the contrast injection system and a lead delivery guide shaped to fit into the target vein and deliver the LV lead. With this telescoping guide system, intubation of the target branch is performed using the vein selector rather than the 0.014-inch wire. The proximal end of the vein selector is attached to a Y-adaptor allowing simultaneous contrast injection and advancement of a 0.014-inch wire. Once contrast injection identifies that the tip of the vein selector is in the target branch, a 0.014-inch wire is advanced deep into the branch. Over this wire, the target vein selector is advanced sufficiently to allow for the lead delivery guide to track over it. Once the lead delivery sheath is into the target branch, the vein selector is removed and the LV lead is advanced over the 0.014-inch wire. Using this technique, tortuosities in the target branch are straightened allowing uninhibited lead advancement (**Fig. 4**). Adoption of an interventional approach to CS cannulation and lead delivery with a telescoping guide system has resulted in shorter procedure times and higher success rates.[7] **Table 1** includes a list of tools commonly used for an "interventional" approach to LV lead delivery.

For patients with a left bundle branch block (LBBB) or chronic right ventricular pacing a lateral CS branch is typically targeted. When multiple lateral branches are available, identification of the optimal target branch may be based on branch characteristics and anticipated interlead distance[13] between LV lead bipoles and the tip of the RV lead. Adequacy of branch selection is confirmed intraprocedurally by measuring the electrical delay from the onset of the QRS complex to the local electrogram at the target site (QLV), with a goal delay of 95 milliseconds or more.[14] It is worth noting that ventricular scar and sodium channel blockers can prolong the QLV because of delayed cell to cell conduction and thus a QLV of greater than 95 milliseconds alone may be insufficient to augment response in these situations.

For patients with non-LBBB and wide LBBB, QLV is measured in candidate branches with a 0.014-inch coronary wire with a unipolar electrode at the distal tip (Visionwire, Biotronik GmbH, Berlin, Germany). This novel wire allows for pacing and sensing along the course of several candidate branches; manipulation with this 0.014-inch wire is typically easier than using an LV lead to perform the same duty. **Fig. 5** depicts an example of how the 0.014-inch wire was used to select a target branch and then subsequently deliver the LV lead.

Difficult CS Lead Delivery

In instances where a 0.014-inch wire is delivered to the target branch but difficulty is encountered delivering the lead (often because of impedance in advancing the lead delivery sheath), snaring of the distal end of the 0.014-inch wire can often provide sufficient support. To perform snaring, the 0.014-inch wire needs to be advanced into the target branch and back to the main body of the CS through collateral vessels. If a 9F catheter CS guide is used, a 4F catheter Gooseneck snare (see **Table 1**) and a lead are accommodated within its lumen. Smaller CS sheaths necessitate separate venous access for snaring and a second point of CS access. Snaring in the right atrium is possible, but much more challenging and time consuming. The use of snares to traction the lead through narrow or tortuous CS branches usually obviates CS tributary venoplasty.[15]

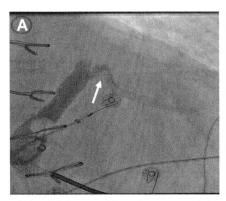
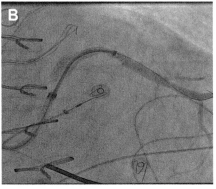

Fig. 4. Use of a lead delivery guide catheter to straighten a tortuous target branch in the CS. (*A*) Sharp bend (*arrow*) in the target branch with occlusive venography. After intubating the branch with a 5F catheter vein selector and 0.014-inch wire, the lead delivery guide catheter is advanced and the bend is straightened (*B*).

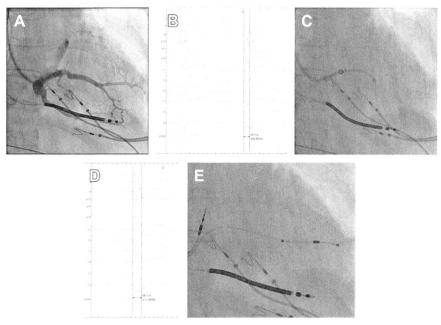

Fig. 5. A local venogram of a posterolateral branch demonstrates a high and a low branch (*A*). The local unipolar signal, measured from the 0.014-inch wire in the lower branch, measures 68 milliseconds from QRS onset to the maximum dV/dT (*B*). The 0.014-inch wire was repositioned into the higher branch (*C*). The local unipolar signal in this higher branch was 98 milliseconds after QRS onset (*D*). Based on the QLV measurement, the LV lead was implanted in the higher branch of the posterolateral vein over the same 0.014-inch wire (*E*).

Right-Sided Cardiac Resynchronization Therapy Implantation

Right-sided LV lead implantation poses a unique challenge given the multiple angles the sheath must take before engaging the CS. For this reason, specific right-sided CS guide catheters are preferred for CS localization. Once the CS is intubated, however, the right-sided guide is exchanged for a standard 9F catheter CS sheath using an extrastiff guidewire, thereby allowing full use of the telescoping inner catheter system or snare (if needed). Once the LV lead is delivered, removal of the CS sheath requires special attention, because the course of the sheath from the right subclavian vein may cause its tip to pull the LV lead superiorly. To avoid this, a 0.035-inch "buddy" wire is placed through the sheath adjacent to the LV lead to maintain a smooth transition from the CS ostium to the right atrium during sheath removal.

POSTPROCEDURE

After device implant, we typically perform brief VV optimization based on the 12-lead electrocardiogram to achieve a QS in lead I, R wave and V1, and maximal QRS narrowing. However, patients with LBBB who receive a device with a dynamic, automated AV and VV programming algorithm are typically programmed with this feature on.[16] Follow-up echocardiograms are ordered 3 to 6 months after the procedure to assess for improvements in LV size and function. Echocardiogram-based optimization is typically performed using the iterative approach and is reserved for CRT nonresponders (by clinical or echocardiographic criteria). Finally, CRT patients who fail to respond despite device optimization are referred to advanced heart failure physicians to assist in augmentation of the medical regimen and consideration of advanced therapies.

SUMMARY

Efficient and effective CRT implantation is achieved with an interventional approach to implantation. This approach relies on a versatile telescoping guide system and high-quality intraprocedural venography rather than sophisticated preprocedural imaging. Competency in subclavian venoplasty and snaring techniques are essential to maintain efficiency and effectiveness during difficult cases. Finally, deliberate follow-up care with echocardiography and timely referral for CRT optimization and/or advanced heart failure is essential for the comprehensive care of CRT patients.

REFERENCES

1. Khan FZ, Virdee MS, Palmer CR, et al. Targeted left ventricular lead placement to guide cardiac resynchronization therapy: the TARGET study: a randomized, controlled trial. J Am Coll Cardiol 2012; 59(17):1509–18.

2. Saba S, Marek J, Schwartzman D, et al. Echocardiography-guided left ventricular lead placement for cardiac resynchronization therapy: results of the Speckle Tracking Assisted Resynchronization Therapy for Electrode Region trial. Circ Heart Fail 2013; 6(3):427–34.

3. Bilchick KC, Kuruvilla S, Hamirani YS, et al. Impact of mechanical activation, scar, and electrical timing on cardiac resynchronization therapy response and clinical outcomes. J Am Coll Cardiol 2014; 63(16):1657–66.

4. Blendea D, Shah RV, Auricchio A, et al. Variability of coronary venous anatomy in patients undergoing cardiac resynchronization therapy: a high-speed rotational venography study. Heart Rhythm 2007; 4(9):1155–62.

5. Truong QA, Szymonifka J, Picard MH, et al. Utility of dual-source computed tomography in cardiac resynchronization therapy: DIRECT study. Heart Rhythm 2018;15(8):1206–13.

6. Worley SJ, Gohn DC, Pulliam RW, et al. Subclavian venoplasty by the implanting physicians in 373 patients over 11 years. Heart Rhythm 2011;8(4):526–33.

7. Jackson KP, Hegland DD, Frazier-Mills C, et al. Impact of using a telescoping-support catheter system for left ventricular lead placement on implant success and procedure time of cardiac resynchronization therapy. Pacing Clin Electrophysiol 2013; 36(5):553–8.

8. Kotter J, Lolay G, Charnigo R, et al. Predictors, morbidity, and costs associated with pneumothorax during electronic cardiac device implantation. Pacing Clin Electrophysiol 2016;39(9):985–91.

9. Chan NY, Kwong NP, Cheong AP. Venous access and long-term pacemaker lead failure: comparing contrast-guided axillary vein puncture with subclavian puncture and cephalic cutdown. Europace 2017;19(7):1193–7.

10. Abu-El-Haija B, Bhave PD, Campbell DN, et al. Venous stenosis after transvenous lead placement: a study of outcomes and risk factors in 212 consecutive patients. J Am Heart Assoc 2015;4(8): e001878.

11. Marcial JM, Worley SJ. Venous system interventions for device implantation. Card Electrophysiol Clin 2018;10(1):163–77.

12. Worley SJ. How to use balloons as anchors to facilitate cannulation of the coronary sinus left ventricular lead placement and to regain lost coronary sinus or target vein access. Heart Rhythm 2009;6(8):1242–6.

13. Heist EK, Fan D, Mela T, et al. Radiographic left ventricular-right ventricular interlead distance predicts the acute hemodynamic response to cardiac resynchronization therapy. Am J Cardiol 2005; 96(5):685–90.

14. Gold MR, Birgersdotter-Green U, Singh JP, et al. The relationship between ventricular electrical delay and left ventricular remodelling with cardiac resynchronization therapy. Eur Heart J 2011;32(20):2516–24.

15. Worley SJ, Gohn DC, Pulliam RW. Goose neck snare for LV lead placement in difficult venous anatomy. Pacing Clin Electrophysiol 2009;32(12):1577–81.

16. Martin DO, Lemke B, Birnie D, et al. Investigation of a novel algorithm for synchronized left-ventricular pacing and ambulatory optimization of cardiac resynchronization therapy: results of the adaptive CRT trial. Heart Rhythm 2012;9(11):1807–14.

Challenging Implants Require Tools and Techniques Not Tips and Tricks

Seth J. Worley, MD

KEYWORDS

- Orthodromic snare technique • Antidromic snare technique • Vein selectors • CS atresia
- Anchor balloon • Amplatz wire • Amplatz support wire technique • CS cannulation

KEY POINTS

- Successful left ventricular (LV) lead implantation requires preparation, tools, and techniques not tips and tricks. The implanting physician must be proactive and not rely on the device company to provide all the necessary tools.
- The Amplatz wire (Cook) + Vertebral Vein Selector is a powerful combination for both initial coronary sinus (CS) cannulation and to implement the support wire technique.
- Patients with CS atresia can be implanted through a persistent vein of Marshall.
- The orthodromic snare technique makes it possible to implant LV leads in small and/or tortuous veins not accessible by other means.
- The antidromic snare technique makes it possible to implant LV leads in target veins where a wire cannot be advanced.

INTRODUCTION

In some cases, left ventricular (LV) lead implantation can be difficult.

This article focuses on specific issues as they appear in the sequence of the implant. Combining the Cook Amplatz (Medical Bloomington, Indiana, USA) wire with the "Vertebral Vein Selector" is useful both for initial coronary sinus (CS) cannulation (**Box 1**, Videos 3 and 4) and to stabilize CS access (**Box 2**, Videos 4, 8, 11, 12, 13, 15). The term "Amplatz Wire-Vertebral Vein Selector technique" refers to the situation whereby the Amplatz wire and the vein selector are used to facilitate CS cannulation, whereas the "Amplatz support wire technique" refers to the situation whereby the wire is used to stabilize CS access (see **Box 2**).

SET UP

The trick is to be prepared by having the necessary equipment in the room readily available on a cart (**Fig. 1**). **Box 3** details the equipment on the cart. Proper table position (**Fig. 2**) and table designed for LV lead implantation (**Fig. 3**) are also important.[1] The proper table is also useful when a subclavian occlusion needs crossed and dilated for venous access.

VENOUS ACCESS

The importance of subclavian venoplasty for venous access is covered in Daniel J. Friedman and Kevin P. Jackson's article, "How to Implant CRT in a Busy Clinical Practice," in this issue of *Cardiac Electrophysiology Clinics*.[2–4]

Disclosure Statement: Royalties from Merit Medical (South Jordan, Utah, USA) and Pressure Products. Consulting Medtronic (Minneapolis, Minnesota, USA), Abbott, Biotronik.
Cardiac Electrophysiology Division, Medstar Heart and Vascular Institute, 110 Irving Street Northwest, Suite 5A-12, Washington, DC 20010, USA
E-mail address: seth@mcworley.com

Card Electrophysiol Clin 11 (2019) 75–87
https://doi.org/10.1016/j.ccep.2018.11.003

Box 1
Amplatz vertebral vein selector coronary sinus cannulation technique step by step

The Amplatz Vertebral Vein Selector CS cannulation tech wire technique works for all catheters used for CS access.

Advance a "Vertebral Vein Selector" over an angled 0.035-in glide wire deep into the CS. When using the Worley sheath, this will be through the braided core.

Keeping the Vertebral Vein Selector deep in the CS, replace the glide wire with a 0.035-in 180-cm J tip Cook Amplatz extra stiff wire. The short taper of the Cook Amplatz is important and not found in J tip Amplatz wires from other companies.

The combination of the Cook Amplatz wire and the Vertebral Vein selector deep in the CS provides a rail over which the sheath can be advanced despite stenosis or tortuosity.

Once the CS is cannulated, the Amplatz wire can be left in place if the 9-French Worley sheath is used for CS access.

Box 2
Amplatz support wire technique step by step

Amplatz wires are stiff and thus do not advance well into the CS but provide excellent support once in place. The Vertebral Vein selector serves as a conduit through which to introduce the Amplatz wire. To avoid perforation, always use a J tip Amplatz wire.

The 9-French internal diameter "Worley" sheath (WOR-CSG-B1-09 Merit Medical) provides the option to use the Amplatz support wire technique. The support wire technique is not an option with 7-French CS access catheters provided by the device companies.

Advance a "Vertebral Vein Selector" over an angled 0.035-in glide wire deep into the CS.

Keeping the Vertebral Vein Selector deep in the CS, replace the glide wire with a 0.035-in 180-cm J tip Cook Amplatz extra stiff wire. The short taper of the Cook Amplatz is important and not found in J tip Amplatz wires from other companies.

Remove the "Vertebral Vein Selector" keeping the Amplatz wire in place.

With the 9-French sheath stabilized by the Amplatz wire, the Vein Selector telescoped inside the subselector is advanced *beside* the Amplatz wire. The shape of the vein selector depends on the takeoff of the target vein. For target veins at the ostium of the CS, the sheath is withdrawn to uncover the target vein without loss of access.

LOCATING THE CORONARY SINUS

Trying to locate the CS with an electrophysiology catheter or wire (poke and pray), although often successful, is intrinsically limited. When you "poke and pray" and do not locate the CS, nothing is learned. Locating the CS via catheter manipulation with contrast injection (described in the video 1) is intrinsically superior but requires a change in approach for many.[5]

Problem = locating the CS for CS Cannulation (**Fig. 4**); solution = contrast injection and catheter manipulation to use the Eustachian ridge and Thebesian valve to facilitate CS cannulation. Watch Video 1 for the details on CS cannulation using the Worley CSG with braided core (https://www.youtube.com/watch?v=OE0yimc13uQ).

Problem = unable to locate the CS despite using contrast and catheter manipulation: possible CS atresia (**Fig. 5**); solution = look for a persistent vein of Marshall through which to implant the LV lead. Watch Video 2 for details of LV lead implantation in a patient with CS atresia and a persistent vein of Marshall (https://www.youtube.com/watch?v=1mLRpwJ1k8A). It is more common than first thought.

CORONARY SINUS CANNULATION ONCE THE CORONARY SINUS IS IDENTIFIED

Problem = difficult to advance into the CS (**Fig. 6**); solution = "Vertebral Vein Selector" combined with the Cook Amplatz wire. Watch Video 3 for details on how to implement the technique (https://www.youtube.com/watch?v=SB4nNBmy-3g).

Problem = difficult CS to advance and unstable CS access with huge right atrium (RA) (**Fig. 7**); solution = Jumbo Worley Sheath and Cook Amplatz support wire. Watch Video 4 to see how (https://www.youtube.com/watch?v=5P7gJltePP8). In many cases just switching from a standard sheath to the Jumbo Worley CSG solves the problem.

Problem = drain pipe CS unable to advance sheath into the CS (**Fig. 8**); solution = the anchor balloon technique.[6] Watch video 5 to learn how to implement the anchor balloon technique for CS cannulation (https://www.youtube.com/watch?v=hmXtcsVjsyw). The anchor balloon can also be used to advance a subselector into a difficult target vein.

Problem = Vieussens valve prevents access to the great cardiac vein (**Fig. 9**); solution = "Vertebral Vein Selector" to advance past the Vieussens valve. Watch Video 6 for details on

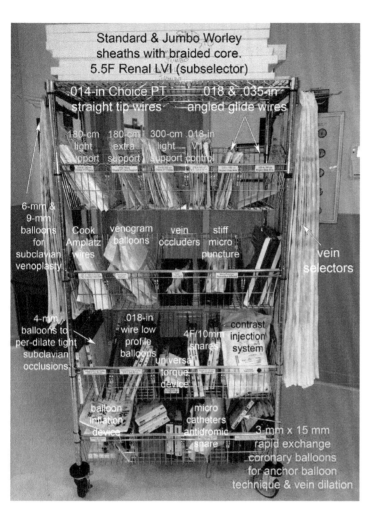

Standard & Jumbo Worley sheaths with braided core.
5.5F Renal LVI (subselector)

.014-in Choice PT .018 & .035-in
straight tip wires angled glide wires

180-cm 180-cm 300-cm .018-in
light extra light V1
support support support control

6-mm & 9-mm balloons for subclavian venoplasty

Cook Amplatz wires

venogram balloons

vein occluders

stiff micro puncture

vein selectors

4-mm balloons to per-dilate tight subclavian occlusions

.018-in wire low profile balloons

universal torque device

4F/10mm snares

contrast injection system

balloon inflation device

micro catheters antidromic snare

3-mm x 15 mm rapid exchange coronary balloons for anchor balloon technique & vein dilation

Fig. 1. Cart with the equipment necessary for both basic and challenging LV lead implantation as well as subclavian venoplasty. (See **Box 1** for complete details.) (*Courtesy of* Seth J. Worley, MD, Washington, DC.)

how to use the "Vertebral Vein Selector" to cross the Vieussens valve (https://www.youtube.com/watch?v=SdTEB3R6W8M&t=5s).

OCCLUSIVE CORONARY SINUS VENOGRAM

Start by using full-strength contrast and a control syringe for an adequate CS venogram. Insure the balloon is occlusive by placing the balloon above the Vieussens valve. Do not assume that it is safe to inflate the balloon because it was advanced over a wire; you could be in the vein of Marshall, so always do a gentle test injection first. Watch for retrograde filling of proximal veins.

Problem = high outputs and phrenic pacing throughout the only viable target vein identified on CS venogram (**Fig. 10**); solution = full-strength contrast injection through a "Vein Selector" advanced over a wire into the branch to demonstrate an alternative target vein off of the CS.

Watch Video 7 for details on selective target vein venography using a Vein Selector (https://www.youtube.com/watch?v=23nhCd2h9Gw).

Problem = high outputs and phrenic pacing throughout the only viable target vein identified on CS venogram (**Fig. 11**); solution = full-strength contrast injection through a "Vein Selector" advanced over a wire into the target vein demonstrates a side branch off the target vein. Watch Video 8 for details (https://www.youtube.com/watch?v=mWVeJIYC92s).

LEFT VENTRICULAR LEAD IMPLANTATION

Problem = using the "poke-and-pray" approach can be difficult to advance a wire into the target vein (**Fig. 12**); solution = 3 vein selector shapes designed to be telescoped into the subselector. Vein selectors attached to the contrast injection system are designed to locate the target vein with a puff of contrast as you might locate the right

Box 3
Implant equipment list

1. Worley Advanced Standard Curve; Order no. WOR-CSG-B1-09 Merit Medical.

2. Worley Advanced Jumbo Curve; Order no. WOR-CSG-B2-09. Merit Medical.

3. Catheters for right side CS access and difficult to locate CS are hand shaped to resemble the braided core. 6-French Boston Scientific (Marlborough, Massachusetts, USA) Runway MP2 (Multipurpose 2) Ref. H74938969390 (Alternative no. 1 = 6 French Boston Scientific Mach 1 MP2 Order 34356-39, Alternative no. 2 = 6 French Medtronic (Minneapolis, Minnesota, USA) MB1 Z2 Guiding Catheter Medtronic Vascular Z26MB1. Alternative no. 3 = 6 French Medtronic Launcher MB2 Ref. LA6MB2. Alternative no. 4 = 6 French Cordis (Milpitas, California USA) Vista Bright Tip MPB 1 Ref. 670-275-00).

4. Worley Standard Vein Selector (5 French × 75 cm) Merit Order no. 57538CS-WOR Merit Medical.

5. Worley Vert Vein Selector (5 French × 75 cm) Merit Order no. 57538CSV-WOR Merit Medical.

6. Worley Hook Vein Selector (5 French × 75 cm) Merit Order no. 57538CSHK-WOR Merit Medical.

7. Contrast Injection System Worley Advanced Kit 1 CAK 1 (comes with contrast bowl and labels) (order no. K12-WORLEY1 Merit Medical).

8. Subselector = 5.5-French ID Worley advanced Telescoping LVI, Order no. WORLVI-75-5-62-55-RE.

9. 5-French micropuncture kit with 0.018 Nitinol wire and stiffened radiopaque dilator Merit Medical. Order no. S-MAK501N15BT.

10. 5-French Impress KA 2 Hydrophilic Angiographic Catheter 5-French 65 cm (Order no. 56538KA2-H Merit Medical) to assist crossing difficult subclavian obstruction.

11. 4-French Impress KA 2 Hydrophilic Angiographic Catheter 4-French 65 cm (Order no. 46538KA2-H Merit Medical).

12. 0.014-in CholCE PT (Polymer Tip) Straight tip Light Support (Order no. 1211-01 Boston Scientific) (see annotated list in later discussion for options).

13. 0.014-in CholCE PT (Polymer Tip) Straight (not angled) Tip Extra Support (Order no. 12161-01 Boston Scientific).

14. 0.014-in CholCE PT (Polymer Tip) Straight (not angled) tip Light Support 300 cm Boston Scientific.

15. 0.018 V-18 Control Wire Guidewire with ICE Coating Polymer Tip Hydrophilic (0.018-in 200-cm short taper) Boston Scientific (Catalog no. 46-852).

16. Cook Amplatz Extra Stiff Wire Guide, 0.035-in, 180-cm, 3-mm tip curve Cook (THSCF-35-180-3-AES) (another ref. no. on the package is G03565) (do not substitute).

17. Angled (not straight) polymer tip hydrophilic wire 0.035 in × 180 cm Laureate wire (Order no. LWSTDA35180 Merit Medical) (Glide wire or Terumo).

18. Angled (not straight) polymer tip hydrophilic wire 0.018 in × 180 cm (Laureate Wire Order no. LWSTDA18180 Merit Medical) (Glide wire or Terumo).

19. Snare (Micro) 10-mm loop/4-French snare catheter Merit One Snare ONE 1000 (snare = 10 mm loop, 120 cm length; catheter = 4-French 100-cm length inside diameter 1.02 mm). This 10-mm snare fits into the 9-French internal diameter CSG Worley beside the vein selector (Order no. ONE100 Merit Medical).

20. Microcatheter for the antidromic technique Merit SureCross Support Catheter (length 90 cm, wire diameter 0.014 in, tip diameter 0.020 in [1.52 French]) Catalog no. SC1490.

21. Subclavian venoplasty balloon 6-mm diameter × 4 cm length × 75 cm. CONQUEST Order no. CQ-7564 Bard (Covington, Georgia, USA) Peripheral Vascular rated burst pressure 30 atm.

22. Subclavian venoplasty 9 mm × 4 cm × 75 cm balloon Order no. CQ-7594 Bard Peripheral Vascular rated burst pressure 26 atm.

23. Cordis Powerflex Pro OTW (0.035-in wire) Balloon Catheter: Balloon 4 mm diameter × 40 mm long; shaft length 80 cm Order no. 4400404S.

24. Noncompliant rapid exchange coronary balloon, for example, NC Sprinter from Medtronic 3.0 mm diameter × 15 mm length, Catalog no. H7493912415300 GITN, no. 08714729783374.

25. Cook Needle's Eye Snare alone = 13-mm. Femoral Snare and straight 12-French sheath without work station; Ref.: G26518, Ref.: LR-SSN001.

26. Cook Needle's Eye Snare alone = 20-mm. Femoral Snare and straight 12-French sheath without work station, Ref.: G26516, Ref: LR-SSN002.

28. 16-French Curved Work Station alone, 16-French Curved Work Station (Femoral Introducer Sheath Set), Ref.: G26566, Ref.: LR-CSS16.

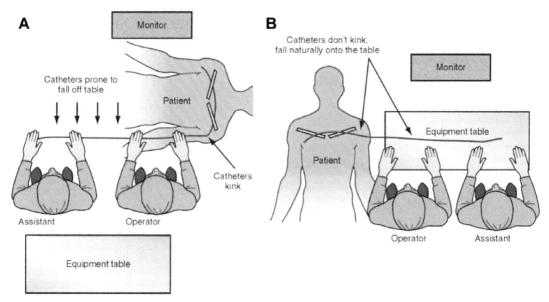

Fig. 2. Importance of table position for successful LV lead implantation. The perpendicular table position improves the ergonomics of catheter and wire exchange; the catheter torque control is improved by removing an acute angle, and wires are less likely to fall off the table. . (*Courtesy of* Seth J. Worley, MD, Washington, DC.)

coronary artery. Once the vein is located, a wire is advanced. The vein selector is then advanced over the wire deep into the target vein. To facilitate advancing the vein selector into a difficult target vein, up to four 0.014-in angioplasty wires can be advanced through the 0.038-in lumen. The subselector is then advanced over the wire stabilized vein selector deep in the target vein. The vein selector is removed, retaining one wire for LV lead delivery. Watch Video 9 for details on the use of the wire stabilized vein selector (https://www.youtube.com/watch?v=IsawLqHGq-g).

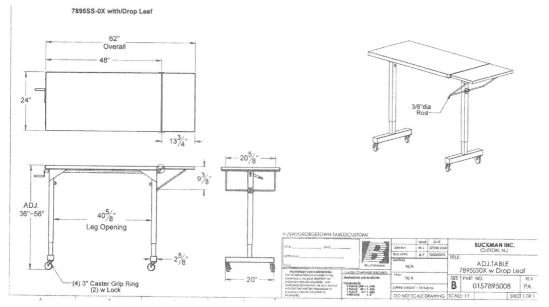

Fig. 3. The table is designed for the interventional approach to device implantation. The table height can be adjusted to the height of the patient table. The extension allows the x-ray tube to be rotated to the right anterior oblique (RAO) without hitting the legs of the table. ADJ, adjustable. (*Courtesy of* Seth J. Worley, MD, Washington, DC.)

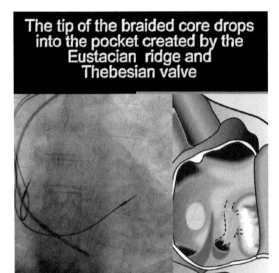

Fig. 4. How to cannulate the CS using catheter manipulation and contrast injection. With counterclockwise torque, the tip of the catheter drops down the annulus into the CS (*arrow*). The Eustachian ridge and Thebesian valve direct the tip of the catheter into the CS. Watch Video 1 for details (https://www.youtube.com/watch?v=OE0yimc13uQ). (*Courtesy of* Seth J. Worley, MD, Washington, DC.)

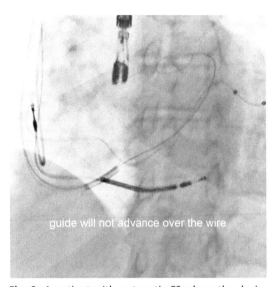

Fig. 6. A patient with a stenotic CS where the device company delivery systems could not be advanced. Using the Merit "Vertebral Vein Selector" and Cook Amplatz wire, CS cannulation was successful. The vein selector/Amplatz wire technique also works well for a tortuous CS. Watch Video 3 for details (https://www.youtube.com/watch?v=SB4nNBmy-3g). (*Courtesy of* Seth J. Worley, MD, Washington, DC.)

Problem = drain pipe target vein (**Fig. 13**); solution = the "Hook Vein Selector" telescoped in the renal lateral vein introducer (LVI) subselector plus the use of multiple wires to advance the vein selector deep into the target vein. For details,

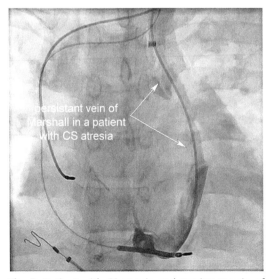

Fig. 5. Patient with CS atresia and persistent vein of Marshall through which the LV lead can be implanted. Watch Video 2 for details (https://www.youtube.com/watch?v=1mLRpwJ1k8A). (*Courtesy of* Seth J. Worley, MD, Washington, DC.)

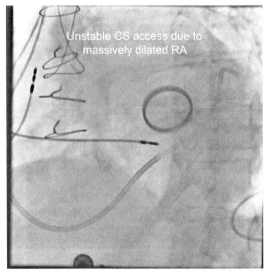

Fig. 7. Using several different device company delivery systems, it was impossible to establish stable CS access in this patient with a massively dilated RA. The Jumbo Worley sheath and Cook Amplatz support provide stable CS access followed by successful LV lead delivery. Sometimes switching from the Standard Worley sheath to the Jumbo Worley sheath facilitates initial CS cannulation. Watch Video 4 for details (https://www.youtube.com/watch?v=5P7gJItePP8). (*Courtesy of* Seth J. Worley, MD, Washington, DC.)

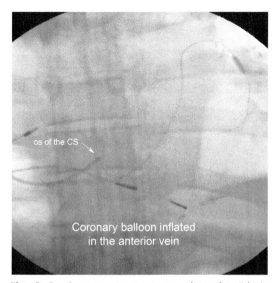

os of the CS

Coronary balloon inflated
in the anterior vein

Fig. 8. Previous attempts to cannulate the "drain pipe" were unsuccessful. As the catheter was advanced, the tip served as a fulcrum and the proximal segment was dropped into the RA. The CS was successfully cannulated using anchor balloon technique. Watch Video 5 for details (https://www.youtube.com/watch?v=hmXtcsVjsyw). (*Courtesy of* Seth J. Worley, MD, Washington, DC.)

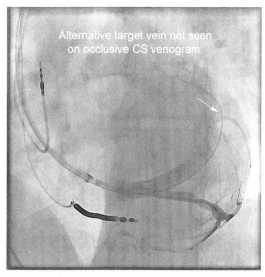

Alternative target vein not seen
on occlusive CS venogram

Fig. 10. Selective venogram using the Vein Selector reveals a CS target vein not seen on occlusive venography. Watch Video 7 for details (https://www.youtube.com/watch?v=23nhCd2h9Gw). (*Courtesy of* Seth J. Worley, MD, Washington, DC.)

watch Video 10 (https://www.youtube.com/watch?v=I9gEdLSNcFg).

Problem = angulated stenotic target vein near the ostium of the CS (**Fig. 14**); solution = the "Hook Vein Selector" telescoped in the renal LVI subselector through the 9-French sheath supported by the Cook Amplatz wire. For details on

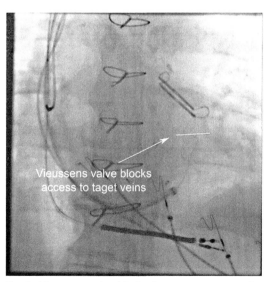

Vieussens valve blocks
access to taget veins

Fig. 9. Vieussens valve blocked access to target veins resulting in 2 failed attempts at LV lead implantation. Using the "Vertebral Vein Selector" and contrast injection system, the valve was crossed, and lead was placed. Watch Video 6 for details (https://www.youtube.com/watch?v=SdTEB3R6W8M). (*Courtesy of* Seth J. Worley, MD, Washington, DC.)

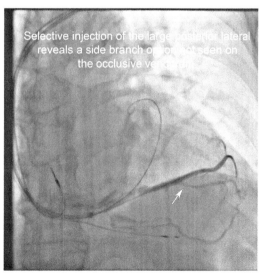

Selective injection of the large posterior lateral
reveals a side branch option not seen on
the occlusive venogram

Fig. 11. Selective venogram using the Vein Selector reveals a side branch off the target vein not seen on occlusive venography. Watch Video 8 for details (https://www.youtube.com/watch?v=mWVeJIYC92s). (*Courtesy of* Seth J. Worley, MD, Washington, DC.)

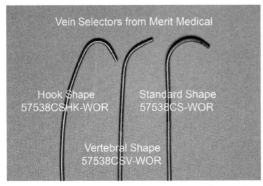

Fig. 12. There are 3 vein selector shapes designed to for specific anatomy. Watch Video 9 for details (https://www.youtube.com/watch?v=IsawLqHGq-g). (*Courtesy of* Seth Worley, MD, Washington, DC; and Merit Medical Systems, Inc, South Jordan, UT.)

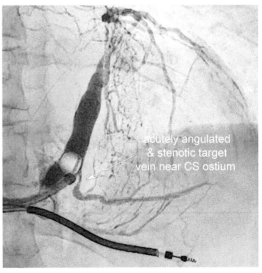

Fig. 14. Target veins with acute angulation near the ostium of the CS can be implanted using the "Hook Vein Selector" telescoped inside the "Renal LVI" subselector with the Worley sheath supported by the Cook Amplatz wire. For details, watch Video 11 (https://www.youtube.com/watch?v=fQynQNB-jp0). (*Courtesy of* Seth Worley, MD, Washington, DC.)

how to use the Hook Vein Selector and Amplatz support wire technique for target veins near the CS os, watch Video 11 (https://www.youtube.com/watch?v=fQynQNB-jp0).

Problem = target vein at the ostium of the CS (**Fig. 15**); solution = the "Vertebral Vein Selector" telescoped in the renal LVI subselector through the 9-French sheath supported by the Cook Amplatz wire. For details on how to use the Amplatz support wire technique for target veins at or near the CS, watch Video 12 (https://www.youtube.com/watch?v=4XYwfi5Ba6U).

Problem = angulated target vein when a subselector cannot be advanced for LV lead delivery (**Fig. 16**); solution = the "Standard Vein Selector" telescoped in the renal LVI subselector

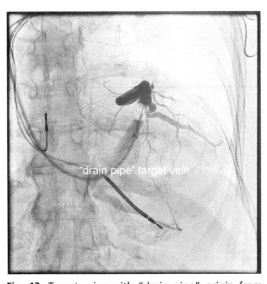

Fig. 13. Target veins with "drain pipe" origin from the CS can be difficult to implant. This patient had a previously failed attempt. The "Hook Vein Selector" telescoped inside the "Renal LVI" subselector makes implantation possible. Watch Video 10 for details (https://www.youtube.com/watch?v=I9gEdLSNcFg). (*Courtesy of* Seth J. Worley, MD, Washington, DC.)

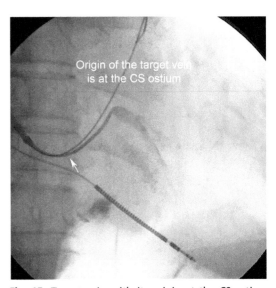

Fig. 15. Target vein with its origin at the CS ostium can be implanted easily using the Cook Amplatz support wire technique and "Vertebral Vein Selector" telescoped inside the "Renal LVI" subselector. Watch Video 12 for details (https://www.youtube.com/watch?v=4XYwfi5Ba6U). (*Courtesy of* Seth Worley, MD, Washington, DC.)

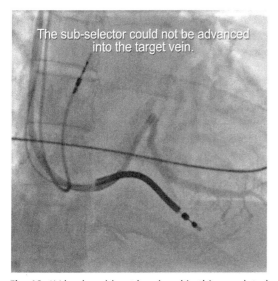

Fig. 16. LV lead could not be placed in this angulated target vein using device company subselector despite multiple attempts by several physicians over the course of several hours. Using the "Standard Vein Selector" telescoped inside the "Renal LVI" subselector, the LV lead was easily placed in 15 minutes. See Video 13 for details (https://www.youtube.com/watch?v=0apbC0kPumo&t=7s). (*Courtesy of* Seth Worley, MD, Washington, DC.)

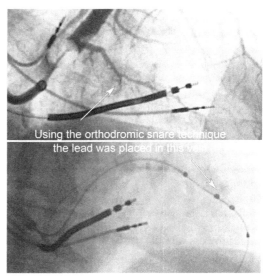

Fig. 17. Target vein too small for LV lead placement using traditional techniques successfully implanted via the orthodromic snare technique. Watch Video 14 for details on how to implement the orthodromic snare technique (https://www.youtube.com/watch?v=tmr8z7bltN0). (*Courtesy of* Seth Worley, MD, Washington, DC.)

Box 4
Sheaths, catheters, and wires required for the orthodromic and antidromic snare technique

1. Worley Advanced Standard Curve; Order no. WOR-CSG-B1-09 Merit Medical or Worley Advanced Jumbo Curve; Order no. WOR-CSG-B2-09. Merit Medical.

2. Worley Standard Vein Selector (5 French × 75 cm) Merit Order no. 57538CS-WOR Merit Medical.

3. Worley Vert Vein Selector (5 French × 75 cm) Merit Order no. 57538CSV-WOR Merit Medical.

4. Worley Hook Vein Selector (5 French × 75 cm) Merit Order no. 57538CSHK-WOR Merit Medical.

5. Contrast Injection System Worley Advanced Kit 1 CAK 1 (comes with contrast bowl and labels) (order no.K12-WORLEY1 Merit Medical).

6. 4-French Impress KA 2 Hydrophilic Angiographic Catheter 4-French 65-cm (Order no. 46538KA2-H Merit Medical).

7. 0.014-in ChoICE PT (Polymer Tip) Straight Tip Light Support 180-cm (order no. 1211-01 Boston Scientific).

8. 0.014-in ChoICE PT (Polymer Tip) Straight (not angled) Tip Light Support 300-cm Boston Scientific.

9. Cook Amplatz Extra Stiff Wire Guide, 0.035 in, 180-cm, 3-mm-tip curve Cook (THSCF-35-180-3-AES) (another ref. no. on the package is G03565) (do not substitute).

10. Snare (Micro) 10-mm loop/4-French snare catheter Merit One Snare ONE 1000 (snare = 10-mm loop, 120-cm length; catheter = 4-French 100-cm length inside diameter 1.02 mm). This 10-mm snare fits into the 9-French internal diameter CSG Worley beside the vein selector (Order no. ONE100 Merit Medical).

11. Microcatheter in case the snared wire gets bent and for the antidromic snare technique Merit Sure-Cross Support Catheter (length 90 cm, wire diameter 0.014 in, tip diameter 0.020 in [1.52 French]) Catalog no. SC1490.

Box 5
Orthodromic snare technique step by step

Engage the target vein with the appropriate shape "Vein Selector."

Advance a straight light support polymer tip wire into the vein (Choice PT Floppy Boston Scientific).

Once the wire is in the vein, advance the vein selector 3 to 7 mm over the wire into the vein.

If the wire becomes bent as it is advanced, it may not traverse the collaterals. Once it is bent, withdrawing the wire back into the vein selector does not straighten the wire. Do not remove the bent wire. Add a second wire. The bent wire orients and supports the vein selector, so the second wire remains straight as it exits into the vein.

The straight second wire is advanced through the collaterals into an adjacent vein (exit vein) and back into the CS.

If there is difficulty advancing the wire through the collaterals, one option is to add a microcatheter as follows: (1) remove the Y adapter from the hub of the injection system; (2) advance a 0.014-in microcatheter (SureCross) over the existing wire; (3) exchange the existing wire for a fresh wire; (4) the microcatheter provides support to advance the fresh wire through the collaterals.

To confirm that the wire is back in the CS, check the left anterior oblique (LAO) and RAO projections.

Once the wire traverses the collaterals, load the 10-mm loop into the 4-French snare catheter.

Holding the vein selector in position, advance the 4-French 10-mm snare into the 9-French sheath beside the 5-French "Vein Selector." (As the snare is advanced, hold the vein selector [or lead] in place; otherwise friction can cause the vein selector [or lead] to advance.)

How the wire is snared depends on the direction the wire takes once it reaches the CS: either (1) up the CS toward the great cardiac vein; or (2) out of the CS into the RA.

1. When the wire turns up into the CS toward the great cardiac vein, the snare is positioned in the body of the CS above the "exit vein" (usually the middle cardiac vein (MCV)) and the wire is advanced into the open loop.

2. When the wire exits into the RA, the vein selector is held in place and the snare is positioned over the ostium of the "exit vein" (usually the MCV). It is critical to check the RAO projection to confirm that the snare is positioned over the MCV. The loop can appear to be properly positioned in the anterior, posterior and LAO projection, but when advanced, the wire is not captured by the snare.

After 15 cm of wire is through the loop, the snare is closed on the wire. It is important to tighten the snare on the stiff part of the wire to avoid bending the wire or pulling off the tip.

To secure the snared wire: (1) the right hand presses the open hemostat against the hub of the snare catheter; (2) the left hand pulls the snare loop tight against the wire; (3) the hemostat is closed on the snare at the hub of the snare catheter.

With wire snared, the sheath is withdrawn into the RA (holding the snare and vein selector in place).

To prevent the snare from being pulled down into the sheath when tension is placed on the wire, a second snap is placed on the snare catheter where it enters the hub of the sheath.

To advance the lead, a rail is created by placing tension on the snared wire.

Tension on the wire creates a rail over which the lead could be advanced despite the stenosis and tortuosity. In some cases, even with the snare, the lead will not advance without venoplasty.

With the wire still snared and the lead in place, thresholds are tested. Thresholds may change slightly once the snare is released and the wire is removed. The presence or absence of phrenic pacing does not change.

Once satisfactory thresholds are achieved, the snare system is removed.

To prevent any chance of lead dislodgment, the sheath is removed with the wire still snared. Again, thresholds may change only slightly once the snare is released and the wire is removed.

To open the snare, the loop is advanced 3 to 5 mm into the snare catheter.

Withdraw the wire through the open snare until the tip is clear of the snare but still in the pacing lead.

With the wire free of the snare, the loop is withdrawn into the snare catheter. Hold the lead in place and remove the snare.

After a final adjustment of slack in the LAO projection, the wire is withdrawn.

Special Situations
Inability to Capture the Wire with the Snare

First, confirm the position of the loop relative to the exit vein in the RAO projection. In some cases, it can be very difficult to snare the wire as it exits the MCV into the RA. One option is to position the snare inside the MCV. To get the snare in the MCV, start by loading a glide wire into the snare catheter. Advance the glide wire/snare catheter into the sheath beside the vein selector. Advance the glide wire into the MCV. Advance the snare catheter over the glide wire into the MCV. Remove the glide wire and load the snare loop into the snare catheter. Deploy the loop in the MCV and advance the wire into the open snare. Alternatively, the snare catheter can be replaced with a 4-French angled catheter (KA2) to aim the loop of the snare in the desired direction.

Wire Becomes Bent by the Snare

On occasion, the snare bends the wire usually when the snared wire is inadvertently pulled back into the sheath. To prevent bending the wire, withdraw the sheath into the RA once the wire is snared. When the wire is bent, it can be impossible to remove from the pacing lead or the bent tip can fracture and embolize. When the wire is bent, follow these steps: (1) keep the wire snared; (2) remove the pacing lead; (3) flush and wipe the wire; (4) advance the microcatheter over the wire through the collaterals up the snare; (4) attach a Y adapter to the hub of the microcatheter, tighten the hemostatic valve, and flush the microcatheter with hepatized saline using a 1- to 3-mL syringe; (5) loosen the hemostatic valve and advance the wire into the microcatheter while the wire is withdrawn into the sheath with the snare; (6) once the bent wire is removed, flush the microcatheter and insert a fresh wire; (7) reinsert the snare into the CS; (8) keeping the wire in place, withdraw the microcatheter and resnare the wire; (8) replace the microcatheter with the pacing lead.

makes it possible to easily advance the subselector into the target vein for LV lead delivery. For details on how the wire-stabilized vein selector is used to augment a subselector, watch Video 13 (https://www.youtube.com/watch?v=0apbC0kPumo&t=7s).

Problem = tortuous small and or stenotic target vein (**Fig. 17**); solution = orthodromic snare technique (**Boxes 4** and **5**).[7] Also watch Video 14 for details on how to implement the orthodromic snare technique (https://www.youtube.com/watch?v=tmr8z7bltN0).

Problem = inability to advance a wire into the target vein (**Fig. 18**); solution = antidromic snare technique (**Boxes 4** and **6**, Video 15). Watch Video 15 for details on how to implement the antidromic

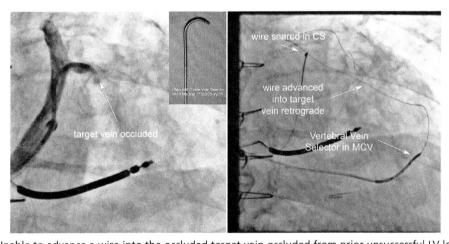

Fig. 18. Unable to advance a wire into the occluded target vein occluded from prior unsuccessful LV lead placement. Wire advanced out of the target vein using collaterals from the middle cardiac vein. Lead placed using the antidromic snare technique and coronary vein venoplasty. Watch Video 15 for details on how to implement the antidromic snare technique (https://www.youtube.com/watch?v=ez4Kvd2iYiE) and (see **Box 6**) for a detailed step by step discussion of the antidromic snare technique. (*Courtesy of* Seth Worley, MD, Washington, DC; and Merit Medical Systems, Inc, South Jordan, UT.)

Box 6
Antidromic snare technique step by step

1. The first step is to engage a branch with collaterals to the target vein, usually the MCV. The 9-French internal diameter "Worley" sheath (WOR-CSG-B1-09 Merit Medical) provides the option to use the support wire technique to easily engage the MCV. The support wire technique is not an option with a 7-French CS access catheter. See the Amplatz support wire technique for details.

2. The shape of the "Vertebral Vein Selector" is well suited for cannulation of the MCV and target veins below the Vieussens valve. Full-strength contrast is injected to define the collaterals to the target vein. A puff of contrast from the injection system confirms the tip of "Vein Selector" has dropped into the MCV. An angled 0.035-in glide wire is advanced into the MCV.

3. With the Worley sheath stabilized by the Cook Amplatz wire, the "Vein Selector" is advanced into the MCV over a glide wire. The glide wire is removed and a puff of contrast is injected to define the collaterals from the MCV to the target vein. In most cases the angle of the "Vertebral Vein Selector" works well with the angle of the collaterals.

4. A 300-cm light support (floppy) straight polymer jacketed angioplasty wire is advanced into the collaterals (Choice PT Floppy).

5. The position of the wire is assessed with a puff of contrast through the vein selector. The 300-cm wire is advanced through the collateral leading to the target vein and then back into the CS.

6. If there is any difficulty advancing the wire through the collaterals, the Y adapter on the vein selector is removed and a SureCross microcatheter is advanced over the wire through the vein selector into the collateral. Because the "Vein Selector" is 75 cm and the SureCross is 90 cm, it is important to remove the Y adapter to load the catheter over the wire.

7. Once the wire is back in the CS, advance the snare catheter over the 180-cm Cook Amplatz to support the wire into the CS. Once the snare catheter is in the mid-CS, the Amplatz wire is removed.

8. With the tip of the 4-French snare catheter in the CS, load the 10-mm loop using the introducer. The 10-mm loop is advanced through the snare catheter until it is deployed in the mid-CS.

9. The angioplasty wire is withdrawn toward the target vein until the tip is beyond the loop of the snare. The wire is then advanced into the open snare. The loop of the snare is closed on the wire by advancing the snare catheter.

10. Once the tip of the wire is secured by the snare, the goal is to use the snare to withdraw 120 cm of the angioplasty wire into the sheath and out into the pocket. However, there is the potential for the cheese cutter effect.

11. To prevent the cheese cutter effect, the wire is covered with a microcatheter. The wire is advanced through the microcatheter, not pulled through the collaterals.

12. The Y adapter is removed, and the SureCross is advanced over the wire, through the vein selector into the collaterals.

Again, because the "Vein Selector" is 75 cm and the SureCross is 90 cm, it is important to remove the Y adapter to load the catheter over the wire.

Hydrophilic microcatheter 90-cm, 0.14-in lumen 1.5-French tip (SureCross Support Catheter Merit Medical).

Alternatively, the vein selector is removed before the microcatheter is advanced through the collaterals.

With the wire snared in the CS, the microcatheter is advanced through the collaterals.

CAUTION: Failure to flush the microcatheter can result in seizure of the wire.

Do not use the snare to pull the wire through the microcatheter.

The distal end of the wire is advanced into the microcatheter while the tip of the lead is withdrawn into the 9-French Worley sheath with the snare.

The wire should advance easily into the microcatheter to provide slack for the snare to withdraw into the sheath.

The process of advancing the proximal end of the wire into the microcatheter and withdrawing the snared end is continued until 80 cm of wire is externalized into the pocket.

The wire should advance easily into the microcatheter to provide slack for the snare to withdraw into the sheath.

If there is any difficulty advancing the wire into the microcatheter's STOP, close the hemostatic valve and flush the microcatheter with a 1- to 2-mL syringe.

The snare is opened, and the bent wire is removed with a pair of scissors.

The cut snared end (tip) of the wire is back-loaded into the tip of the pacing lead.

The proximal end of the wire is secured at the hub of the Y adapter used to flush the microcatheter.

With tension on the distal end of the wire, the pacing lead is advanced into the target vein.

Before advancing the pacing lead, be certain the sheath is out of the CS. The sheath can get jammed into the crux between the MCV (wire exit vein and the CS) preventing the lead from advancing.

In some cases, the lead may not advance because there is too much tension on the wire.

Temporarily relaxing tension while advancing can help the lead to advance, particularly around tight curves.

Another situation where there can be difficulty advancing the LV lead is when you forget to withdraw the tip of the microcatheter back into the microcatheter.

To allow the lead to advance, the microcatheter must be withdrawn into the collaterals.

Once the lead is in place and thresholds confirmed, the sheath is peeled away. The wire is removed through the microcatheter.

If there is any difficulty moving the wire, close the hemostatic valve and flush the microcatheter.

Also flush the leads as described below.

Special Cases

1. In some patients, the "Vertebral Vein Selector" is not the correct shape to engage the collateral to the target vein. When this occurs, switch to a "standard" or "hook" vein selector.

2. Although the collaterals leading to the target vein are often found in the MCV, they may be found connecting to other adjacent veins.

3. If the microcatheter will not advance through the collaterals (rare with the 0.014-in SureCross), the microcatheter can be exchanged for an over-the-wire 1.25-mm coronary balloon. Once the balloon is through the collaterals into the CS, the lumen of the balloon is used as the conduit through which to advance the wire.

4. Usually the wire is snared in the CS before the microcatheter is advanced. However, sometimes the wire traverses the collaterals to the target vein but will not advance from the target vein into the CS. To get the wire to exit the target vein, the Y adapter is removed and the 0.014-in microcatheter is advanced over the wire through the collaterals into the target vein. The support of the microcatheter facilitates wire passage out of the target vein into the CS. Once the microcatheter is in the target vein, a bent wire can be replaced without the risk of not being able to cross the collaterals.

5. The "Vein Selector" can be replaced with the 0.014-in microcatheter and advanced through the collaterals into the target vein to facilitate wire passage out of the target vein into the CS. The microcatheter provides support to advance the wire and/or the bent wire can be replaced with a new wire. The wire can then be advanced into the open snare and secured.

snare technique (https://www.youtube.com/watch?v=ez4Kvd2iYiE).

REFERENCES

1. [Chapter 30] Worley SJ. Coronary Sinus Lead Implantation. In: Ellenbogen KA, Wilkoff BL, Kay GN, et al, editors. Coronary sinus lead implantation in: clinical cardiac pacing, defibrillation and resynchronization therapy. 45th edition. Philadelphia (PA): Elsevier; 2017.

2. Worley SJ, Gohn DC, Pulliam RW, et al. Subclavian venoplasty by the implanting physicians in 373 patients over 11 years. Heart Rhythm 2011;8(4):526–33.

3. [Chapter 13] Worley SJ. How to perform venoplasty for access. In: Worley SJ, editor. How-to manual for pacemaker and ICD devices: procedures and programming. Hoboken (NJ): John Wiley & Sons. Inc; 2017. p. 97–109.

4. Marcial JM, Worley SJ. Venous system interventions for device implantation. Card Electrophysiol Clin 2018;10(1):163–77.

5. Jackson KP, Hegland DD, Frazier-Mills C, et al. Impact of using a telescoping-support catheter system for left ventricular lead placement on implant success and procedure time of cardiac resynchronization therapy. Pacing Clin Electrophysiol 2013;36(5):553–8.

6. Worley SJ. How to use balloons as anchors to facilitate cannulation of the coronary sinus left ventricular lead placement and to regain lost coronary sinus or target vein access. Heart Rhythm 2009;6(8):1242–6.

7. Worley SJ, Gohn DC, Pulliam RW. Goose neck snare for LV lead placement in difficult venous anatomy. Pacing Clin Electrophysiol 2009;32:1577–81.

Following CRT Patients Long-term

Optimizing Cardiac Resynchronization Therapy Devices in Follow-up to Improve Response Rates and Outcomes

Jose María Tolosana, MD, PhD[a], Josep Brugada, MD, PhD[b],*

KEYWORDS

- Cardiac resynchronization therapy • Percentage of biventricular pacing • Response rate
- Device programming • Medical treatment optimization

KEY POINTS

- Structured follow-up with regular visits to device and heart failure specialists is mandatory to improve outcomes and response to cardiac resynchronization therapy (CRT).
- Device programming should aim to reach 100% of complete and effective biventricular pacing.
- Postimplant optimization of the device still remains a challenge. Suboptimal device programming is one of the main reasons for the lack of favorable CRT response.
- Atrioventricular and interventricular intervals optimization may be useful to improve the beneficial effects of CRT.

BACKGROUND

Cardiac resynchronization therapy (CRT) in appropriately selected heart failure (HF) patients has been shown to induce left ventricular (LV) reverse remodeling and improve both functional capacity and quality of life, thus decreasing hospital admissions and mortality.[1]

Although CRT will improve symptoms and survival in most patients, about one-third (30%) of CRT recipients do not obtain clinical benefit from the therapy and are considered clinical nonresponders. The percentage reaches 40% when the criterion is echocardiographic response to CRT, defined as significant LV reverse remodeling.[2]

The lack of response to CRT depends on multiple factors, starting with patient selection followed by factors related to the implant procedure and the optimization of the therapy, including appropriate drugs and device programming during follow-up (FU).

The main goal of CRT FU is to assess that HF status of the patients is optimized and that the CRT device is programmed to maximize the benefits of the therapy.

A systematic effort should be done to identify and treat reversible causes that may cause a poor response to CRT. This effort includes optimization of medical therapy, checking for appropriate and effective biventricular (BiV) pacing, and treatment of arrhythmias and other reversible causes of deterioration.[3]

Disclosure Statement: J. Brugada: Advisory contracts with Abbott, Biotronik, and Boston Scientific. J.M. Tolosana: Advisory contracts with Boston Scientific, Abbot, Medtronic, and Biotronik.
a Cardiovascular Institute, Hospital Clínic, Arrhythmia Unit Hospital Clinic, University of Barcelona, Villarroel 170, Barcelona 08036, Spain; b Pediatric Arrhythmia Unit, Cardiovascular Institute, Hospital Clínic, Hospital Sant Joan de Déu, University of Barcelona, Barcelona, Spain
* Corresponding author.
E-mail address: josep@brugada.org

Card Electrophysiol Clin 11 (2019) 89–98
https://doi.org/10.1016/j.ccep.2018.11.010

The authors review how to optimize the CRT device during FU, highlighting the different aspects to keep in mind to improve the benefits and outcomes of the patients treated with CRT.

CARDIAC RESYNCHRONIZATION THERAPY DEVICE FOLLOW-UP

After CRT device implantation, conventional care requires patients to regularly attend calendar-based in-clinic FU visits to monitor and to check the proper functioning of the device and to assess patient's health status.[3] Patients will require FU services for as long as they have their device implanted, which is usually lifelong.

Device testing includes interrogation of battery status, lead impedances, amplitudes of intrinsic cardiac signals in atrium, right and left ventricle, and pacing threshold testing in all chambers.

Loss of LV or right ventricular (RV) pacing capture that can be restored by reprogramming occurs in 12% of patients and constitutes an important cause of CRT interruption[4] (**Fig. 1**).

Data from CRT counters, although useful, could be misleading because counters may overestimate the percentage of BiV pacing. Ineffective sensing and pacing cannot be detected directly from counter data.

During motorization, special attention should be paid to detect the presence of arrhythmias, such as atrial fibrillation (AF) or premature ventricular beats (PVCs), which as discussed later could reduce the percentage of BiV pacing.

TWELVE-LEAD SURFACE ELECTROCARDIOGRAM

The 12-lead surface electrocardiogram (ECG) plays an important role in the FU for CRT patients. Although representing only a snapshot in time, the ECG may provide useful information to complement the device evaluation (**Box 1**, **Fig. 2**).

Loss of LV capture is a recognized complication of CRT implantation. Changes in QRS width and morphology and axis observed on ECG recorded can be confirmed by device threshold testing. Several ECG algorithms, with sensitivity and specificity of 95% for the identification of loss of LV capture, have focused on the QRS polarity in lead V1 and the presence of a q/Q wave in lead I.[3]

EXERCISE TEST

The exercise test can be used to quantify the functional capacity of CRT patients and may be useful to detect intermittent sensing or pacing problems or rhythm changes that interrupt CRT, such as, (a) sinus tachycardia above upper tracking limit; (b) shortening of the intrinsic atrioventricular (AV) interval during exercise; (c) rapid and noncontrolled intrinsic ventricular rate in AF (above sensor rate); or (d) loss of ventricular tracking due to P-wave sensing in the postventricular atrial refractory period.[5]

ECHOCARDIOGRAM AFTER THE IMPLANT

An echocardiogram at 3 or 6 months after CRT implant should be carried out to assess for the

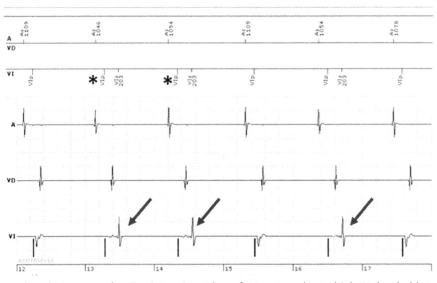

Fig. 1. Intracardiac electrograms showing intermittent loss of LV capture due to high LV threshold. A, atrial electrogram; VD, RV electrogram; VI, LV electrogram; red arrow, loss of LV capture; asterisks, channel marker. Loss of LV capture is classified as LV pacing by the device.

presence of LV reverse remodeling and improvement in left ventricular ejection fraction (LVEF). In patients with poor response to CRT, the different AV and VV intervals may be optimized by echocardiography.

IMPORTANCE OF EFFECTIVE BIVENTRICULAR PACING IN CARDIAC RESYNCHRONIZATION THERAPY

Sustained and effective BiV pacing is necessary to achieve response to CRT. Koplan and colleagues[6] demonstrated a 44% reduction in the composite end point of mortality and HF hospitalization in patients receiving ≥93% of BiV pacing, compared with those receiving 92% or less. These results were supported by data obtained from a large cohort of CRT patients, which described the greatest reduction in mortality when the percentage of BiV pacing achieved 98% or more.[7] However, in the "real world," 40% of the patients treated with CRT exhibited less than 98% of ventricular pacing.[8] Therefore, optimal device programming should aim to reach 100% of ventricular pacing in order to provide the most benefit.

Different causes for lost ventricular pacing are summarized in **Table 1**. When loss of CRT pacing is seen, it often occurs as a result of intrinsic ventricular activation superseding BiV resynchronization. The main causes for lost ventricular pacing in patients treated with CRT are due to programming of an inappropriately long AV interval delay (34%), atrial tachycardia, mainly AF (31%), or frequent PVCs.[8,9]

Long atrioventricular Interval

Most of the patients who receive CRT have preserved intrinsic AV nodal conduction. AV delay programming in CRT devices is usually performed at rest and may therefore overestimate the optimal interval for pacing during exercise or sympathetic activation. When the intrinsic AV conduction is faster than the programmed sensed or paced AV intervals, CRT is inhibited. CRT loss because of inappropriately programmed sensed and paced atrioventricular intervals (SAV/PAV) can be readily resolved by modifying the programmed SAV/PAV

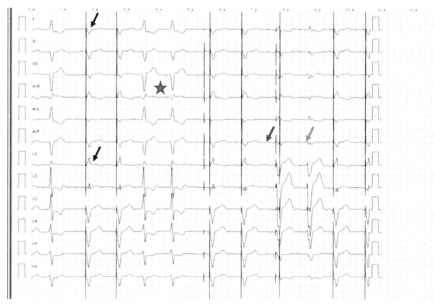

Fig. 2. Twelve-lead surface ECG showing different causes of loss of BiV pacing: star, inhibition of CRT pacing due to PVCs; red arrow, atrial undersensing; green arrow, CRT inhibition of CRT pacing due to atrial undersensing; blue arrow, BiV paced QRS (Q wave in lead I and R wave in lead V1).

Table 1
Causes of loss of cardiac resynchronization therapy pacing

Device programming	Suboptimal AV timing
	High LV threshold
	Low upper tracking rate
	Atrial undersensing.
	RV oversensing
	LV oversensing
Arrhythmia	AF
	Atrial flutter
	Frequent PVCs
	Junctional rhythm

intervals. If intrinsic AV conduction is present and causes pseudofusion, the AV delay should be shortened (**Fig. 3**).

Atrial Fibrillation

One-fifth of patients who receive CRT in Europe are in AF.[10] Furthermore, the incidence of paroxysmal and persistent AF in patients treated with CRT may reach 20% to 42%.[11,12]

Patients in AF have fast and irregular ventricular rates, which may interfere with complete BiV pacing delivery. Moreover, the percentage of BiV pacing alone as recorded by the CRT device may be an ineffective surrogate of complete and consistent BiV capture. Fusion and pseudofusion beats resulting from an interaction between intrinsically conducted and paced beats may be responsible for ineffective pacing, despite apparent delivery of CRT as assessed by a high percentage of BiV pacing.[10]

In patients with AF, a great effort should be made to reach 100% of ventricular pacing. There are several options to manage AF in patients treated with CRT, from reestablishing normal sinus rhythm either with antiarrhythmic drugs or with AF catheter ablation to atrioventricular junctional (AVJ) ablation in cases of permanent and refractory AF.

Despite the complex risk profile of this cohort, studies have shown that complication rates in patients with HF undergoing AF ablation are not different from patients with a structurally normal heart.[13] Recently, the multicenter randomized study AATAC showed that AF catheter ablation was superior to medical treatment in achieving freedom from AF at long-term FU. Moreover, in comparison with medical treatment, catheter AF ablation reduced unplanned hospitalization and mortality in patients with HF and persistent AF.[14,15]

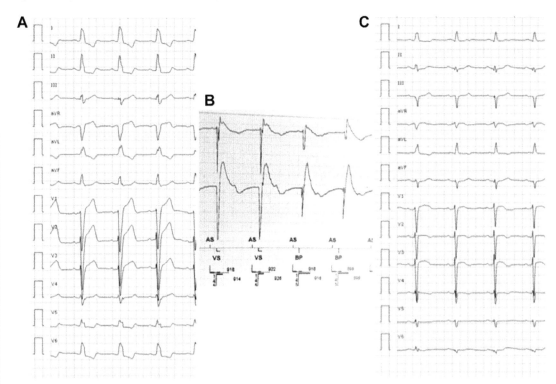

Fig. 3. CRT inhibition due to long AV interval programming: (*A*) 12-lead surface ECG showing inhibition of CRT pacing; (*B*) intracardiac electrograms. *, RV ECM; ¶, far field shock electrogram; channel marker: BP, BiV pacing. (*C*) 12-lead surface ECG after AV interval optimization.

AVJ ablation should be considered in all CRT patients when AF engenders a fast ventricular rate despite adequate doses of AV nodal-negative chronotropic drugs, when such drugs are not tolerated, or when antiarrhythmic medications are ineffective or contraindicated.[16,17]

Remote monitoring of CRT devices with regular transmissions of data, such as atrial/ventricular arrhythmia burden, percentage of BiV pacing, or heart rate histograms, allows for a faster detection of problems that could reduce the response to CRT.

Premature Ventricular Complexes

The rate of PVCs is another factor that frequently reduces the percentage of BiV pacing. Data from the MADIT-CRT study showed that even low frequencies of PVCs reduce the percentage of BiV pacing, resulting in less reverse remodeling and increased risk of HF, ventricular tachyarrhythmias, and death.[18] At 3 years FU, a burden of greater than 10 PVCs per hour has been associated with a high risk of HF, mortality, ventricular tachycardia (VT), and ventricular fibrillation as compared with patients with low VPC burden.[19] Radiofrequency catheter ablation of VT or frequent PVCs should be offered to such patients that fail medical therapy.[20,21]

CRT loss from atrial undersensing, ventricular oversensing, or nontracking pacing modes can be resolved by appropriate device programming or lead revisions. Regarding the upper rate limit, it is reasonable to consider programming a rate that is 80% of the maximal age predicted heart rate. Programming a low upper tracking rate in a patient with intrinsic conduction may lead to a high risk of symptomatic loss of BiV capture during exercise.[8]

RATE RESPONSE VENTRICULAR PACING

Chronotropic incompetence is a common finding in patients with advanced chronic HF.[22]

Some studies have shown that in patients who failed to achieve 70% of the predicted maximal heart rate (220 − patient's age) on a treadmill test, programming a DDDR mode at 50 to 140 bpm resulted in increased exercise time, metabolic equivalents, and Vo_{2max} compared with the DDD mode.[23,24]

OPTIMIZATION OF CARDIAC RESYNCHRONIZATION THERAPY PROGRAMMING AFTER THE IMPLANT AND DURING FOLLOW-UP

Nowadays, postimplant optimization of the device remains a clinical challenge. Postimplant device optimization includes individualized programming of the AV and interventricular (VV) timings and other additional variables, such as the AV delay offset of atrial-sensed (AS) versus atrial-paced (AP) events. Altogether, this increases the complexity of CRT programming.

There is a lack of consensus regarding CRT optimization. The European Society of Cardiology guidelines have not recommended it as part of routine clinical care.[1] However, the suboptimal programming of the AV or VV timings may limit the response to CRT.[9] For this reason, evaluation and optimization of AV and VV delay are often recommended to correct suboptimal device settings.

The value of trying to optimize AV or VV intervals after implantation using echocardiographic or electrocardiographic criteria or blood pressure response is uncertain but may be considered for patients who have had a disappointing response to CRT.

Echocardiography Optimization

Echocardiography has traditionally been considered the gold standard for CRT optimization.[25] A recent meta-analysis of 13 controlled studies found a small but significant improvement in LVEF when CRT was optimized by echocardiogram in patients with HF.[26]

The most common echocardiographic optimization technique for AV delay is assessing mitral inflow, which can be done through application of the Ritter method, the iterative method, or the aortic velocity time integral. VV optimization is typically assessed through echocardiography by measuring the septal-posterior wall motion delay or tissue Doppler imaging.[27] Optimizing VV delay can also be facilitated by other techniques, like speckle-tracking echocardiography or real-time 3-dimensional echocardiography.[28]

However, the aforementioned methods are complex, require expertise, and are time consuming. Because of its limited feasibility and large interobserver and intraobserver variability, only a minority of clinicians perform echocardiography CRT optimization in routine clinical practice. As a result, at CRT implant, nearly 58% of the investigators do not optimize the device, and nominal programming is chosen as the first option, leaving CRT optimization of nonresponders at FU visits or during hospital admissions.[29,30]

The development of a less time-consuming and easier optimization method might enable a more systematic optimization of the AV and VV delays at routine FU visits in all recipients of CRT systems.

Automatic Algorithms of Cardiac Resynchronization Therapy Programming

Ideally, the device should be able to evaluate the optimal setting automatically. Therefore, in an attempt to simplify CRT optimization, the CRT manufacturing companies have developed several intracardiac automated electrogram-based algorithms with conflicting results. The QuickOpt algorithm (St. Jude Medical) failed to demonstrate clear benefit compared with usual clinical practice.[31] The SmartDelay algorithm was developed to optimize the AV delay by the Boston Scientific CRT system. When compared with a fixed nominal AV delay or echocardiography optimized AV delay, The SmartDelay algorithm failed to show a significant benefit as well.[32] The Adapted CRT developed by Medtronic provides dynamic optimization of both the AV and the VV timings. The algorithm uses intrinsic intervals to provide RV-synchronized LV pacing when AV conduction is normal or BiV pacing otherwise. Adapted CRT was found to be as effective as BiV pacing with echocardiographic optimization in clinical composite scores. Patient outcomes improved when synchronized LV pacing was $\geq$50%.[33,34] SonR developed by SORIN optimizes the AV and VV intervals guided by a contractility sensor guide placed in the atrial lead. The RESPOND-CRT trial[35] described better clinical response and outcomes in patients randomized to automatic CRT optimization by sonR compared with echocardiogram-guided optimization.

Electrocardiogram-QRS–Based Optimization

Paced QRS shortening has been linked to clinical response and echocardiographic improvement.[36,37] Therefore, shortening the paced QRS duration could be a simple and widely applicable optimization method.

Previous studies have shown that optimization of the VV guided by QRS width has a good correlation with echocardiographic optimization.[38] Furthermore, when comparing echocardiographic and electrocardiographic optimization, the best acute hemodynamic improvements and greater LV reverse remodeling were obtained by selecting the VV value yielding the narrowest QRS measured from the earliest deflection and not from the stimulus artifact.[39,40]

On the other hand, there are some data demonstrating that patients showing fusion between BiV pacing with intrinsic conduction may obtain more benefit from CRT, probably by shortening the LV activation time.[41]

The authors recently described a simple and easily performed method of QRS-based optimization called fusion optimized intervals (FOI).[42] FOI uses fusion with intrinsic conduction to achieve the shortest pacing QRS. The idea behind fusion-guided BiV pacing with the intrinsic rhythm is to allow partial or complete intrinsic depolarization of the VV septum (fusion pacing), which creates 3 activation fronts instead of 2 during pure BiV pacing.

The FOI method was as follows: To find the "fusion band," during AS, the AV interval was progressively shortened with LV pacing only, starting with the longest AV interval that allowed LV capture, and followed by 20-millisecond decrements until the AV interval produced only LV capture. The AV interval that provided the narrowest QRS was selected and considered as the fusion optimized AV interval. This procedure was repeated during AP at 10 bpm above the intrinsic sinus rhythm. Once the AV interval during AS and AP was selected, the VV interval was adjusted during AS, comparing QRS duration in different configurations: simultaneous RV and LV pacing (VV: 0 milliseconds), LV preexcitation of 30 milliseconds (LV: 30 milliseconds), and RV preexcitation of 30 milliseconds (RV: 30 milliseconds). These VV intervals were chosen because in previous studies most patients had the best VV value within this range.[30] The VV value that obtained the narrowest QRS was considered the optimal VV interval (**Figs. 4** and **5**).

In comparison with nominal settings, patients optimized by FOI had a narrower paced QRS, a better LV dP/dt$_{max}$, and a better correction of the different parameters of intraventricular LV asynchrony.[41] Long-term benefits of optimizing by FOI were demonstrated in a randomized study by Trucco and colleagues.[43] The investigators compared the percentage of clinical and echocardiographic LV responders to CRT optimizing by FOI versus nominal settings. At 12 months, there were no differences in the percentage of clinical responders. However, significant LV reverse remodeling was achieved in a larger proportion of the FOI group (74% vs 53%, respectively [odds ratio: 2.02 (95% confidence interval: 1.08–3.76)]; $P = .026$). There was a correlation ($r = 0.23$; $P = .01$) between response and the degree of QRS narrowing; patients with the most QRS narrowing experienced the greatest benefit, as measured by echocardiographic remodeling. In addition, after 12 months of CRT, fewer patients in the FOI group were classified as negative responders to the therapy (11% vs 24% in the nominal settings group; $P = .041$).

Therefore, FOI is a simple method for CRT optimization that may be recommended for patients in sinus rhythm with left bundle branch block and normal AV nodal conduction.

FOI method is not applicable for patients with AV block, AF, or prolonged AV interval, because the intrinsic conduction cannot be included in the

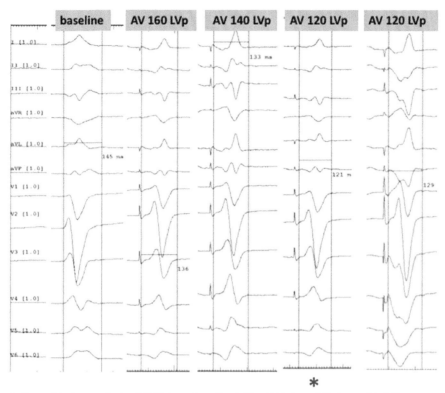

Fig. 4. Description of fusion-optimized AV interval method. The AV interval that provided the narrowest QRS is selected and considered as the fusion-optimized AV interval. The 12 leads of the surface ECG are recorded simultaneously and displayed in vertical alignment on the screen.

equation. Perhaps ECG-based optimization adjusting the VV interval may be useful in this subgroup of patients in order to obtain the narrowest paced QRS.[36,37]

LEFT VENTRICULAR MULTISITE PACING

The concept of MultiPoint pacing (MPP) arose from the fact that the LV activation pattern is heterogeneous among patients with conduction block. Pacing from 2 different sites from the LV allows for a faster and more homogeneous LV activation. Recently, the advent of a quadripolar LV lead has led to MPP.

Compared with standard BiV pacing, MPP resulted in an additional reduction in QRS duration, a decrease in total endocardial activation time, and an increase in LV dp/dt$_{max}$.[44] Pappone and colleagues[45] showed in a select cohort of patients that pressure volume loop-guided multipoint LV pacing resulted in greater LV reverse remodeling and increased LV function at 12 months compared with pressure volume loop-guided conventional CRT.

The MultiPoint Pacing (MPP) trial was planned to assess the safety and efficacy of pacing 2 LV

sites with a quadripolar lead in patients treated with CRT.[46] There were no differences in system-related complications between the standard BiV arm and the MPP arm. If the MPP arm was programmed with maximal anatomic separation (distance between the 2 cathodal LV electrodes ≥30 mm) and the shortest intraventricular timing delay of 5 ms, patients had a significantly higher response rate to CRT than the conventional group (87% vs 65%, $P = .003$).

The MORE-CRT MPP (MOre REsponse on Cardiac Resynchronization Therapy with MultiPoint Pacing; NCT02006069) is a prospective, randomized, double-blind, international multicenter study, enrolling 1250 patients with a standard CRT indication to assess the impact of the MPP feature at 12 months in the treatment of patients not responding to standard CRT after 6 months. Results of this trial may explain if MPP might be a solution for CRT nonresponse.

MEDICAL OPTIMIZATION

The European Society of Cardiology and the American Heart Association recommend drug

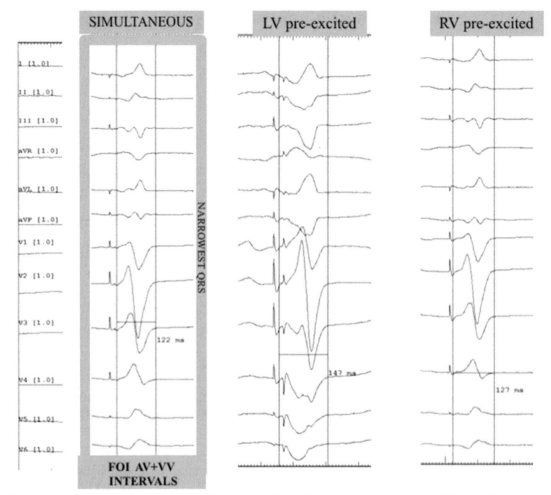

Fig. 5. Description of fusion-optimized VV interval method. Once the fusion-optimized AV interval is selected, the optimal VV interval is adjusted during AS. The optimal VV interval is then chosen by comparing the QRS duration in LV preexcited, simultaneous BiV or RV preexcited configuration.

optimization before and after implantation of a CRT device.[1]

Patients treated with CRT should continue optimal medical therapy and undergo appropriate uptitration of medications to the maximal tolerable dosage. However, up to 24% of CRT patients do not take one of their guideline-directed HF medications, thereby worsening the response and outcomes in these patients.[9]

In mild HF patients treated with CRT, the continuation of angiotensin-converting enzyme inhibitor or angiotensin receptor blocker and the discontinuation of diuretics result in improvements in LV reverse remodeling.[47]

SUMMARY

Nonresponse to CRT therapy is still a major issue. A better understanding of device programming during FU, together with a multidisciplinary

approach and an optimal FU of the patients, may reduce the percentage of nonresponders.

REFERENCES

1. Brignole M, Auricchio A, Baron-Esquivias G, et al, ESC Committee for Practice Guidelines (CPG). 2013 ESC Guidelines on cardiac pacing and cardiac resynchronization therapy: the Task Force on cardiac pacing and resynchronization therapy of the European Society of Cardiology (ESC). Developed in collaboration with the European Heart Rhythm Association (EHRA). Eur Heart J 2013;34(29):2281–329.
2. YU CM, Hayes DL. Cardiac resynchronization therapy. Eur Heart J 2013;34(19):1396–403.
3. Daubert JC, Saxon L, Adamson PB, et al. 2012 EHRA/HRS expert consensus statement on cardiac resynchronization therapy in heart failure: implant and follow-up recommendations and management. Europace 2012;14(9):1236–86.

4. Knight BP, Desai A, Coman J, et al. Long-term retention of cardiac resynchronization therapy. J Am Coll Cardiol 2004;44:72–7.

5. Barold SS, Ilercil A, Leonelli F, et al. First-degree atrioventricular block. Clinical manifestations, indications for pacing, pacemaker management & consequences during cardiac resynchronization. J Interv Card Electrophysiol 2006;17:139–52.

6. Koplan BA, Kaplan AJ, Weiner S, et al. Heart failure decompensation and all-cause mortality in relation to percent biventricuar pacing in patient with heart failure: is a goal of 100% biventricular pacing necessary? J Am Coll Cardiol 2009;53:355–60.

7. Hayes DL, Boehmer J, Day J. Cardiac resynchronization therapy and relationship of percent biventricular pacing. Heart Rhythm 2011;8(9):1469–75.

8. Cheng A, Landman SR, Stadler RW, et al. Reasons for loss of cardiac resynchronization therapy pacing: insights from 32 844 patients. Circ Arrhythm Electrophysiol 2012;5:884.

9. Mullens W, Grimm RA, Verga T, et al. Insights from a cardiac resynchronization optimization clinic as part of a heart failure disease management program. J Am Coll Cardiol 2009;53:765–73.

10. Kamath G, Cotiga D, Koneruja Y, et al. The utility of 12 lead holter monitoring in patients with permanent atrial fibrillation for the identification of non-responders after cardiac resynchronization therapy. J Am Coll Cardiol 2009;53(12):1050–5.

11. Leclercq C, Padeletti L, Cihák R, et al, CHAMP Study Investigators. Incidence of paroxysmal atrial tachycardias in patients treated with cardiac resynchronization therapy and continuously monitored by device diagnostics. Europace 2010;12: 71–7.

12. Puglisi A, Gasparini M, Lunati M, et al, on behalf of InSync III Italian Registry Investigators. Persistent atrial fibrillation worsens heart rate variability, activity and heart rate, as shown by a continuous monitoring by implantable biventricular pacemakers in heart failure patients. J Cardiovasc Electrophysiol 2008; 19:693–701.

13. Cappato R, Calkins H, Chen SA, et al. Updated worldwide survey on the methods, efficacy, and safety of catheter ablation for human atrial fibrillation. Circ Arrhythm Electrophysiol 2009;3(1):32–8.

14. Di Biase L, Mohanty P, Mohanty S, et al. Ablation vs. Amiodarone for treatment of persistent atrial fibrillation in patients with congestive heart failure and implanted device: results from the AATAC multicenter randomized trial. Circulartion 2016;133(17): 1637–44.

15. Marrouche NF, Brachmann J, Andresen D, et al. Catheter ablation for atrial fibrillation with heart failure. N Engl J Med 2018;378(5):417–27.

16. Gasparini M, Leclercq C, Lunati M, et al. Cardiac resynchronization therapy in patients with atrial fibrillation: the CERTIFY study (Cardiac Resynchronization Therapy in Atrial Fibrillation Patients Multinational Registry). JACC Heart Fail 2013;1(6): 500–7.

17. Tolosana JM, Trucco E, Khatib M, et al. Complete atrioventricular block doe nor reduce long term mortality in patietns with permanent atrial fibrillation treated with CRT. Eur J Heart Fail 2013;15(12): 1412–8.

18. Ruwald MH, Mittal S, Ruwald AC, et al. Association between frequency of atrial and ventricular ectopic beats and biventricular pacing percentage and outcomes in patients with cardiac resynchronization therapy. J Am Coll Cardiol 2014; 64(10):971.

19. Ruwald AC, Aktas MK, Ruwald MH, et al. Postimplantation ventricular ectopic burden and clinical outcomes in cardiac resynchronization therapy-defibrillator patients: a MADIT-CRT substudy. Ann Noninvasive Electrocardiol 2018;23(2): e12491.

20. Yamada T, Tabereaux PB, McElderry HT, et al. Successful catheter ablation of epicardial ventricular tachycardia worsened by cardiac resynchronization therapy. Europace 2010;12(3):437–40.

21. Herczku C, Kun C, Edes I, et al. Radiofrequency catheter ablation of premature ventricular complexes improved left ventricular function in a nonresponder to cardiac resynchronization therapy. Europace 2007;9(5):285–8.

22. Witte KK, Cleland JG, Clark AL. Chronic heart failure, chronotropic incompetence, and the effects of beta blockade. Heart 2006;92:481–6.

23. Sims DB, Mignatti A, Colombo PC, et al. Rate responsive pacing using cardiac resynchronization therapy in patients with chronotropic incompetence and chronic heart failure. Europace 2011;13: 1459–63.

24. Tse HF, Siu CW, Lee KL, et al. The incremental benefit of rate-adaptive pacing on exercise performance during cardiac resynchronization therapy. J Am Coll Cardiol 2005;46:2292–7.

25. Cazeau S, Gras D, Lazarus A, et al. Multisite stimulation for correction of cardiac asynchrony. Heart 2000;84:579–81.

26. Kosmala W, Marwick TH. Meta-analysis of effects of optimization of cardiac resynchronization therapy on left ventricular function, exercise capacity, and quality of life in patients with heart failure. Am J Cardiol 2014;113:988–94.

27. Brabham William W, Gold MR. The role of AV and VV optimization for CRT. J Arrhythm 2013;29(3): 153–61.

28. Bertini M, Delgado V, Bax JJ, et al. Why, how and when do we need to optimize the setting of cardiac resynchronization therapy? Europace 2009; 11(Suppl 5):v46–57.

29. Lunati M, Magenta G, Cattafi G, et al. Clinical relevance of systematic CRT device optimization. J Atr Fibrillation 2014;31(7):1077.

30. Gras D, Gupta MS, Boulogne E, et al. Optimization of AV and VV delays in the real-world CRT patient population: an international survey on current clinical practice. Pacing Clin Electrophysiol 2009; 32(Suppl 1):S236–9.

31. Abraham WT, Gras D, Yu CM, et al, FREEDOM Steering Committee. Rationale and design of a randomized clinical trial to assess the safety and efficacy of frequent optimization of cardiac resynchronization therapy: the Frequent Optimization Study Using the QuickOpt Method (FREEDOM) trial. Am Heart J 2010;159:944–8.e1.

32. Stein KM, Ellenbogen KA, Gold MR, et al. SmartDelay determined AV optimization: a comparison of AV delay methods used in cardiac resynchronization therapy (SMART-AV): rationale and design. Pacing Clin Electrophysiol 2010;33:54–63.

33. Singh JP, Abraham WT, Chung ES, et al. Clinical response with adaptive CRT algorithm compared with CRT with echocardiography-optimized atrioventricular delay: a retrospective analysis of multicentre trials. Europace 2013;15:1622–8.

34. Birnie D, Lemke B, Aonuma K, et al. Clinical outcomes with synchronized left ventricular pacing: analysis of the adaptive CRT trial. Heart Rhythm 2013;10:1368–74.

35. Brugada J, Delnoy PP, Brachmann J, et al, RESPOND CRT Investigators. Contractility sensor-guided optimization of cardiac resynchronization therapy: results from the RESPOND-CRT trial. Eur Heart J 2017;38:730–8.

36. LecoQ G, Lecler C, Leray E, et al. Clinical and electrocardiographic predictors of a positive response to cardiac resynchronization therapy in advanced heart failure. Eur Heart J 2005;26:1094–100.

37. Hsin JM, Selzman KA, Leclercq C, et al. Paced left ventricular QRS width and ECG parameters predict outcomes after cardiac resynchronization therapy: PROSPECT-ECG sub-study. Circ Arrhythm Electrophysiol 2011;4:851–7.

38. Vidal B, Tamborero D, Mont L, et al. Electrocardiographic optimization of interventricular delay in cardiac resynchronization therapy: a simple method to optimize the device. J Cardiovasc Electrophysiol 2007;18:1252–7.

39. Tamborero D, Mont L, Sitges M, et al. Optimization of the interventricular delay in cardiac resynchronization therapy using the QRS width. Am J Cardiol 2009;104:1407–12.

40. Tamborero D, Vidal B, Tolosana JM, et al. Electrocardiographic versus echocardiographic optimization of the interventricular pacing delay inpatien undergoing cardiac resynchronization therapy. J Cardiovasc Electrophysiol 2011;22:1129–34.

41. Vatasescu R, Berruezo A, Mont L, et al. Midterm "super-response" to cardiac resynchronization therapy by biventricular pacing with fusion: insights from electro-anatomical mapping. Europace 2009;11: 1675–82.

42. Arbelo E, Tolosana JM, Trucco E, et al. Fusion-optimized intervals (FOI): a new method to achieve the narrowest QRS for optimization of the AV and VV intervals in patients undergoing cardiac resynchronization therapy. J Cardiovasc Electrophysiol 2014; 25:283–92.

43. Trucco E, Tolosana JM, Arbelo E, et al. Improvement of reverse remodeling using electrocardiogram fusion-optimized intervals in cardiac resynchronization therapy: a randomized study. JACC Clin Electrophysiol 2018;4(2):181–9.

44. Menardi E, Ballari GP, Goletto C, et al. Characterization of ventricular activation pattern and acute hemodynamics during multipoint left ventricular pacing. Heart Rhythm 2015;12:1762–9.

45. Pappone C, Ćalović Ž, Vicedomini G, et al. Improving cardiac resynchronization therapy response with multipoint left ventricular pacing: twelve-month follow-up study. Heart Rhythm 2015; 12:1250–8.

46. Niazi I, Baker J 2nd, Corbisiero R, et al. Safety and efficacy of multipoint pacing in cardiacresynchronization therapy: the MultiPoint Pacing Trial. JACC Clin Electrophysiol 2017;3(13):1510–8.

47. Penn J, Goldenberg I, McNitt S, et al. Changes in drug utilization and outcome with cardiac resynchronization therapy: a MADIT-CRT Substudy. J Card Fail 2015;21(7):541.

Benefits of Multisite/Multipoint Pacing to Improve Cardiac Resynchronization Therapy Response

Bernard Thibault, MD*, Blandine Mondésert, MD,
Julia Cadrin-Tourigny, MD, Marc Dubuc, MD,
Laurent Macle, MD, Paul Khairy, MD, PhD

KEYWORDS

• Cardiac resynchronization therapy • Biventricular pacing • Multisite pacing • Multipoint pacing

KEY POINTS

- Nonresponse to therapy remains a major concern for heart failure treatment with biventricular implanted devices.
- Small-scale clinical studies showed some potential benefits from multisite pacing and multipoint pacing to overcome this serious and unfortunate limitation. However, the more recent and larger multicenter randomized trials have failed to confirm these promises.
- Multipoint pacing offers some advantages over multisite pacing in terms of ease of device programming and device-related adverse events.
- Multipoint pacing programmed with the largest left ventricular pacing vector and simultaneously (MPP-AS) may present some benefits. The phase II of the MORE-CRT-MPP trial will attempt to assess if MPP-AS can succeed in converting nonresponders into responders.

Cardiac resynchronization therapy (CRT) has undeniably been one of the major advances of the 21st century in the treatment of heart failure (HF). It has shown benefits above and beyond optimal medical management in terms of providing patients with HF with improvements in symptoms, quality of life, and exercise capacity, along with a decrease in hospitalizations for HF and better survival.[1–3] However, consistent across studies, including the most recent clinical trials, a substantial proportion of patients ($\leq$40%) do not derive the desired benefits from this therapy and are deemed nonresponders or suboptimal responders (Leclercq C, Burri H, Curnis A, et al. CRT nonresponders to responder conversion rate in the more response to CRT with MultiPoint pacing (MORE-CRT-MPP) study: results from phase I. Eur Heart J, submitted).[4] Multiple strategies have been described to maximize the response to therapy with the objective of

Disclosure statement: B. Thibault received research support and honoraria for presentation from Abbott and Medtronic. B. Mondésert received support and honoraria for presentations from Abbott, Boston Scientific and Medtronic. J. Cadrin-Tourigny has no disclosures. M. Dubuc received support and honoraria for presentations from Medtronic. L. Macle received support and honoraria for presentations from Abbott and Medtronic. P. Khairy has no disclosures.
Department of Cardiology, Montréal Heart Institute, University of Montréal, 5000 Bélanger Street, Montréal, Québec, H1T 1C8, Canada
* Corresponding author. 5000 Belanger Street, Montreal, Quebec H1T 1C8, Canada.
E-mail address: bernard.thibault@umontreal.ca

Card Electrophysiol Clin 11 (2019) 99–114
https://doi.org/10.1016/j.ccep.2018.11.016

improving patient well-being and prognosis,[5,6] including approaches that focus on optimizing the left ventricular (LV) lead. To deliver effective resynchronization, it is important for the LV lead to reach the "sweet spot" of latest activation, where myocardium is captured with an adequate pacing output while avoiding scar and phrenic nerve stimulation, both acutely and over the long term. Within this context, the quadripolar LV leads represent the latest advancement. They are widely accessible (as opposed to endocardial LV pacing, for example) with proven advantages over bipolar LV leads, including improved survival.[7] These benefits essentially reflect greater flexibility resulting from the additional possible pacing configurations that can be critical in overcoming issues during follow-up, without the need for reintervention or, worse, abandoning resynchronization therapy.[8–11]

The purposes of this article are to provide a general overview of the underlying mechanisms that support pacing from more discrete points and/or a wider vector to improve LV resynchronization, to provide a critical overview of the current literature, and to identify remaining knowledge gaps to spur further research. It is not our goal to provide a systematic review with a comprehensive bibliography, but rather to focus on selected publications that, in our opinion, have either expertly reviewed a specific aspect of CRT or have been landmark studies in the field.

MULTISITE PACING AND MULTIPOINT PACING: SOME DEFINITIONS

The expression "multisite pacing" (MSP) generally refers to biventricular (BiV) pacing from 3 ventricular leads[12]: either with 2 right ventricular (RV) + 1 LV lead[13] or 2 LV+ 1 RV lead.[14] Strictly speaking, because the normal human heart has only 2 ventricles, the "triventricular" expression seems to be misleading, such that we prefer the "trifocal" designation. In patients with complex congenital heart disease, the term MSP has also been used to refer to resynchronization of a single ventricle by means of 2 ventricular leads.

In contrast, multipoint pacing (MPP) refers to pacing from more than one pole of a multipolar LV lead.[15] Physiologically, this also results in "multifocal" or "trifocal" stimulation, albeit from only 2 leads. A few authors have reported that it is possible to achieve some form of MPP with anodal capture, either from a bipolar RV lead,[16] from a bipolar LV lead,[17] or a quadripolar LV lead,[18–20] with the latter option providing more potential points for MPP.

RESYNCHRONIZATION WITH MULTISITE PACING AND MULTIPOINT PACING

The ultimate goals of resynchronization therapy are to improve the clinical condition of patients and to keep them alive and out of hospital. Indications for CRT were integrated into management guidelines after large, randomized trials demonstrated and confirmed such benefits. A few thousand patients enrolled in MADIT-CRT[21] and RAFT[22] trials were required to demonstrate efficacy. It is unlikely that any trial with the end point of mortality and/or HF hospitalizations will be performed in the near future comparing MSP/MPP with BiV pacing. This is considering the large sample size that would be required to detect the smaller projected incremental benefits. Consequently, the best evidence we currently have are from studies that rely on surrogate/mechanistic end points.

MULTISITE PACING AND MULTIPOINT PACING TO CORRECT ELECTRICAL ASYNCHRONY

CRT works mainly in patients with electrical LV dyssynchrony, as expressed by a left bundle branch block with a prolonged QRS duration. CRT provides better results when it shortens QRS duration, but this is not an absolute prerequisite.[23,24]

Comparing MSP/MPP with BiV, animal models (**Table 1**) showed that pacing the LV from a greater number of electrodes resulted in a faster LV activation time and shorter QRS duration.[25–28]

In clinical studies, MSP and MPP were inconsistently reported to further reduce LV activation time and/or QRS duration (by 0–20 ms) compared with standard BiV pacing.[13,16,29–36] In theory, it is biologically plausible that recruiting myocardium from more sites and/or a wider pacing vector can shorten LV electrical activation, but this may be impeded by slow cell-to-cell activation from the epicardium and areas of slow conduction, functional block, or scar.[31]

Recently, Engels and colleagues[37] suggested that the mechanisms involved in the response to MPP-CRT extend beyond a reduction in QRS duration. They introduced the concept that a more "LV-dominant" activation sequence, as reflected by QRS area and/or maximal QRS vector, can play an important role.

The narrowest QRS obtained with the best MPP configuration remains approximately 135 to 140 ms on average.[31,35,36] Narrower QRS durations (123 ± 12 ms) were recently reported with an algorithm that optimizes the atrioventricular delay by aiming to fuse BiV pacing with intrinsic

Table 1
Computer and animal models

First Author, Year	Model	Comparison	Main Finding(s)
Niederer et al,[69] 2012	Electroanatomical biophysical model	BiV-MPP vs BiV	BiV-MPP improves LV dP/dt$_{max}$ in the presence of posterolateral scar
Bordachar et al,[25] 2012	Canine model with ischemic HF + LBBB	LV epi vs LV endo vs BiV epi vs BiV endo vs trifocal	BiV endo provides best results overall. Trifocal is not superior to BiV epi, may even be worse than "best/optimized BiV"
Ploux et al,[26] 2014	Canine model with LBBB	Single LV vs Multiple epi LV (up to 7 sites)	Multi-LV provides shorter LV total activation time and dispersion of repolarization. LV dP/dt$_{max}$ improved only when single LV provides suboptimal response
Qiu et al,[27] 2017	Canine model with HF	BiV vs MSP (4 epi sites)	MSP provides shorter QRS, better synchrony, and higher LV dP/dt$_{max}$. MSP is better than BiV in 60% of instances. Best MSP is different between animals
Huntjens et al,[28] 2018 + editorial by Waks et al,[70] 2018	Computer simulation (CircAdapt)	LV dP/dt$_{max}$	In scar-free LBBB condition, interventricular asynchrony is the predominant component driving response to (BiV) CRT. This suggests futility of MSP/MPP in this condition

Abbreviations: BiV, biventricular; endo, endocardial (pacing); dP/dt$_{max}$, maximal rate of rise of left ventricular pressure; epi, epicardial (pacing); HF, heart failure; LBBB, left bundle branch block; LV, left ventricle (left ventricular); MPP, multipoint pacing; MSP, multisite pacing; trifocal, instead of triventricular.

conduction over the His-Purkinje system.[38] This was achieved with standard BiV pacing and would itself qualify as another form of MSP/MPP. This algorithm remains to be tested on the long term and with MPP from a quadripolar LV lead to determine its impact on decreasing the QRS duration.

MULTISITE PACING AND MULTIPOINT PACING TO CORRECT MECHANICAL DYSSYNCHRONY AND IMPROVE LEFT VENTRICULAR EJECTION FRACTION

It is presumed that electrical dyssynchrony (left bundle branch block + prolonged QRS) gives rise to mechanical dyssynchrony. There are (at least) 3 components to electrically induced mechanical dyssynchrony.

1. Prolonged atrioventricular delay on the left side with prolonged PR intervals (>200–230 ms)[39] and/or left bundle branch block with prolonged QRS duration[40] results in suboptimal LV diastolic function, LV filling timings, and patterns. This sequence in turns contributes to depressed LV systolic function.[41] Even in the presence of a normal QRS duration, first-degree atrioventricular block may lead to deleterious effects, with the potential for presystolic mitral regurgitation.[39]

2. Left bundle branch block is associated with interventricular (RV–LV) dyssynchrony, also leading to abnormal filling timings and patterns, as well as a decreased LV systolic function. This finding appeals to the concepts of interdependence between the 2 ventricles that share the same pericardial space[42] and ventricular septal contraction abnormalities.[40]

3. Left bundle branch block generates intraventricular dyssynchrony with significant dispersion in peak contraction of the different LV segments. This finding was observed time and again in both nonischemic and ischemic cardiomyopathy, recognizing that, in ischemic cardiomyopathy, areas of scar from prior myocardial infarction also play a role.[43] Interestingly, intra-LV mechanical dyssynchrony may even exist in the absence of QRS prolongation, suggesting that, at least in a subset of patients with HF, electromechanical coupling may be defective.[44]

It remains unclear which of these 3 mechanisms predominate(s) in any given patient. In the recent 15 to 20 years of research in the field, the focus was primarily on the intra-LV component. However, the importance of intraventricular dyssynchrony was recently challenged by negative studies such as PROSPECT[45] and ECHO-CRT.[46] The topic is complex, with intricate interactions likely to be at play between the 3 components.[28,47]

Considering these mechanisms, LV pacing from a wider vector (more sites/points) is expected to improve resynchronization mostly (only) at the third level, by recruiting more segments simultaneously. In theory, this could be most pronounced when LV pacing sites overcome areas of conduction block, either functional or owing to scar.[48]

MULTISITE PACING AND MULTIPOINT PACING TO IMPROVE LEFT VENTRICULAR CONTRACTILITY

Acute hemodynamic response is most often evaluated invasively and represents global effects of CRT on the failing LV. Although this measure seems sensible, the relationship between acute hemodynamic response at the time or shortly after implant and later response to CRT or prognosis is not well-established. In 2011 (before the era of MPP), Duckett and colleagues[49] nevertheless reported that acute hemodynamic response to LV pacing predicts LV remodeling on follow-up.

There are serious caveats to these metrics, be they maximal rate of rise of LV pressure (dP/dt_{max}) or pressure–volume loops. The measurements are difficult to perform reliably and subject to potential contamination from internal and external factors as we[50] and Niederer and colleagues[51] have previously described. This factor limits the number of pacing configurations that can be tested in a reasonable period of time, favoring repeated measurements, in random order, and after steady state is obtained.

Bearing these limitations in mind, most series have understandably included a limited number of patients. Nonetheless, MSP and MPP were generally associated with superior LV performance measures.[15,29–31,33,34,37,52–54] In contrast, a few studies have reported discordant results with no or limited benefits from MPP compared with BiV pacing.[17,32,35,48,55]

We had the privilege of reporting the first series of acute hemodynamic response with MPP.[15] Our findings seem to have forecasted what was to become the future of MPP in CRT. **Fig. 1** provides an overview of the different types of responses that we observed. These were categorized into

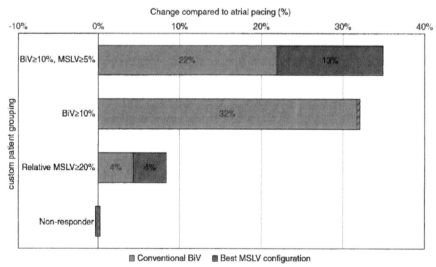

Fig. 1. The 4 types of acute hemodynamic response with biventricular pacing (BiV; *green*) and multipoint pacing (MPP; *red*), observed at the time of implant. One group of patients did well with BiV pacing and were improved further with MPP. One group of patients did very well with BiV and for whom MPP did not bring further benefits. One group of patients responded partially to BiV pacing and were somewhat helped by MPP, but did not reach the response threshold of 10% improvement in maximal rate of rise of LV pressure (dP/dt_{max}). A fourth group of patients did not improve at all with either BiV pacing or MPP. With a small number of patients (19 with analyzed data), it was impossible to identify markers to predict the type of response. MSLV, multi-site left ventricle; Mean percent change in LV dP/dt_{max} in groups of patients categorized by response to BiV and multisite pacing. (*Data from* Thibault B, Ansalone G, Ricci R, et al. Acute haemodynamic comparison of multisite and biventricular pacing with a quadripolar left ventricular lead. Europace 2103;15(7):989; with permission.)

4 groups: (1) those who improved with BiV pacing and further benefited from MPP; (2) those who responded very well to BiV and were not helped by MPP (in 1 instance, MPP even proved to be deleterious), (3) those in whom BiV pacing provided suboptimal results with modest improvements gained with MPP that fell short of meeting the response criterion (10% improvement in LV maximal rate of rise of LV pressure), and (4) those with no improvement at all, despite any pacing configuration. We could not predict which patients would fall into which categories such that the matter still remains unresolved.

MULTISITE PACING AND MULTIPOINT PACING TO IMPROVE CLINICAL RESPONSE TO CARDIAC RESYNCHRONIZATION THERAPY

A limited number of randomized trials have compared MSP/MPP with BiV pacing over time (Tables 2–4). All but one were small-scale studies, in general with fewer than 100 patients. Conflicting results were reported with superior outcomes associated with MSP/MPP in some,[12,53,56–60] whereas others noted no or limited impact.[61,62] In a recent metaanalysis, Zhang and colleagues[63] nevertheless concluded that MSP provided some benefits over BiV pacing in terms of LVEF and functional capacity, especially in patients with QRS duration of greater than 155 ms.

The MPP study is the largest clinical trial published on the topic so far. It randomized 381 patients after 3 months of resynchronization.[64] Two primary end points were evaluated at 9 months (6 months after randomization). The safety end point, which consisted of freedom from system-related complications, was 93.2% with MPP. The primary efficacy end point of a noninferior response rate was also met, with 30% nonresponders with MPP compared with 25% with BiV. Clinical response was defined by means of a clinical composite score (Packer's score[65]).

CONVERTING A NONRESPONDER TO CARDIAC RESYNCHRONIZATION THERAPY INTO A RESPONDER

Evidence suggests that MSP/MPP may play a more important role when response to BiV pacing is suboptimal.[26,48] This issue was specifically addressed in 2 recent published randomized, multicenter trials, one with MSP, one with MPP.

The V[3] trial[66] included 84 patients who were nonresponders to resynchronization therapy. They were randomized to a second LV lead (upgrading to MSP) versus continued standard BiV pacing. After 2 years, adding a second LV lead was associated with a 20% rate of complications with no benefit with regard to New York Heart Association functional class, HF hospitalizations, and LV ejection fraction.

The MORE-CRT-MPP trial was presented at the European Heart Association meeting in March 2018, with publication of the article pending (Leclercq C, Burri H, Curnis A, et al. CRT nonresponders to responder conversion rate in the more response to CRT with MultiPoint pacing (MORE-CRT-MPP) study: results from phase I. Eur Heart J, submitted). The study randomized 467 nonresponders (after 6 months of resynchronization) to MPP versus continued BiV pacing. The primary end point was also the proportion of responders with both modalities after 6 months of therapy, with response defined as a greater than 15% decrease in LV end-systolic volume assessed by a blinded independent core laboratory. The primary end point was not met: the conversion rate from nonresponder to responder was 31.8% with MPP versus 33.8% with BiV.

Interestingly, both the MPP and MORE-CRT-MPP studies found that how MPP is programmed matters. In both studies, it was left at the discretion of the investigator. In exploratory analyses, the subgroup of patients programmed with an LV1–LV2 distance of 30 mm or greater and a minimal delay of 5 ms (labeled MPP-AS) outperformed those with other MPP configurations. Whether MPP-AS can improve the conversion rate when compared with BiV is being assessed in phase II of the MORE-CRT-MPP study.

MULTISITE PACING VERSUS MULTIPOINT PACING: A QUESTION OF PRACTICALITY

With regard to safety and practicality, the V[3] trial suggests a prohibitively high adverse event rate (20%) associated with adding a second LV lead. In this regard, MPP offers a clear advantage over MSP, because it can easily be programmed ON or OFF at any time, with no invasive reintervention. Currently, there exists MPP-capable devices with the possibility of programming outputs according to each specific threshold (RV, LV1, and LV2). There are no MSP-specific devices. For patients in permanent atrial fibrillation, BiV devices have been used with the atrial pole used for a ventricular lead. Otherwise, 2 LV leads can be connected by means of a Y adaptor. This precludes individual programming of LV1–LV2 outputs (forcing programming according to the highest threshold) and generates a lower impedance. In their series of 20 patients, Behar and colleagues[67] reported nonfunctional MSP systems in 100% after 2 years, with problems mostly related to high thresholds

Table 2
MSP studies with 2 RV leads + 1 LV lead

First Author, Year	Type of Study Number of Patients	Comparison	Main Finding(s)
Bulava et al,[16] 2004	Observational study Single-center 39 patients 19/39 had anodal capture with proximal RV lead ring	"Virtual bifocal RV" + LV vs BiV	"Virtual" bifocal RV + LV shortens QRS by 10–20 ms and provides better LV synchrony (tissue Doppler)
Yamasaki et al,[29] 2011	Acute hemodynamic comparative study Single-center 32 patients	2 RV + 1 LV vs BiV	Trifocal better than BiV: shorter QRS duration, better LV dP/dt$_{max}$ and cardiac output Only 10/32 patients improves with trifocal compared with BiV 4/14 nonresponders with BiV become responders Baseline LVEDVol predicts better response to trifocal
Rogers et al,[12] 2012	Randomized cross-over echocardiographic study Single center 43 patients	Group A: 2 LV + 1 RV Group B: 2 RV + 1 LV vs BiV	Trifocal better than BiV: 6MWTD, LVEF, and LVESVol Similar results in both groups (2 LV + 1 LV and 2 RV + 1 LV)
Providencia[71] (2016) Follow-up from Rogers study (2012)	Retrospective study 34 patients with trifocal vs 34 BiV (propensity score matching)	Best trifocal (2 LV + 1 RV or 2 RV + 1 LV) vs BiV	Lower all-cause mortality/heart transplantation and higher percent of freedom from appropriate ICD therapy with trifocal vs BiV Similar safety profile (lead dislodgment, infection, phrenic nerve capture)
Anselme et al,[62] 2016	Pilot safety/feasibility randomized study Multicenter 76 patients	2 RV + 1 LV vs BiV	Primary end point: no difference in MACE at 6 mo (34% vs 26%; $P = .425$) No difference in 6MWTD, QOL, and LV function by echo at 6 mo Subgroup with 12-month follow-up: Better LVEF and higher percent of responders with trifocal
Marques et al,[13] 2016	Acute observational Single-center 40 patients with permanent AF and LVEV of <40%	2 RV + 1 LV vs BiV	Trifocal provides shorter QRS duration, better LVEF and cardiac output than BiV (Flotrac system) Trifocal was better than BiV in 33/40 patients
Marques et al,[72] 2018	Prospective observational study 6- and 12-month follow-up from previous study 40 patients (33 trifocal, 7 BiV)	Best pacing configuration chosen from previous	LVEF improved from 26% to 39% at 6 mo and 41% at 12 mo With trifocal: Response rate was 59% (6 mo) and 79% (12 mo), with 9% and 16% of superresponders With BiV: Response rate was 60% (6 mo) and 60% (12 mo) with no superresponders

Abbreviations: 6MWTD, 6-minute walk test distance; AF, atrial fibrillation; BiV, biventricular; dP/dt$_{max}$, maximal rate of rise of left ventricular pressure; LV, left ventricular; LVEDVol, left ventricle end-diastolic volume; LVESVol, left ventricle end-systolic volume; LVEF, left ventricular ejection fraction; MACE, major adverse cardiac event; MSP, multisite pacing; QOL, quality of life; RV, right ventricular.

Table 3
MSP studies with 2 LV leads + 1 RV lead

First Author, Year	Type of Study Number of Patients	Comparison	Main Finding(s)
Lenarczyk et al,[73] 2007	Observational feasibility study Single-center 26 patients	2 LV + 1 RV vs BiV	22/26 successful implants After 3 mo: trifocal improved NYHA functional class, Vo_{2max}, 6MWTD, LVEF, and LV synchrony (by echo) Response rate: 95.4%
Leclercq et al,[61] 2008; TRIP-HF study	Randomized, cross-over Multicenter 40 patients in permanent AF with pacemaker indication for slow ventricular response	2 LV + 1 RV vs BiV 3 mo each mode, randomized order	34/40 successful implants, and 26 patients with data No difference in primary end point: ventricular synchrony (Z ratio) Secondary end points: better LVEF and LVESVol with trifocal vs BiV No difference in procedure related morbidity/mortality
Lenarczyk et al,[57] 2009	Retrospective analysis Single center 54 patients	2 LV + 1 RV vs BiV (historical controls + 4 failures)	27/31 success rate (including 22 patients from 2007 report) Follow-up at 3 mo Trifocal improved NYHA functional class, Vo_{2max}, 6MWTD, LVEF, and LV synchrony (by echo) Response rate: 96.3% vs 62.9%
Lenarczyk et al,[58] 2012; TRUST-CRT study	Prospective randomized study Single center 100 patients	2 LV + 1 RV vs BiV	Follow-up at 12 mo (implant 94% success rate) Incidence of serious CRT-related adverse events 30% with trifocal vs 21% with BiV ($P = .3$) Trifocal improved more NYHA functional class vs to BiV
Ginks et al,[31] 2012	Acute comparative study in EP laboratory Single center 10 patients	BiV vs BiV-LV endo vs LV endo vs 2 LV + 1 RV	Trifocal provides better LV dP/dt_{max} and LV endocardial activation time Nonischemic patients respond well to BiV and do not benefit from other modalities Benefits observed mainly in ischemic patients with suboptimal response to standard BiV
Rogers et al,[12] 2012	Randomized cross-over echocardiographic study Single center 43 patients	Group A: 2 LV + 1 RV Group B: 2 RV + 1 LV vs BiV	Trifocal better than BiV: 6MWTD, LVEF, and LVESVol Similar results in both groups (2 LV + 1 LV and 2 RV + 1 LV)
Ogano et al,[52] 2013	Acute hemodynamic study with follow-up (mean, 481 d) Single center 58 patients	2 LV + 1 RV vs BiV (based on best AHR)	40/58 implant success rate 22/40 trifocal provided better LV dP/dt_{max} Hemodynamically guided trifocal prevented ventricular arrhythmias at long term and better repolarization (QTc, JTc, and TDRc)

(continued on next page)

Table 3
(continued)

First Author, Year	Type of Study Number of Patients	Comparison	Main Finding(s)
Behar et al,[67] 2015	Observational Single center 20 patients	2 LV leads with Y connector (no comparator)	19/20 implant success rate 2 patients with LV 2 turned OFF at implant (high threshold) 2 patients with LV 2 turned OFF at discharge (high threshold and/or hemodynamic deterioration) All 15 patients left had LV 2 turned OFF after 255 d High current (high voltage + low impedance) results in generator longevity diminished 3.5 y (vs estimated 5 y)
Providencia et al,[71] 2016; Follow-up from Rogers study (2012)	Retrospective study 34 patients with trifocal vs 34 BiV (propensity score matching)	Best trifocal (2 LV + 1 RV or 2 RV + 1 LV) vs BiV	Lower all-cause mortality/heart transplantation and higher percent of freedom from appropriate ICD therapy with trifocal vs BiV Similar safety profile (lead dislodgment, infection, phrenic nerve capture)
Jackson et al,[74] 2018; iSPOT study	Acute hemodynamic comparative study Multicenter 24 patients with LBBB And CMR-LGE with scar evaluation	BiV vs MSP (2 LV + 1 RV) vs MPP	Neither MSP nor MPP improves LV dP/dt$_{max}$ overall However, in 6 patients (25%) with scar burden >8.5% (by MRI): MPP (but not MSP) provided improved acute hemodynamic response
Bordachar et al,[66] 2018; V³ study	Randomized study Multicenter 84 nonresponders to CRT	Adding second LV lead vs continuing with BiV	90% implant success rate at first try 80% functioning system after 2 y 20% procedure or system-related complications At 12 and 24 mo: no benefits in terms of NYHA functional class, HF hospitalizations, LVEF
Zanon et al,[30] 2018	Acute hemodynamic comparative study Single center 15 patients with ischemic cardiomyopathy and permanent AF	BiV vs 2 LV + 1 RV vs MPP vs MPP + 2 LV + 1 RV	MPP-trifocal provided best LV dP/dt$_{max}$, and shortest QRS duration followed by MPP, then trifocal, then BiV

Abbreviations: 6MWTD, 6-minute walk test distance; AF, atrial fibrillation; AHR, acute hemodynamic response; BiV, biventricular; CMR-LGE, cardiac magnetic resonance with late gadolinium enhancement; CRT, cardiac resynchronization therapy; dP/dt$_{max}$, maximal rate of rise of left ventricular pressure; EP, electrophysiology; HF, heart failure; ICD, implantable cardioverter-defibrillator; LV, left ventricular; LVESVol, left ventricle end-systolic volume; LVEF, left ventricular ejection fraction; MPP, multipoint pacing; MSP, multisite pacing; NYHA, New York Heart Association; RV, right ventricular.

Table 4
MPP studies

First Author, Year	Type of Study Number of Patients	Comparison	Main finding(s)
Thibault et al,[15] 2013	Acute hemodynamic comparative study Single center 21 patients	Multiple MPP configurations vs BiV	19/21 patients with data 84% patients had better LV dP/dt$_{max}$ with MPP vs BiV Best MPP with largest LV pacing vector in 74% patients
Rinaldi et al,[75] 2013; Rinaldi et al,[76] 2014	Acute comparative echocardiographic study Multicenter 52 patients	Multiple MPP configurations vs BiV	41/52 patients with data MPP provides better LV synchrony: standard deviation of peak contraction of 12 and peak radial strain (obtained by tissue Doppler imaging in 40 patients)
Shetty et al,[32] 2014	Acute comparative hemodynamic study Single-center 15 patients	BiV vs BiV- endo vs MSP vs MPP	BiV endo provided best LV dP/dt$_{max}$ MSP and MPP provides nonsignificant improvement in LV dP/dt$_{max}$ compared with BiV LV activation time does not predict acute hemodynamic response
Pappone et al,[53] 2014	Acute comparative hemodynamic study Single center 40 patients	MPP vs BiV PV loop study	MPP better than BiV for LV dP/dt$_{max}$, stroke work, stroke volume, and LVEF MPP also provided better diastolic parameters: LV dP/dt$_{min}$, relaxation time constant and end-diastolic pressure
Pappone et al,[59,60] 2015	Randomized study Single center 44 patients	Best MPP vs best BiV (from previous study)	Follow-up at 3 and 12 mo MPP provides better NYHA functional class, LVEF, LVESVol Response rate: 76% vs 57% at 12 mo
van Gelder and Bracke,[17] 2015	Acute comparative study Single center 17 patients	"Virtual MPP" with anodal capture from second LV electrode vs BiV	Difference observed in LV dP/dt$_{max}$ between 2 LV pacing electrodes No difference between "best BiV" and "virtual" MPP
Sohal et al,[48] 2015	Acute hemodynamic comparative study Single center 16 patients with quartet lead	BiV vs BiV alternative vs MSP vs MPP	9/16 patients respond well to BiV and are not improved by other modalities (LV dP/dt$_{max}$) MSP and MPP help essentially in nonresponders Nonresponders do not exhibit strict criteria for LBBB and do not have functional line of conduction block (endocardial mapping)
Zanon et al,[33] 2015	Acute hemodynamic comparative study Single center 29 patients with LBBB	MPP vs BiV (multiple veins tested)	Compared with BiV, MPP provided slightly better LV dP/dt$_{max}$ and slightly shorter QRS duration There was a correlation between QRS duration reduction and AHR with MPP

(continued on next page)

Table 4
(continued)

First Author, Year	Type of Study Number of Patients	Comparison	Main finding(s)
Menardi et al,[34] 2015	Acute hemodynamic comparative study Single center 10 patients with nonischemic cardiomyopathy	MPP vs BiV	Compared with BiV, MPP provided improved more LV dP/dt$_{max}$ (by 30% vs 25%) further QRS duration reduction (-22% vs -11%) with better LV activation time reduction (-25% vs -10%) MPP captures a greater LV surface during first 25 and 50 ms
Osca et al,[77] 2016	Acute comparative echocardiographic study Single center 27 patients	MPP vs BiV	MPP provides better LVEF, cardiac index, and LV synchrony
Umar et al,[54] 2016; MAESTRO study	Acute hemodynamic comparative study 16 patients with ischemic cardiomyopathy LV lead straddling LV scar	MPP vs BiV	8 responders among 10 patients Best LV dP/dt$_{max}$ with MPP in 5/8 patients LV dP/dt$_{max}$ similar with MPP and BiV$_{apical}$
Sterlinski et al,[35] 2016; iSPOT study	Acute hemodynamic comparative study Multicenter 24 patients with LBBB	MPP vs BiV	No difference in LV dP/dt$_{max}$ MPP provided better LV dP/dt$_{max}$ in only 2/24 patients No difference in QRS duration No correlation overall between QRS duration reduction, Q-LV timing and Q-LV ratio and improvement in LV dP/dt$_{max}$
Zanon et al,[78] 2016	Retrospective study Single center 110 patients	BiV vs BiV$_{opt}$ vs MPP$_{opt}$	1-year follow-up MPP provides a greater percent ($\leq 90\%$) of responders (LVESVol and NYHA)
Forleo et al,[36] 2017; IRON-MPP study	Multicenter registry 507 patients	MPP vs BiV	Follow-up at 6 mo MPP provides better LVEF (39% vs 34%) more clinical (composite score) responders (56% vs 38%) and shorter QRS (135 ms vs 141 ms) Benefits observed mainly in patients with LBBB (vs non-LBBB), QRS >150 ms (vs <150 ms) Benefits similar for ischemic and nonischemic patients
Niazi et al,[64] 2017; MPP study	Randomized study Multicenter 469 patients	MPP vs BiV After 3 mo of BiV pacing	Primary end point: freedom from system-related complication met (MPP noninferior to BiV) No difference in terms of responders at 9 mo MPP with largest LV pacing vector and shorter LV1-LV2 delay (MPP-AS) showed higher percent of responders compared with other MPP configuration (35% vs 13% responders)

(continued on next page)

Table 4
(continued)

First Author, Year	Type of Study Number of Patients	Comparison	Main finding(s)
Siciliano et al,[79] 2017	Acute comparative echocardiographic study Single center 11 patients	MPP vs BiV	3D echocardiography and particle imaging velocimetry MPP provided better LV remodeling (LVED and LVESVol) vs BiV but no difference in strain
Akerstrom et al,[68] 2018	Observational study 2 centers 46 patients with MPP programmed ON	Impact on device longevity	With pacing output ≤1.5 V (24% patients), no impact on estimated device longevity However, with output ≤4.0 V, estimated longevity diminished from >8 y to 7.4 y And with output ≤6.0 V, estimated longevity = 7.0 y
Ciconte et al,[80] 2018	Acute noninvasive hemodynamic study (SphygmoCor CVMS) Single center 19 patients	MPP vs BiV	MPP with largest pacing configuration provided better preejection period and ejection duration than BiV in 17/19 patients
Jackson et al,[74] 2018; iSPOT study	Acute hemodynamic comparative study Multicenter 24 patients with LBBB And CMR-LGE with scar evaluation	BiV vs MSP (2 LV + 1 RV) vs MPP	Neither MSP nor MPP improves LV dP/dt$_{max}$ overall However, in 6 patients (25%) with scar burden >8.5% (by MRI): MPP (but not MSP) provided improved acute hemodynamic response
Socie et al,[81] 2018	Acute noninvasive hemodynamic study Starling SV monitoring system Single center 22 patients	MPP vs BiV	MPP did not provide better cardiac output compared with BiV AVV and VV optimization further improved cardiac output compared with nonoptimized BiV
Lercher et al,[82] 2018	Acute noninvasive feasibility study Finometer MIDI + 6-mo follow-up (echocardiography) Multicenter 42 patients	MPP vs BiV	29/37 patients did better with MPP than with BiV (increase in systolic blood pressure) 23/27 responders at 6 mo (LVESVol) vs 4/5 with BiV
van Everdingen et al,[83] 2018	Acute hemodynamic study (PV loop) Single center 44 patients	MPP vs BiV	Optimization of pacing site through a quadripolar LV lead is more important than programming MPP
Engels et al,[37] 2018	Acute hemodynamic comparative study Single center 26 patients	MPP vs BiV	MPP provides better acute hemodynamic response vs BiV Despite similar QRS duration and area 5/26 had smaller QRS area, 17/26 had rotation of maximal vector indicating a more LV dominant activation sequence

(continued on next page)

Table 4
(continued)

First Author, Year	Type of Study Number of Patients	Comparison	Main finding(s)
Leclercq C, Burri H, Curnis A, et al. CRT nonresponders to responder conversion rate in the more response to cardiac resynchronization therapy with MultiPoint pacing (MORE-CRT-MPP) study: results from phase I. Eur Heart J, submitted	MORE-CRT-MPP Randomized study Multicenter 1921 patients	MPP vs BiV in nonresponders after 6 mo	467 randomized patients 32% conversion to responders with MPP vs 34% with BiV (*P* = NS) MPP with largest pacing vector and shorter LV1-LV2 delay (MPP-AS) provided higher conversion rate: 46% vs 26% with other MPP configurations Difference with BiV did not reach significance (*P* = .10)

Abbreviations: 3D, 3-dimensional; AHR, acute hemodynamic response; AV, atrio-ventricular; BiV, biventricular; CMR-LGE, cardiac magnetic resonance with late gadolinium enhancement; dP/dt$_{max}$, maximal rate of rise of left ventricular pressure; endo, endocardial (pacing); LBBB, left bundle branch block; LV, left ventricle (left ventricular); LVEF, left ventricle ejection fraction; LVESVol, left ventricle end-systolic volume; MPP, multipoint pacing; MSP, multisite pacing; NYHA, New York Heart Association functional class; PV, pressure–volume loops; RV, right ventricle (right ventricular); trifocal, instead of triventricular; VV, inter-ventricular.

and an inability to capture LV2 at the maximal output. Longevity was shorter than expected with implanted devices (42 vs 58 months). Longevity can also be impacted by MPP. According to Alkerstrom and colleagues,[68] the effect of MPP on longevity is marginal at a pacing output 1.5 V or less, but may be decrease by approximately 1 year (out of estimated >8-year devices) at with outputs of 1.5 to 4.0 V.

SUMMARY

Despite advances in resynchronization over the past 20 years, many unanswered questions remain. Nonresponse or suboptimal response to CRT is a lingering major concern that can be improved by restricting CRT indications to patients with left bundle branch block and a prolonged QRS duration (>150 ms). However, narrowing inclusion criteria to improve the response rate necessarily reduces the pool of eligible patients that may derive some benefit. This article specifically addressed the issue of whether resynchronization could be further improved by MSP or MPP, with an advantage for MPP over MSP with regard to safety and practicality of use. Although there are promising data, confirmation from large randomized trials is still required. If the second phase of the MORE-CRT-MPP trial yields positive results, it would be the first time a strategy to convert nonresponders into responders would be achieved in the context of a large multicenter study. Such

results would be a great step forward and provide the impetus for further research to determine whether MPP may prove superior to BiV pacing from the onset in patients with less clear indications for CRT.

REFERENCES

1. McAlister FA, Ezekowitz JA, Wiebe N, et al. Systematic review: cardiac resynchronization in patients with symptomatic heart failure. Ann Intern Med 2004;141(5):381–90.
2. Adabag S, Roukoz H, Anand IS, et al. Cardiac resynchronization therapy in patients with minimal heart failure: a systematic review and meta-analysis. J Am Coll Cardiol 2011;58(9):935–41.
3. Leyva F, Nisam S, Auricchio A. 20 years of cardiac resynchronization therapy. J Am Coll Cardiol 2014; 64(10):1047–58.
4. Brugada J, Delnoy PP, Brachmann J, et al. Contractility sensor-guided optimization of cardiac resynchronization therapy: results from the RESPOND-CRT trial. Eur Heart J 2017;38(10):730–8.
5. Mullens W, Kepa J, De Vusser P, et al. Importance of adjunctive heart failure optimization immediately after implantation to improve long-term outcomes with cardiac resynchronization therapy. Am J Cardiol 2011;108(3):409–15.
6. Auricchio A, Heggermont WA. Technology advances to improve response to cardiac resynchronization therapy: what clinicians should know. Rev Esp Cardiol (Engl Ed) 2018;71(6):477–84.

7. Turakhia MP, Cao M, Fischer A, et al. Reduced mortality associated with quadripolar compared to bipolar left ventricular leads in cardiac resynchronization therapy. JACC Clin Electrophysiol 2016;2(4):426–33.

8. Thibault B, Karst E, Ryu K, et al. Pacing electrode selection in a quadripolar left heart lead determines presence or absence of phrenic nerve stimulation. Europace 2010;12(5):751–3.

9. Sperzel J, Danschel W, Gutleben KJ, et al. First prospective, multi-centre clinical experience with a novel left ventricular quadripolar lead. Europace 2012;14(3):365–72.

10. Boriani G, Connors S, Kalarus Z, et al. Cardiac resynchronization therapy with a quadripolar electrode lead decreases complications at 6 months: results of the MORE-CRT randomized trial. JACC Clin Electrophysiol 2016;2(2):212–20.

11. Rijal S, Wolfe J, Rattan R, et al. Lead related complications in quadripolar versus bipolar left ventricular leads. Indian Pacing Electrophysiol J 2017;17(1): 3–7.

12. Rogers DP, Lambiase PD, Lowe MD, et al. A randomized double-blind crossover trial of triventricular versus biventricular pacing in heart failure. Eur J Heart Fail 2012;14(5):495–505.

13. Marques P, Nobre Menezes M, Lima da Silva G, et al. Triple-site pacing for cardiac resynchronization in permanent atrial fibrillation - acute phase results from a prospective observational study. Rev Port Cardiol 2016;35(6):331–8.

14. Lenarczyk R, Kowalski O, Sredniawa B, et al. Triple-site versus standard cardiac resynchronization therapy study (TRUST CRT): clinical rationale, design, and implementation. J Cardiovasc Electrophysiol 2009;20(6):658–62.

15. Thibault B, Dubuc M, Khairy P, et al. Acute haemodynamic comparison of multisite and biventricular pacing with a quadripolar left ventricular lead. Europace 2013;15(7):984–91.

16. Bulava A, Ansalone G, Ricci R, et al. Triple-site pacing in patients with biventricular device-incidence of the phenomenon and cardiac resynchronization benefit. J Interv Card Electrophysiol 2004;10(1): 37–45.

17. van Gelder BM, Bracke FA. Acute hemodynamic effects of single- and dual-site left ventricular pacing employing a dual cathodal coronary sinus lead. Pacing Clin Electrophysiol 2015;38(5):558–64.

18. Morishima I, Tomomatsu T, Morita Y, et al. Intentional anodal capture of a left ventricular quadripolar lead enhances resynchronization equally with multipoint pacing. HeartRhythm Case Rep 2015;1(5):386–8.

19. Occhetta E, Dell'Era G, Giubertoni A, et al. Occurrence of simultaneous cathodal-anodal capture with left ventricular quadripolar leads for cardiac resynchronization therapy: an electrocardiogram evaluation. Europace 2017;19(4):596–601.

20. Dell'Era G, De Vecchi F, Prenna E, et al. Feasibility of cathodic-anodal left ventricular stimulation for alternative multisite pacing. Pacing Clin Electrophysiol 2018;41(6):597–602.

21. Moss AJ, Hall WJ, Cannom DS, et al. Cardiac-resynchronization therapy for the prevention of heart-failure events. N Engl J Med 2009;361(14):1329–38.

22. Tang AS, Wells GA, Talajic M, et al. Cardiac-resynchronization therapy for mild-to-moderate heart failure. N Engl J Med 2010;363(25):2385–95.

23. Coppola G, Ciaramitaro G, Stabile G, et al. Magnitude of QRS duration reduction after biventricular pacing identifies responders to cardiac resynchronization therapy. Int J Cardiol 2016;221:450–5.

24. Bryant AR, Wilton SB, Lai MP, et al. Association between QRS duration and outcome with cardiac resynchronization therapy: a systematic review and meta-analysis. J Electrocardiol 2013; 46(2):147–55.

25. Bordachar P, Grenz N, Jais P, et al. Left ventricular endocardial or triventricular pacing to optimize cardiac resynchronization therapy in a chronic canine model of ischemic heart failure. Am J Physiol Heart Circ Physiol 2012;303(2):H207–15.

26. Ploux S, Strik M, van Hunnik A, et al. Acute electrical and hemodynamic effects of multisite left ventricular pacing for cardiac resynchronization therapy in the dyssynchronous canine heart. Heart Rhythm 2014; 11(1):119–25.

27. Qiu Q, Yang L, Mai JT, et al. Acute effects of multisite biventricular pacing on dyssynchrony and hemodynamics in canines with heart failure. J Card Fail 2017;23(4):304–11.

28. Huntjens PR, Ploux S, Strik M, et al. Electrical substrates driving response to cardiac resynchronization therapy: a combined clinical-computational evaluation. Circ Arrhythm Electrophysiol 2018; 11(4):e005647.

29. Yamasaki H, Seo Y, Tada H, et al. Clinical and procedural characteristics of acute hemodynamic responders undergoing triple-site ventricular pacing for advanced heart failure. Am J Cardiol 2011; 108(9):1297–304.

30. Zanon F, Marcantoni L, Baracca E, et al. Hemodynamic comparison of different multisites and multipoint pacing strategies in cardiac resynchronization therapies. J Interv Card Electrophysiol 2018; 53(1):31–9.

31. Ginks MR, Shetty AK, Lambiase PD, et al. Benefits of endocardial and multisite pacing are dependent on the type of left ventricular electric activation pattern and presence of ischemic heart disease: insights from electroanatomic mapping. Circ Arrhythm Electrophysiol 2012;5(5):889–97.

32. Shetty AK, Sohal M, Chen Z, et al. A comparison of left ventricular endocardial, multisite, and multipolar epicardial cardiac resynchronization: an acute

haemodynamic and electroanatomical study. Europace 2014;16(6):873–9.

33. Zanon F, Baracca E, Pastore G, et al. Multipoint pacing by a left ventricular quadripolar lead improves the acute hemodynamic response to CRT compared with conventional biventricular pacing at any site. Heart Rhythm 2015;12(5):975–81.

34. Menardi E, Ballari GP, Goletto C, et al. Characterization of ventricular activation pattern and acute hemodynamics during multipoint left ventricular pacing. Heart Rhythm 2015;12(8):1762–9.

35. Sterlinski M, Sokal A, Lenarczyk R, et al. In heart failure patients with left bundle branch block single lead multispot left ventricular pacing does not improve acute hemodynamic response to conventional biventricular pacing. A multicenter prospective, interventional, non-randomized study. PLoS One 2016;11(4):e0154024.

36. Forleo GB, Santini L, Giammaria M, et al. Multipoint pacing via a quadripolar left-ventricular lead: preliminary results from the Italian registry on multipoint left-ventricular pacing in cardiac resynchronization therapy (IRON-MPP). Europace 2017;19(7):1170–7.

37. Engels EB, Vis A, van Rees BD, et al. Improved acute haemodynamic response to cardiac resynchronization therapy using multipoint pacing cannot solely be explained by better resynchronization. J Electrocardiol 2018;51(6S):S61–6. https://doi.org/10.1016/j.jelectrocard.2018.07.011.

38. Varma N, O'Donnell D, Bassiouny M, et al. Programming cardiac resynchronization therapy for electrical synchrony: reaching beyond left bundle branch block and left ventricular activation delay. J Am Heart Assoc 2018;7(3) [pii:e007489].

39. Salden F, Kutyifa V, Stockburger M, et al. Atrioventricular dromotropathy: evidence for a distinctive entity in heart failure with prolonged PR interval? Europace 2018;20(7):1067–77.

40. Grines CL, Bashore TM, Boudoulas H, et al. Functional abnormalities in isolated left bundle branch block. The effect of interventricular asynchrony. Circulation 1989;79(4):845–53.

41. Auricchio A, Ding J, Spinelli JC, et al. Cardiac resynchronization therapy restores optimal atrioventricular mechanical timing in heart failure patients with ventricular conduction delay. J Am Coll Cardiol 2002;39(7):1163–9.

42. Hoit BD. Pathophysiology of the pericardium. Prog Cardiovasc Dis 2017;59(4):341–8.

43. Bax JJ, Ansalone G, Breithardt OA, et al. Echocardiographic evaluation of cardiac resynchronization therapy: ready for routine clinical use? A critical appraisal. J Am Coll Cardiol 2004;44(1):1–9.

44. Yu CM, Lin H, Zhang Q, et al. High prevalence of left ventricular systolic and diastolic asynchrony in patients with congestive heart failure and normal QRS duration. Heart 2003;89(1):54–60.

45. Chung ES, Leon AR, Tavazzi L, et al. Results of the predictors of response to CRT (PROSPECT) trial. Circulation 2008;117(20):2608–16.

46. Ruschitzka F, Abraham WT, Singh JP, et al. Cardiac-resynchronization therapy in heart failure with a narrow QRS complex. N Engl J Med 2013;369(15):1395–405.

47. Jones S, Lumens J, Sohaib SMA, et al. Cardiac resynchronization therapy: mechanisms of action and scope for further improvement in cardiac function. Europace 2017;19(7):1178–86.

48. Sohal M, Shetty A, Niederer S, et al. Mechanistic insights into the benefits of multisite pacing in cardiac resynchronization therapy: the importance of electrical substrate and rate of left ventricular activation. Heart Rhythm 2015;12(12):2449–57.

49. Duckett SG, Ginks M, Shetty AK, et al. Invasive acute hemodynamic response to guide left ventricular lead implantation predicts chronic remodeling in patients undergoing cardiac resynchronization therapy. J Am Coll Cardiol 2011;58(11):1128–36.

50. Thibault B, Dubuc M, Karst E, et al. Design of an acute dP/dt hemodynamic measurement protocol to isolate cardiac effect of pacing. J Card Fail 2014;20(5):365–72.

51. Niederer S, Walker C, Crozier A, et al. The impact of beat-to-beat variability in optimising the acute hemodynamic response in cardiac resynchronisation therapy. Clin Trials Regul Sci Cardiol 2015;12:18–22.

52. Ogano M, Iwasaki YK, Tanabe J, et al. Antiarrhythmic effect of cardiac resynchronization therapy with triple-site biventricular stimulation. Europace 2013;15(10):1491–8.

53. Pappone C, Calovic Z, Vicedomini G, et al. Multipoint left ventricular pacing improves acute hemodynamic response assessed with pressure-volume loops in cardiac resynchronization therapy patients. Heart Rhythm 2014;11(3):394–401.

54. Umar F, Taylor RJ, Stegemann B, et al. Haemodynamic effects of cardiac resynchronization therapy using single-vein, three-pole, multipoint left ventricular pacing in patients with ischaemic cardiomyopathy and a left ventricular free wall scar: the MAESTRO study. Europace 2016;18(8):1227–34.

55. van Everdingen WM, Zweerink A, Salden OAE, et al. Pressure-volume loop analysis of multipoint pacing with a quadripolar left ventricular lead in cardiac resynchronization therapy. JACC Clin Electrophysiol 2018;4(7):881–9.

56. Lenarczyk R, Kowalski O, Pruszkowska-Skrzep P, et al. Triple site biventricular pacing in a patient with congestive heart failure and severe mechanical dyssynchrony. J Interv Card Electrophysiol 2007;18(2):187–90.

57. Lenarczyk R, Kowalski O, Kukulski T, et al. Mid-term outcomes of triple-site vs. conventional cardiac resynchronization therapy: a preliminary study. Int J Cardiol 2009;133(1):87–94.

58. Lenarczyk R, Kowalski O, Sredniawa B, et al. Implantation feasibility, procedure-related adverse events and lead performance during 1-year follow-up in patients undergoing triple-site cardiac resynchronization therapy: a substudy of TRUST CRT randomized trial. J Cardiovasc Electrophysiol 2012;23(11):1228–36.

59. Pappone C, Calovic Z, Vicedomini G, et al. Improving cardiac resynchronization therapy response with multipoint left ventricular pacing: twelve-month follow-up study. Heart Rhythm 2015; 12(6):1250–8.

60. Pappone C, Calovic Z, Vicedomini G, et al. Multipoint left ventricular pacing in a single coronary sinus branch improves mid-term echocardiographic and clinical response to cardiac resynchronization therapy. J Cardiovasc Electrophysiol 2015;26(1): 58–63.

61. Leclercq C, Gadler F, Kranig W, et al. A randomized comparison of triple-site versus dual-site ventricular stimulation in patients with congestive heart failure. J Am Coll Cardiol 2008;51(15):1455–62.

62. Anselme F, Bordachar P, Pasquie JL, et al. Safety, feasibility, and outcome results of cardiac resynchronization with triple-site ventricular stimulation compared to conventional cardiac resynchronization. Heart Rhythm 2016;13(1):183–9.

63. Zhang B, Guo J, Zhang G. Comparison of triple-site ventricular pacing versus conventional cardiac resynchronization therapy in patients with systolic heart failure: a meta-analysis of randomized and observational studies. J Arrhythm 2018;34(1): 55–64.

64. Niazi I, Baker J 2nd, Corbisiero R, et al. Safety and efficacy of multipoint pacing in cardiac resynchronization therapy: the multipoint pacing trial. JACC Clin Electrophysiol 2017;3(13):1510–8.

65. Packer M. Proposal for a new clinical end point to evaluate the efficacy of drugs and devices in the treatment of chronic heart failure. J Card Fail 2001; 7(2):176–82.

66. Bordachar P, Gras D, Clementy N, et al. Clinical impact of an additional left ventricular lead in cardiac resynchronization therapy nonresponders: the V(3) trial. Heart Rhythm 2018; 15(6):870–6.

67. Behar JM, Bostock J, Ginks M, et al. Limitations of chronic delivery of multi-vein left ventricular stimulation for cardiac resynchronization therapy. J Interv Card Electrophysiol 2015;42(2): 135–42.

68. Akerstrom F, Narvaez I, Puchol A, et al. Estimation of the effects of multipoint pacing on battery longevity in routine clinical practice. Europace 2018;20(7): 1161–7.

69. Niederer SA, Shetty AK, Plank G, et al. Biophysical modeling to simulate the response to multisite left ventricular stimulation using a quadripolar pacing lead. Pacing Clin Electrophysiol 2012; 35(2):204–14.

70. Waks JW, Perez-Alday EA, Tereshchenko LG. Understanding mechanisms of cardiac resynchronization therapy response to improve patient selection and outcomes. Circ Arrhythm Electrophysiol 2018; 11(4):e006290.

71. Providencia R, Rogers D, Papageorgiou N, et al. Long-term results of triventricular versus biventricular pacing in heart failure: a propensity-matched comparison. JACC Clin Electrophysiol 2016;2(7): 825–35.

72. Marques P, Nobre Menezes M, Lima da Silva G, et al. Triple-site pacing for cardiac resynchronization in permanent atrial fibrillation: follow-up results from a prospective observational study. Europace 2018; 20(6):986–92.

73. Lenarczyk R, Kowalski O, Kukulski T, et al. Triple-site biventricular pacing in patients undergoing cardiac resynchronization therapy: a feasibility study. Europace 2007;9(9):762–7.

74. Jackson T, Lenarczyk R, Sterlinski M, et al. Left ventricular scar and the acute hemodynamic effects of multivein and multipolar pacing in cardiac resynchronization. Int J Cardiol Heart Vasc 2018; 19:14–9.

75. Rinaldi CA, Kranig W, Leclercq C, et al. Acute effects of multisite left ventricular pacing on mechanical dyssynchrony in patients receiving cardiac resynchronization therapy. J Card Fail 2013;19(11): 731–8.

76. Rinaldi CA, Leclercq C, Kranig W, et al. Improvement in acute contractility and hemodynamics with multipoint pacing via a left ventricular quadripolar pacing lead. J Interv Card Electrophysiol 2014; 40(1):75–80.

77. Osca J, Alonso P, Cano O, et al. The use of multisite left ventricular pacing via quadripolar lead improves acute haemodynamics and mechanical dyssynchrony assessed by radial strain speckle tracking: initial results. Europace 2016;18(4): 560–7.

78. Zanon F, Marcantoni L, Baracca E, et al. Optimization of left ventricular pacing site plus multipoint pacing improves remodeling and clinical response to cardiac resynchronization therapy at 1 year. Heart Rhythm 2016;13(8): 1644–51.

79. Siciliano M, Migliore F, Badano L, et al. Cardiac resynchronization therapy by multipoint pacing improves response of left ventricular mechanics and fluid dynamics: a three-dimensional and particle

image velocimetry echo study. Europace 2017; 19(11):1833–40.

80. Ciconte G, Calovic Z, Vicedomini G, et al. Multi-point pacing improves peripheral hemodynamic response: noninvasive assessment using radial artery tonometry. Pacing Clin Electrophysiol 2018; 41(2):106–13.

81. Socie P, Squara F, Semichon M, et al. Combination of the best pacing configuration and atrioventricular and interventricular delays optimization in cardiac resynchronization therapy. Pacing Clin Electrophysiol 2018;41(4):362–7.

82. Lercher P, Lunati M, Rordorf R, et al. Long-term reverse remodeling by cardiac resynchronization therapy with multipoint pacing: a feasibility study of noninvasive hemodynamics-guided device programming. Heart Rhythm 2018. https://doi.org/10.1016/j.hrthm.2018.06.032.

83. van Everdingen WM, Zweerink A, Salden OAE, et al. Atrioventricular optimization in cardiac resynchronization therapy with quadripolar leads: should we optimize every pacing configuration including multi-point pacing? Europace 2018. https://doi.org/10.1093/europace/euy138.

Gender-Based Differences in Cardiac Resynchronization Therapy Response

Marin Nishimura, MD[a], Ulrika Birgersdotter-Green, MD[b],*

KEYWORDS

- Cardiac resynchronization therapy • Gender • QRS • LBBB

KEY POINTS

- Studies have demonstrated that women tend to derive greater therapeutic benefit from cardiac resynchronization therapy (CRT) compared with men.
- Women were noted to derive benefit at a lesser degree of QRS prolongation than men, below the generally accepted cutoff of QRS ≥150 milliseconds.
- Given the difference in response to CRT based on QRS duration between genders, further refinement in the current selection criteria may be considered.

INTRODUCTION

Heart failure (HF) is a leading cause of significant morbidity and mortality worldwide. HF affects both genders equally, and at 40 years of age, the lifetime risk of developing HF for both men and women is 1 in 5.[1] Cardiac resynchronization therapy (CRT) has been shown to improve quality of life and functional status, reduce risk of HF admission, and improve survival, and it is the standard of care for select patients with systolic HF.[2,3] Current guidelines make recommendations for CRT predominantly based on the factors that reflect ventricular dyssynchrony: QRS duration and morphology. However, recent studies have demonstrated that gender may also play an important role in determining response to CRT. In this review, the authors aim to summarize female representation in the pivotal clinical trials, to review current knowledge on gender-based differences in CRT response, and to offer possible explanations for the disparate responses between genders.

BACKGROUND

Impaired electromechanical coupling is commonly seen with progression of HF and portends worse outcome. Prolonged QRS duration occurs in approximately one-third of patients with advanced HF and can be associated with ventricular dyssynchrony.[4] Such dyssynchrony can result in reduced left ventricular (LV) systolic function, functional mitral regurgitation, and adverse metabolic and structural remodeling.[5,6] CRT, by allowing simultaneous pacing of the ventricles, restores ventricular synchrony and can have immediate and long-term favorable effects on the diseased heart; it has been shown to enhance reverse remodeling,

Disclosure Statement: None.
[a] Division of Cardiovascular Medicine, Department of Medicine, University of California, San Diego, 9500 Gilman Drive, Mail Code 7411, La Jolla, CA 92037-7411, USA; [b] Pacemaker and ICD Services, Cardiac Electrophysiology Section, Division of Cardiology, Department of Medicine, University of California, San Diego, 9444 Medical Center Drive, MC 7411, La Jolla, CA 92037, USA
* Corresponding author.
E-mail address: ubgreen@ucsd.edu

Card Electrophysiol Clin 11 (2019) 115–122
https://doi.org/10.1016/j.ccep.2018.11.015
1877-9182/19/© 2018 Elsevier Inc. All rights reserved.

leading to improvement in systolic function and LV dimensions in some patients.[6–8] Robust data from multiple randomized control trials (RCTs) have established the clinical benefit of CRT in improving functional status, quality of life, HF readmission rate, and most importantly, mortality.[9–12]

Patient selection for CRT in the current guidelines is primarily based on factors reflective of severity of electromechanical uncoupling and LV dyssynchrony: duration of the QRS and the morphology of QRS (left bundle branch block [LBBB] vs non-LBBB).[2,3] The current 2012 American College of Cardiology (ACC)/American Heart Association (AHA)/Heart Rhythm Society (HRS) focused update on the guidelines for device-based therapy gives class I recommendation for CRT in HF patients with ejection fraction (EF) ≤35%, LBBB with a QRS duration ≥150 milliseconds, and New York Heart Association (NYHA) class II, III, or ambulatory IV symptoms (Level of Evidence [LOE]: A for NYHA class III/IV; LOE: B for NYHA class II).[2] A weaker, class IIa recommendation was given to patients with QRS duration 120 to 149 milliseconds and NYHA class II, III, or ambulatory IV symptoms (LOE: B) and to patients with non-LBBB pattern with QRS duration ≥150 milliseconds and NYHA class III/ambulatory IV symptoms (LOE: A).[2] The 2016 European Society of Cardiology (ESC) guidelines similarly give class I recommendation for patients with LBBB with QRS duration ≥150 milliseconds (LOE: A), but also give class I recommendation for patients with

LBBB with QRS 130 to 149 milliseconds with a lower LOE (LOE: B).[13] These QRS duration cutoffs and recommendation on QRS morphologies are based on COMPANION (Comparison of Medical Therapy, Pacing, and Defibrillation in Heart Failure), MIRACLE (Multicenter InSync Randomized Clinical Evaluation), CARE-HF (Cardiac Resynchronization-Heart Failure), REVERSE (Resynchronization reVErses Remodeling in Systolic left vEntricular dysfunction), MADIT-CRT (Multicenter Automatic Defibrillator Implantation Trial with Cardiac Resynchronization Therapy), and RAFT (Resynchronization-Defibrillation for Ambulatory Heart Failure Trial), which have firmly established the role of CRT in the management of patients with HF.[9–12,14,15]

However, the ability to extrapolate findings from clinical trials into clinical practice becomes limited when the study population did not represent the patient at hand. One patient population that was underrepresented in the CRT clinical trials was women. The study populations of MIRACLE, REVERSE, MADIT-CRT, and RAFT, for example, were 77%, 79%, 75%, and 83% men, respectively (**Fig. 1**).[10–12,15] A systematic review of 183 clinical trials and registries of CRT found that female representation in these studies ranged from 2% to 60%.[16] Ninety percent of the studies had ≤35% women; half of the studies had ≤23% women.[16] This underrepresentation of women in these practice-changing clinical trials makes the direct extrapolation into clinical practice more problematic.

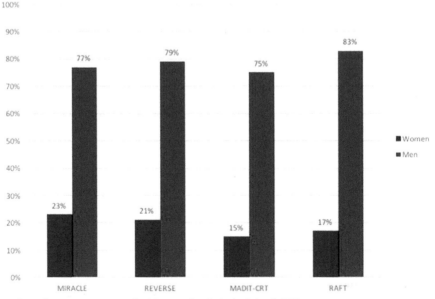

Fig. 1. Proportion of women compared with men in clinical trials of CRT.

CARDIAC RESYNCHRONIZATION THERAPY RESPONSE IN WOMEN

However, when women receive CRT, do they respond differently? Recent studies have demonstrated that there in fact seems to be clear gender-based differences in structural, symptomatic, and mortality outcomes in response to CRT (**Table 1**).[17–22]

Reverse Cardiac Remodeling

Women appear to derive greater reverse cardiac remodeling with CRT than men. In the post hoc analysis of the MADIT-CRT, best-subset regression analysis was performed to identify factors associated with reverse remodeling (as defined by reduction in left ventricular end diastolic volume [LVEDV] at 1 year); female gender emerged as one of the few independent predictors of reverse remodeling following CRT.[23] In another analysis of the MADIT-CRT, predictors of superresponse to CRT as defined by top quartile of left ventricular ejection fraction (LVEF) change were investigated; as a result, female gender was identified as an independent predictor of CRT superresponse (odds ratio [OR] 1.96; $P = .001$).[17] In a meta-analysis of 72 studies involving 33,434 patients, changes in echocardiographic parameters following CRT were compared between genders. Women were noted to have greater improvement in LVEF (+9.4% and +7.6% in women and in men, respectively, $P<.001$) as well as improvement in LV dimensions with CRT compared with men (left ventricular end systolic volume [LVESV]: -24.8 vs -13.5 in women vs men, $P<.001$; LVEDV: -22.7 vs -10.9 in women vs men, $P<.001$).[18] Another meta-analysis comprising 11 studies with a total of 149,259 patients similarly found that women underwent greater improvement in LVEF (standard mean difference [SMD] 0.25; 95% confidence interval [CI]: 0.07–0.43) and reduction in left ventricular end diastolic dimension (SMD: -0.27; 95% CI -0.39 to -0.25) following CRT compared with men.[24] No significant gender-based differences in change in LV volumes with CRT were noted in this study.

Clinical Outcomes

Studies suggest women derive at least equivalent, if not greater clinical therapeutic benefit following initiation of CRT compared with men. For example, COMPANION (women: 33%) and CARE-HF (women: 25%) studies found that although CRT was associated with significant clinical benefit in both men and women, they did not find difference in benefit between genders.[9,14] At the same time, however, numerous studies have also demonstrated greater clinical benefit of CRT in women. In the prespecified subgroup analysis of MADIT-CRT, Cardiac Resynchronization Therapy-Defibrillator (CRT-D) was associated with a greater benefit in the composite outcome of mortality and nonfatal HF events in women (hazard ratio [HR]: 0.37; 95% CI: 0.22–0.61) compared with men (HR: 0.76; 95% CI: 0.59–0.97) with significant interaction between gender and treatment ($P = .01$).[15] In a sex-specific outcome analysis of the MADIT-CRT, women had better clinical outcome from CRT-D compared with implantable cardioverter-defibrillator (ICD) alone than in men, with a significant 69% reduction in composite of death or HF (HR: 0.31 and $P<.001$ in women; HR: 0.72 and $P<.01$ in men; interaction $P<.01$).[19] Whereas CRT was associated with significant reduction in mortality in women ($P = .02$), similar mortality reduction was not seen in men.[19] Another subgroup analysis of the MADIT-CRT study limited to subjects with LBBB morphology similarly demonstrated greater clinical benefit of CRT in women with significant 71% reduction in HF or death (HR: 0.29; $P<.001$) and 77% reduction in HF alone (HR: 0.23; $P<.001$) compared with 41% reduction in HF or death (HR: 0.59; $P<.01$) and 50% reduction in HF alone (HR: 0.50, $P<.001$; interaction $P<.05$).[20]

The greater benefit conferred to women with CRT is also evident outside of the clinical trials. In an observational analysis of a large real-world patient population from the National Cardiovascular Data Registry, Zusterzeel and colleagues[21] examined sex-specific death risk in 75,079 patients with NYHA III or IV HF, reduced LVEF, and prolonged QRS receiving either CRT-D or ICD. Using propensity score analysis, women receiving CRT-D were found to have lower mortality risk than those receiving ICD (absolute difference: 11%; HR: 0.77; 95% CI 0.72–0.82; $P<.001$). Men receiving CRT-D also had lower risk of mortality compared with those with ICD, although to a lesser degree (absolute difference: 7%; HR: 0.88; 95% 0.85–0.92; $P<.001$); statistically significant difference in mortality was noted between sexes ($P<.001$). Furthermore, in a recent meta-analysis including 11 studies comprising 149,259 patients, women were demonstrated to have lower all-cause mortality with CRT than men (OR: 0.50; 95% CI 0.36–0.70).[24]

QRS Duration and Gender

Another important aspect in terms of gender difference in CRT response is that the effect of QRS duration on CRT response appears to be dependent on gender. In the previously mentioned sex-specific analysis of MADIT-CRT, women with

Table 1
Key studies demonstrating gender based differences in cardiac resynchronization therapy response

Author, y	Study Design	Title	Findings
Cheng et al,[18] 2014	Meta-analysis of 72 studies, 33,434 patients	More favorable response to cardiac resynchronization therapy in women than in men	Women had better outcomes from CRT compared with men: 33% reduction in mortality (HR 0.67, P<.001), 20% reduction in death or hospitalization for HF (HR 0.80, P<.001), and 41% reduction in cardiac mortality (HR 0.59, P<.001). Women demonstrated greater improvement in EF (+9.4% vs +7.6% in women vs men) and LV dimension (LVESV: −24.8 vs −13.5 in women vs men, P<.001; LVEDV: −22.7 vs −10.9 in women vs men, P<.001) with CRT compared with men
Arshad et al,[19] 2011	Sex-specific analysis of MADIT-CRT (n = 1820)	Cardiac resynchronization therapy is more effective in women than in men: The MADIT-CRT trial	Women had significantly better results from CRT than men with 69% reduction in death or HF (HR: 0.31, P<.001) and 70% reduction in HF alone (HR: 0.30, P<.001). Women with QRS <150 ms were found to derive clinical benefit in reduction in composite of death or HF (HR: 0.30, P<.01) with CRT while men did not (HR: 1.09; P<.66; interaction P<.01).
Biton et al,[20] 2015	Subgroup analysis of MADIT-CRT limited to LBBB	Sex Differences in Long-Term Outcomes with Cardiac Resynchronization Therapy in mild HF patients with left bundle branch block	Women experienced 71% reduction in HF or death (HR: 0.29; P<.001) and 77% reduction in HF alone (HR: 0.23; P<.001) compared with 41% reduction in HF or death (HR: 0.59; P<.01) and 50% reduction in HF alone in men (HF: 0.50; P<.001). Women with CRT-D had significant reduction in HF or mortality with QRS duration both below the 150 ms cutoff (HR: 0.32; 95% CI 0.14–0.76; P<.01) and above (HR: 0.27; 95% CI 0.17–0.45; P<.001). Men only showed improvement in outcomes when QRS duration was greater than or equal to 150 ms
Zusterzeel et al,[21] 2015	Large, real-world population of 7,509 patients with HF and prolonged QRS	Cardiac resynchronization therapy in women vs men: observational comparative effectiveness study from the national cardiovascular data registry	In a large real-world cohort with LBBB, women receiving CRT-D had lower risk of mortality compared those receiving ICD (absolute difference 11%; HR 0.74; 95% CI 0.68–0.81). Lower mortality with CRT-D compared with ICD in men was less pronounced (absolute difference 9%; HR 0.84, sex × device interaction P = .0025)
Varma et al,[22] 2014; Varma et al,[31] 2018	Retrospective analysis of 212 patients with NICM undergoing CRT	Probability and magnitude of response to cardiac resynchronization therapy according to QRS duration and gender in nonischemic cardiomyopathy and LBBB	86% of women vs 36% of men (P<.001) responded in the QRS <150 ms cohort; 83% vs 69% response rate in women and men, respectively, when QRS ≥150 ms (P = .05)

Abbreviation: NICM, nonischemic cardiomyopathy.

QRS less than 150 milliseconds were found to derive clinical benefit in reduction in composite of death or HF (HR: 0.30, P<.01) with CRT, whereas men did not (HR: 1.09; P<.66; interaction P<.01).[19] Analysis limited to patients with LBBB morphology also revealed that women with CRT-D had significant reduction in HF or mortality with QRS duration both below (HR: 0.32; 95% CI 0.14–0.76; P<.01) and above (HR: 0.27; 95% CI 0.17–0.45; P<.001) the 150-milliseconds cutoff.[20] Men, on the other hand, again only showed improvement in outcomes when QRS duration was greater than or equal to 150 milliseconds.[20] In an analysis of 212 patients with nonischemic cardiomyopathy and LBBB, Varma and colleagues[22] compared echocardiographic response to CRT on the basis of QRS duration and gender. In the overall cohort, a significantly higher response rate was seen with QRS ≥150 milliseconds compared with less than 150 milliseconds (76% vs 58%, respectively, P-.009). However, echoing the findings in the subgroup analyses of MADIT-CRT, the response rates on the basis of QRS differed between genders in this analysis. Eighty-six percent of women versus 36% of men (P<.001) responded in the QRS <150 milliseconds cohort; 83% versus 69% response rate in women and men, respectively, when QRS ≥150 milliseconds (P = .05).[22] Hence, although men, composing most of the study population, primarily showed benefit with CRT when QRS ≥150 milliseconds, women had a significant reduction in the composite outcome with therapy at both QRS <150 milliseconds and QRS ≥150 milliseconds.

WHY WOULD WOMEN RESPOND GREATER TO CARDIAC RESYNCHRONIZATION THERAPY?

It is not entirely clear why women would demonstrate greater benefit from CRT than men. It is also not clear whether female gender itself leads to improved outcome, or whether a characteristic more often associated with the female gender leads to the differences observed in response to CRT. Because nonischemic cardiomyopathy has been linked to more effective reverse remodeling in response to CRT, female preponderance for nonischemic cardiomyopathy has been suggested to explain improved therapeutic response seen in women.[25–27]

Another possible explanation for the gender-based difference in CRT response is the difference in baseline QRS duration between genders.[28] On average, healthy women have QRS duration that is 6 milliseconds shorter than men.[29] Accordingly, women have also been shown to have LBBB and LV dyssynchrony at narrower QRS duration compared with men.[28] Hence, at any given QRS duration, women might have more conduction disturbance and LV dyssynchrony than men, which are the target substrates for CRT explaining the improved clinical benefit seen in women.

It is also important to note that prolonged QRS may occur not only in the context of reduced conduction velocity but also from increased chamber dimension, which increases the "travel distance" of the propagating wavefront.[30,31] Stewart and colleagues[32] found that each 10-millisecond increase in QRS duration was associated with 8.3% increase in LV mass and 9.2% increase in LVEDV. QRS duration also has been also shown to correlate with body size.[32] Hence, by the virtue of large LV dimension and mass as well as body size, men may demonstrate prolonged QRS without LV dyssynchrony.

Whereas LBBB is associated with improved therapeutic response to CRT, one-third of patients diagnosed with LBBB by conventional criteria may not have true complete LBBB, and this miscategorization occurs more commonly in men.[33,34] This miscategorization combined with higher prevalence of LBBB in women has been hypothesized as another possible explanation for the gender-specific response to CRT.[28] In an analysis of MADIT-CRT limited to patients with LBBB, however, the clinical benefit of CRT-D was still greater among women, suggesting that female sex and not LBBB contributed to the observed benefit.[20]

However, in a recent meta-analysis of 5 RCTs, QRS duration and height, but not gender, were identified to be independent predictors of CRT benefit.[35] This study suggests that average shorter height of women and not the gender itself contributes to the improved outcome following CRT in women.

SHOULD WOMEN HAVE DIFFERENT SELECTION CRITERIA FOR CARDIAC RESYNCHRONIZATION THERAPY THAN MEN?

CRT has been shown to have a multitude of beneficial effects in a select patient with systolic HF: by enhancing reverse remodeling, improving quality of life and functional status, reducing risk of HF admission, and most importantly, by improving survival. Thus, there is a strong clinical mandate for the appropriate use of CRT in eligible patients. Nonetheless, echocardiographic and clinical responses to CRT are not uniform, and approximately one-third of recipients were considered nonresponders in clinical trials. Hence, refinement in the selection criteria to more accurately capture the group of patients most likely to respond to CRT is urgently needed.

As with many similar device-related trials in the past, the clinical trials on CRT also suffered from underrepresentation of women. However, women included in the study were found to derive greater benefit from CRT compared with men. Another highly clinically relevant point in terms of gender-based difference in response to CRT was that women benefited from CRT with QRS duration both above and below 150 milliseconds, whereas therapeutic benefit in men were limited to those with QRS duration greater than 150 milliseconds. Given that men comprised the significant majority of the study population in these clinical trials, the overall finding was a strong signal of benefit with CRT above QRS duration of 150 milliseconds.

Based on the clinical trials data, the current 2012 ACC/AHA/HRS guideline gives class I indication for CRT in patients with QRS duration ≥150 milliseconds, whereas giving a lower class II indication for those with QRS between 120 and 149 milliseconds.[2] The 2016 ESC guideline gives class I indication for both QRS duration ≥150 milliseconds and QRS 130 to 149 milliseconds, although with lower LOE for the latter recommendation.[13] Hence, these selection criteria, if followed strictly, have the potential to miss female patients with shorter QRS duration that have been demonstrated to benefit from CRT. Therefore, a refinement in the selection criteria for CRT is likely warranted based on the current evidence.

SUMMARY

CRT has been shown to have a multitude of beneficial effects in a select patient with systolic HF, by enhancing reverse remodeling, improving quality of life and functional status, reducing risk of HF admission, and most importantly, improving survival. Although women were relatively underrepresented in the clinical trials, they were demonstrated to derive greater therapeutic benefit from CRT compared with men. Importantly, women were noted to derive benefit at a smaller degree of QRS prolongation than men, well below the now generally accepted cutoff of QRS ≥150 milliseconds. Given the difference in response to CRT based on QRS duration between genders, further refinement in the current selection criteria may be considered.

REFERENCES

1. Lloyd-Jones DM, Wang TJ, Leip EP, et al. Lifetime risk for development of atrial fibrillation: the framingham heart study. Circulation 2004;110(9):1042–6.

2. Tracy CM, Epstein AE, Darbar D, et al. 2012 ACCF/AHA/HRS focused update incorporated into the ACCF/AHA/HRS 2008 guidelines for device-based therapy of cardiac rhythm abnormalities: a report of the American college of cardiology foundation/American heart association task force on practice guide. J Am Coll Cardiol 2013;61(3): e6–75.

3. Ponikowski P, Voors AA, Anker SD, et al. 2016 ESC guidelines for the diagnosis and treatment of acute and chronic heart failure: the Task Force for the diagnosis and treatment of acute and chronic heart failure of the European Society of Cardiology (ESC)Developed with the special contribution of the Heart Failure Association (HFA) of the ESC. Eur Heart J 2016;37(27): 2129–200.

4. Khan NK, Goode KM, Cleland JGF, et al. Prevalence of ECG abnormalities in an international survey of patients with suspected or confirmed heart failure at death or discharge. Eur J Heart Fail 2007;9(5): 491–501.

5. Masci PG, Marinelli M, Piacenti M, et al. Myocardial structural, perfusion, and metabolic correlates of left bundle branch block mechanical derangement in patients with dilated cardiomyopathy: a tagged cardiac magnetic resonance and positron emission tomography study. Circ Cardiovasc Imaging 2010; 3(4):482–90.

6. Ukkonen H, Sundell J, Knuuti J. Effects of CRT on myocardial innervation, perfusion and metabolism. Europace 2008;10(Supplement 3):iii114–7.

7. Yu C-M, Chau E, Sanderson JE, et al. Tissue Doppler echocardiographic evidence of reverse remodeling and improved synchronicity by simultaneously delaying regional contraction after biventricular pacing therapy in heart failure. Circulation 2002;105(4):438–45. Available at: http://www.ncbi.nlm.nih.gov/pubmed/11815425. Accessed August 11, 2018.

8. Saxon LA, De Marco T, Schafer J, et al. Effects of long-term biventricular stimulation for resynchronization on echocardiographic measures of remodeling. Circulation 2002;105(11):1304–10.

9. Bristow MR, Saxon LA, Boehmer J, et al. Cardiac-resynchronization therapy with or without an implantable defibrillator in advanced chronic heart failure. N Engl J Med 2004;350(21):2140–50.

10. Tang ASL, Wells GA, Talajic M, et al. Cardiac-resynchronization therapy for mild-to-moderate heart failure. N Engl J Med 2010;363(25):1757–65.

11. Linde C, Abraham WT, Gold MR, et al. Randomized trial of cardiac resynchronization in mildly symptomatic heart failure patients and in asymptomatic patients with left ventricular dysfunction and previous heart failure symptoms. J Am Coll Cardiol 2008; 52(23):1834–43.

12. Young JB, Abraham WT, Smith AL, et al. Combined cardiac resynchronization and implantable cardioversion defibrillation in advanced chronic heart failure. JAMA 2003;289(20):2685.

13. Ponikowski P, Voors A, Anker S, et al. 2016 ESC guidelines for the diagnosis and treatment of acute and chronic heart failure: the task force for the diagnosis and treatment of acute and chronic heart failure of the European Society of Cardiology (ESC). Developed with the special contribution of the Heart Failure Association (HFA) of the ESC. Eur J Heart Fail 2016;18:891–975.

14. Cleland JGF, Daubert J-C, Erdmann E, et al. The effect of cardiac resynchronization on morbidity and mortality in heart failure. N Engl J Med 2005;352(15):1539–49.

15. Moss AJ, Hall WJ, Cannom DS, et al. Cardiac-resynchronization therapy for the prevention of heart-failure events. N Engl J Med 2009;361(14):1329–38.

16. Herz ND, Engeda J, Zusterzeel R, et al. Sex differences in device therapy for heart failure: utilization, outcomes, and adverse events. J Womens Health 2015;24(4):261–71.

17. Hsu JC, Solomon SD, Bourgoun M, et al. Predictors of super-response to cardiac resynchronization therapy and associated improvement in clinical outcome: the MADIT-CRT (Multicenter Automatic Defibrillator Implantation Trial with Cardiac Resynchronization Therapy) study. J Am Coll Cardiol 2012;59(25):2366–73.

18. Cheng Y-J, Zhang J, Li W-J, et al. More favorable response to cardiac resynchronization therapy in women than in men. Circ Arrhythm Electrophysiol 2014;7(5):807–15.

19. Arshad A, Moss AJ, Foster E, et al. Cardiac resynchronization therapy is more effective in women than in men: the MADIT-CRT (multicenter automatic defibrillator implantation trial with cardiac resynchronization therapy) trial. J Am Coll Cardiol 2011;57(7):813–20.

20. Biton Y, Zareba W, Goldenberg I, et al. Sex differences in long-term outcomes with cardiac resynchronization therapy in mild heart failure patients with left bundle branch block. J Am Heart Assoc 2015;4(7). https://doi.org/10.1161/JAHA.115.002013.

21. Zusterzeel R, Spatz ES, Curtis JP, et al. Cardiac resynchronization therapy in women versus men: observational comparative effectiveness study from the national cardiovascular data registry. Circ Cardiovasc Qual Outcomes 2015;8:S4–11.

22. Varma N, Manne M, Nguyen D, et al. Probability and magnitude of response to cardiac resynchronization therapy according to QRS duration and gender in nonischemic cardiomyopathy and LBBB. Heart Rhythm 2014;11(7):1139–47.

23. Goldenberg I, Moss AJ, Hall WJ, et al. Predictors of response to cardiac resynchronization therapy in the multicenter automatic defibrillator implantation trial with cardiac resynchronization therapy (MADIT-CRT). Circulation 2011;124(14):1527–36.

24. Yin F-H, Fan C-L, Guo Y-Y, et al. The impact of gender difference on clinical and echocardiographic outcomes in patients with heart failure after cardiac resynchronization therapy: a systematic review and meta-analysis. Plos One 2017;12(4):e0176248.

25. Gasparini M, Regoli F, Ceriotti C, et al. Remission of left ventricular systolic dysfunction and of heart failure symptoms after cardiac resynchronization therapy: temporal pattern and clinical predictors. Am Heart J 2008;155(3):507–14.

26. Woo GW, Petersen-Stejskal S, Johnson JW, et al. Ventricular reverse remodeling and 6-month outcomes in patients receiving cardiac resynchronization therapy: analysis of the MIRACLE Study. J Interv Card Electrophysiol 2005;12(2):107–13.

27. Frazier CG, Alexander KP, Newby LK, et al. Associations of gender and etiology with outcomes in heart failure with systolic dysfunction. A pooled analysis of 5 randomized control trials. J Am Coll Cardiol 2007;49(13):1450–8.

28. Linde C, Stahlberg M, Benson L, et al. Gender, underutilization of cardiac resynchronization therapy, and prognostic impact of QRS prolongation and left bundle branch block in heart failure. Europace 2015;17:424–31.

29. Macfarlane PW, McLaughlin SC, Devine B, et al. Effects of age, sex, and race on ECG interval measurements. J Electrocardiol 1994;27(Suppl):14–9. Available at: http://www.ncbi.nlm.nih.gov/pubmed/7884351. Accessed August 12, 2018.

30. Surawicz B, Childers R, Deal BJ, et al. AHA/ACCF/HRS recommendations for the standardization and interpretation of the electrocardiogram. Part III: intraventricular conduction disturbances a scientific statement from the American Heart Association Electrocardiography and Arrhythmias Committee. J Am Coll Cardiol 2009;53(11):976–81.

31. Varma N, Sogaard P, Bax JJ, et al. Interaction of left ventricular size and sex on outcome of cardiac resynchronization therapy among patients with a narrow QRS duration in the EchoCRT trial. J Am Heart Assoc 2018;7(11). https://doi.org/10.1161/JAHA.118.009592.

32. Stewart RA, Young AA, Anderson C, et al. Relationship between QRS duration and left ventricular mass and volume in patients at high cardiovascular risk. Heart 2011;97(21):1766–70.

33. Strauss DG, Selvester RH, Wagner GS. Defining left bundle branch block in the era of cardiac resynchronization therapy. Am J Cardiol 2010;107(6):927–34.

34. Loring Z, Caños DA, Selzman K, et al. Left bundle branch block predicts better survival in women than men receiving cardiac resynchronization therapy: long-term follow-up of ~145,000 patients. JACC Heart Fail 2013;1(3): 237–44.

35. Linde C, Cleland JGF, Gold MR, et al. The interaction of sex, height, and QRS duration on the effects of cardiac resynchronization therapy on morbidity and mortality: an individual-patient data meta-analysis. Eur J Heart Fail 2018;20(4): 780–91.

Increasing Role of Remote Monitoring of Cardiac Resynchronization Therapy Devices in Improving Outcomes

Suneet Mittal, MD

KEYWORDS

• Cardiac resynchronization therapy • Outcomes • Remote monitoring

KEY POINTS

- Remote monitoring has become an essential component of the care of patients with a cardiac implantable electronic device, including those undergoing CRT-D implantations.
- It allows for earlier detection of battery- and lead-related issues, atrial and ventricular arrhythmias, and may facilitate early identification of patients at risk for developing an exacerbation of heart failure.
- Some randomized studies have shown no benefit in comparison with usual in-office follow-up, whereas other randomized and large observational studies have shown favorable benefits with respect to stroke, appropriate and inappropriate shocks, prevention of heart failure–related hospitalizations, overall health care use, and survival.
- Additional studies are ongoing to determine how best to detect heart failure in these patients and how best to manage these patients based on the information.

INTRODUCTION

Current guidelines from the Heart Rhythm Society advocate that all patients with a cardiac implantable electronic device should be offered remote monitoring as part of the standard follow-up management strategy.[1] Virtually all cardiac implantable electronic devices are capable of remote follow-up; increasingly, all devices being implanted are capable of wireless remote monitoring. There is now a wealth of scientific data supporting the clinical value of remote monitoring in patients with a cardiac implantable electronic device; as a result, in the United States there is a well-defined reimbursement policy for remote follow-up and/or monitoring. This article reviews the increasing role of remote monitoring of cardiac resynchronization therapy (CRT) devices in improving patient outcomes.

CASE PRESENTATION

A 64-year-old man with mild hypertension presented with acute decompensated heart failure. His presenting electrocardiogram (ECG) showed sinus tachycardia with left bundle branch block; the QRS duration was 162 milliseconds (**Fig. 1**). Laboratory data were unremarkable. Echocardiography showed severe global left ventricular (LV) dysfunction; cardiac catheterization showed elevated filling pressure, but no underlying coronary disease. The patient was diuresed and begun on guideline-directed medical therapy with carvedilol, spironolactone, and sacubitril/valsartan, which were uptitrated to the maximal tolerated doses. However, 3 months later, the patient had persistent class II heart failure symptoms and repeat imaging showed persistent LV dysfunction. He was referred for implantation of a CRT-defibrillator (CRT-D).

Relevant disclosures: Consultant to Abbott, Boston Scientific, and Medtronic.
Electrophysiology Laboratory, The Valley Hospital, Valley Health System, Snyder Center for Comprehensive Atrial Fibrillation, 223 North Van Dien Avenue, Ridgewood, NJ 07450, USA
E-mail address: mittsu@valleyhealth.com

Card Electrophysiol Clin 11 (2019) 123–130
https://doi.org/10.1016/j.ccep.2018.11.011
1877-9182/19/© 2018 Elsevier Inc. All rights reserved.

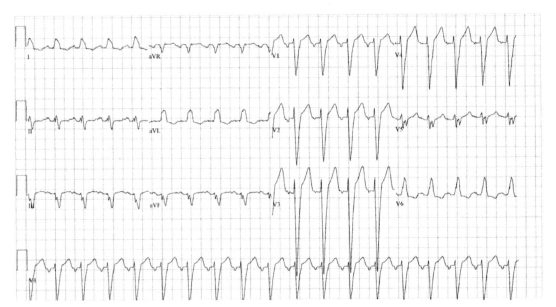

Fig. 1. Electrocardiogram. The underlying rhythm is sinus. The patient has left bundle branch block with a QRS duration of 162 milliseconds.

LEFT VENTRICULAR REVERSE REMODELING

Proper patient selection for CRT, optimal LV lead location, and evidence-based device programming are critical to achieve LV reverse remodeling, which has been associated with improved patient outcomes.[2,3] However, this cannot be achieved in a significant number of patients. Common reasons for a suboptimal response include improper device programming, suboptimal medical treatment, arrhythmias (eg, atrial fibrillation, ventricular ectopy), inappropriate lead position, or poor patient selection.[4] Thus, proper patient follow-up is an essential component of the care of the post-CRT patient. Increasingly, it is being recognized that continuous remote monitoring of these devices and patients, as opposed to relying on a calendar-based follow-up strategy, is associated with improved clinical outcomes.

THE EVOLUTION OF THE REMOTE MONITORING STORY

Initial randomized studies were designed to demonstrate that remote monitoring could shorten the time from the occurrence of clinical events to ability of clinicians to act on these events. The CONNECT (Clinical Evaluation of Remote Notification to Reduce Time to Clinical Decision) trial was designed to determine the impact of wireless remote monitoring with automatic clinician alerts on the time from clinical events to clinical decisions and on health care utilization.[5] In this multicenter, prospective, randomized clinical trial, 1997 patients from 136 centers implanted with an implantable cardioverter defibrillator (ICD) with or without CRT were randomized to undergo wireless remote monitoring versus standard in-office follow-up and followed for 15 months. Remote monitoring was associated with a significant decrease in the median time from clinical event to clinical decision (22 to 4.6 days; P<.001) and mean length of stay per cardiovascular hospitalization (from 4 to 3.3 days; P = .002). However, no data were provided about whether a difference was observed between patients who underwent an ICD implant and those who underwent a CRT-D implant.

The ALTITUDE survival (observational) study compared survival between ICD and CRT-D patients followed solely in-office and patients who were regularly transmitted remote data from the device to a central network on an average of four times monthly.[6] The study included 30,010 CRT-D patients using remote monitoring and 47,741 CRT-D patients who were undergoing in-office follow-up only. Patients on the network had a 55% lower mortality than nonnetworked patients (hazard ratio [HR], 0.45; 95% confidence interval [CI], 0.388–0.532; P<.001).

This directionality was confirmed in the IN-TIME study, which was a prospective, randomized clinical trial.[7] This trial randomized 664 patients (390 [59%] patients with a CRT-D) at 36 clinical centers; patients had chronic heart failure, no permanent atrial fibrillation, and a recent dual chamber ICD or CRT-D. Patients were randomized to undergo telemonitoring or not and followed for a year. The primary endpoint was a composite clinical score combing all-cause death, overnight hospital admission for heart failure, change in New York Heart Association class, and a change in patient global self-assessment. The telemonitoring group had a significantly lower composite score (18.9% vs 27.2% in the control group; P = .013).

A subsequent large observational study confirmed the association between remote monitoring and survival in patients with an implanted device; of the 269,471 patients evaluated, a CRT-D was present in 61,475 (23%) patients.[8] Overall, only 48% of the CRT-D patients were enrolled into remote monitoring. The study showed that the highest survival was observed in patients who were enrolled in remote monitoring and were highly adherent (>75%) with as assessed by weekly connectivity. During a mean follow-up of 2.91 years, CRT-D patients with high adherence to remote monitoring had greater survival than patients with low adherence (HR, 1.28; 95% CI, 1.20–1.36; P<.001) and those that were not remotely monitored at all (HR, 2.11; 95% CI, 2.00–2.22; P<.001).

Many of these survival studies have included patients implanted with devices from a single manufacturer. Thus, there has been an unmet clinical need to understand the impact of remote monitoring in a population of patients being implanted with devices from all manufacturers. The Contemporary Modalities In Treatment of Heart Failure Registry (COMMIT-HF) is a prospective observational registry designed to answer this question. The authors recently reported on 1429 consecutive patients with heart failure who were enrolled in the registry; 822 patients with initial implant of an ICD (~70%) or CRT-D (~30%) were selected for further analysis.[9] They ultimately matched 287 patients on remote monitoring to an equal number of patients not on remote monitoring. In this study, 5.1% of patients were remotely monitored on the (Medtronic Carelink system, Minneapolis, MN), 72% of patients were remotely monitored on the (St. Jude Medical Merlin system, St. Paul, MN), and 22.9% of patients were remotely monitored on the (Biotronik Home Monitoring system, Berlin, Germany). The 1- and 3-year mortality was significantly lower in the remote monitoring group (2.1% remote monitoring [+] vs 11.5% remote monitoring [-], P<.0001; and 4.9% remote monitoring [+] vs 22.3% remote monitoring [-], P<.0001, respectively.)

Remote monitoring has also been shown to reduce health care use. A recent study evaluated 92,566 patients who underwent device implantation; this included 10,230 (11%) patients with a CRT device.[10] Only 37% of the total cohort was enrolled into remote monitoring; these patients had lower risk of all-cause hospitalization (adjusted HR, 0.82; 95% CI, 0.80–0.84; P<.001), shorter mean length of hospitalization (5.3 vs 8.1 days; P<.001), and 30% reduction in hospitalization costs. The benefit of remote monitoring was greatest in the CRT-D patients who underwent remote monitoring. As compared with patients who did not undergo remote monitoring, CRT-D patients undergoing remote monitoring had a lower hospitalization cost per patient-year ($12,425 vs $22,574; P<.001), lower hospitalizations per patient-year (0.46 vs 0.65; P<.001), lower days in hospital per patient-year (2.8 vs 4.7; P<.001), and adjusted HR for hospitalization (0.72; 95% CI, 0.67–0.77; P<.001).

MECHANISM OF BENEFIT
Lead Complications

Remote monitoring can assist with early identification of lead-related complications (**Table 1**). In a recent study, a median of 1224 ICD patients, 30% of whom had a CRT-D device, were remotely monitored with comprehensive analysis of all transmitted materials.[11] During a follow-up of 4457 patient years there were 64 lead failures (10 caused by failure of the high-voltage component and 54 caused by failure of the pace-sense component). Use of remote monitoring allowed a diagnosis to be made before occurrence of a clinical complication in 61 (95%) patients; delivery of an inappropriate shock was prevented in nearly every patient. However, reliance on impedance-based alerts is insufficient to detect all types of lead failures. In fact, lead failure may be more likely to present as an arrhythmic event, highlighting the need to carefully adjudicate all stored alert electrograms.[12]

Atrial Arrhythmias

Atrial fibrillation is noted in 20% to 40% of patient following implantation of a CRT-D.[13] Atrial fibrillation contributes to suboptimal response to CRT by decreasing the percentage of effective LV pacing. In addition, patients with atrial fibrillation have a higher incidence of inappropriate and appropriate shocks. In many patients, atrioventricular (AV) junction ablation becomes necessary to ensure proper response to CRT.[14] Thus, early recognition of the occurrence of atrial fibrillation may be of value in these patients.

As an example, the HomeGuide study enrolled 1650 patients, a quarter of whom had either a CRT-D or CRT-pacemaker, who were monitored using a daily transmission remote monitoring system with automatic alerts for atrial fibrillation.[15] During the study period, 810 episodes of atrial

Table 1
Value proposition of remote monitoring in cardiac resynchronization therapy–defibrillator patients

Parameter	Finding	Troubleshooting
Battery	End of life Malfunction	Assess need for generator replacement
Lead-related issues	Significant change in pacing impedance Significant change in pacing threshold Detection of noise	Assess integrity of leads
Percentage left ventricular pacing	High % LV pacing, high % effective LV pacing High % LV pacing, low % effective LV pacing Low % LV pacing, low % effective LV pacing	Optimal, desired state Identify cause for fusion or pseudofusion Reprogram AV interval, consider AV junction ablation in AF patients, suppress ventricular ectopy
Arrhythmia-related issues	Atrial tachyarrhythmias Premature ventricular ectopy Sustained ventricular arrhythmias	Assess for need for antiarrhythmic medications and/or catheter ablation
Heart failure exacerbation	Vendor dependent	Precise management algorithm remains yet undefined

Abbreviations: AF, atrial fibrillation; AV, atrioventricular.

fibrillation or tachycardia were observed in 18% of patients (two-thirds of whom had no prior history of atrial fibrillation); 93% of these episodes were detected via remote monitoring. Medical interventions occurred in 305 episodes; the incidence of thromboembolism was low, less than half of what was expected based on the patient's underlying CHA_2DS_2-VASc profile.

Loss of Left Ventricular Pacing

A basic premise for CRT is that near 100% LV pacing must be delivered to ensure maximal response.[16] Even slight reductions in the percentage of LV pacing delivered can significantly adversely impact patient outcomes. Factors associated with reduced LV pacing include the following: (1) intrinsic AV conduction "faster" than programmed sensed/paced AV interval; (2) arrhythmias, such as atrial fibrillation and ventricular ectopy[17–19]; and (3) loss of LV pacing because of dislodgment, suboptimal pacing vector, or lack of capture of the LV lead. Newer algorithms can differentiate between the overall percentage of pacing that effectively captures the LV from ineffective pacing (**Fig. 2**); furthermore, automated algorithms have the ability to perturb the pacing rate during atrial fibrillation to ensure maximal effective LV pacing.[20,21]

Heart Failure Decompensation

Multiple attempts have been made to identify patients with a defibrillator who may be at high risk for heart failure decompensation. However, initial trials relied on a single parameter (eg, transthoracic impedance as a surrogate for lung fluid accumulation; weight and blood pressure) as a marker of the high-risk patient and have largely failed to demonstrate a conclusive benefit. As an example, a recent trial evaluated 18,289 patients implanted with an ICD or CRT-D; 10,908 (60%) of these patients had a CRT-D device.[22] These patients were significantly more likely to be undergoing assessment of weight and blood pressure. However, this assessment failed to decrease cardiovascular, heart failure, or all-cause hospitalization or mortality.

In contrast, a multiparametric approach seems to be more promising. A recent study assessed heart rate, accelerator-based heart sounds, respiration rate, relative tidal volume, activity, and intrathoracic impedance in CRT-D patients.[23] Patients were considered to have had a heart failure event if they were admitted and incurred a calendar day change or received one or more intravenous medications. A proprietary algorithm was developed based on an initial sample and then tested in an independent sample; it had a sensitivity of 70% to

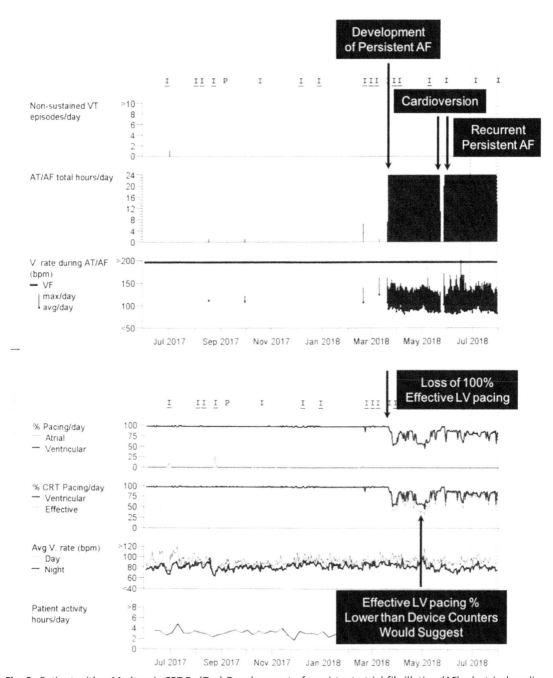

Fig. 2. Patient with a Medtronic CRT-D. (*Top*) Development of persistent atrial fibrillation (AF); electrical cardioversion was able to maintain sinus rhythm for only a few days. (*Bottom*) The development of AF results in an immediate decline in LV pacing percentage. The actual percentage of effective LV pacing (*dashed line*) is even lower than that suggested by the percentage of LV pacing diagnostic alone (*solid line*).

detect worsening heart failure at a median of 34 days *before* to onset of the event. Additional studies are ongoing to determine the impact of this algorithm on clinical outcomes in high-risk patients, such as those undergoing CRT-D implantation.

Case Vignette

A 68-year-old morbidly obese man (6 foot, 3 inches; 390 pounds; body mass index, 48.7) with hypertension was referred in October 2014 for evaluation and management of persistent atrial

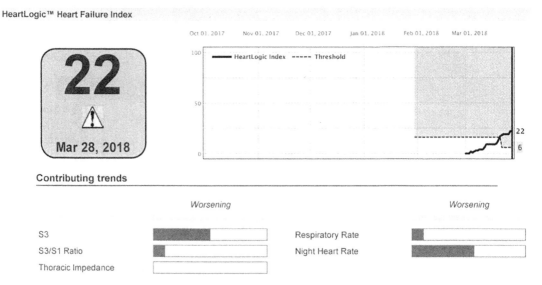

Fig. 3. Elevated HeartLogic heart failure index. This patient underwent implantation of a CRT-D on January 30, 2018. On March 28, 2018, a remote monitoring alert was received because the heart failure index had crossed the prespecified threshold of 16. The largest contributors to the index seemed to be the S3 and nighttime heart rate.

fibrillation. He had previously undergone electrical cardioversion in December 2011 and September 2014; in both instances, sinus rhythm held for a while, but then persistent atrial fibrillation recurred. Importantly, the patient had no symptoms referable to atrial fibrillation.

At his visit in October 2014, his ECG showed atrial fibrillation with a ventricular rate of 98 bpm. There was left axis deviation. The corrected QT interval was 480 milliseconds; thus, amiodarone was considered the only viable antiarrhythmic drug option. An echocardiogram showed mild mitral regurgitation and normal LV function. Following an extensive shared medical decision regarding the pros and cons of the various therapeutic options, a decision was made to pursue rate control, anticoagulation, and bariatric surgery for weight loss.

The patient underwent gastric sleeve surgery in November 2014. By July 2015, he had lost 108 pounds. ECG showed atrial fibrillation; however, the corrected QT interval was now normal. In addition, for the first time, the patient complained of fatigue. Thus, in August 2015, he was admitted for initiation of dofetilide. The maximal tolerated dose was 125 µg every 12 hours; he was successfully cardioverted to sinus rhythm. A month later, he remained in sinus rhythm but reported no change in his symptoms. Atrial fibrillation recurred in January 2016; dofetilide was stopped.

He did well until August 2017 when he reported worsening fatigue. A 24-hour Holter showed atrial fibrillation with controlled ventricular rates. An echocardiogram showed severe mitral regurgitation. He underwent successful percutaneous clipping of his mitral valve; a follow-up echocardiogram showed no significant mitral regurgitation and new LV dysfunction (ejection fraction, 35%), despite ongoing therapy with metoprolol and lisinopril. He was referred for ICD implantation for primary prevention of sudden death. A single-chamber transvenous system was implanted on January 30, 2018. The device contained a multiparametric sensor for detection of heart failure decompensation.

On March 22, 2018, an alert was received because the sensor (HeartLogic Heart Failure Index, Boston Scientific, St. Pula, MN) had crossed its prespecified threshold of 16. The patient was referred to the heart failure service, where was seen a week later by which time the sensor showed further deterioration (from 18 to 22; **Fig. 3**). This was largely driven by two parameters: the S3 and nighttime heart rate. The patient was transitioned from lisinopril to sacubitril/valsartan, which was then up-titrated to maximal tolerated dose. On April 21, 2018, the sensor returned to normal (index = 3). The patient could be managed on an outpatient basis throughout this process.

A second study reported similar findings. The TRIAGE-HF study assessed 100 patients, 69 (69%) of whom had a CRT-D device.[24] A low- (heart failure hospitalization rate of 0.6% in the next 30 days), medium- (heart failure hospitalization rate of 1.3% in the next 30 days), or high-risk (heart failure hospitalization rate of 6.8% in the next 30 days) heart failure risk score was generated for each patient using the following parameters: thoracic impedance, patient activity, night heart rate, heart rate variability, percent LV pacing, atrial fibrillation/flutter burden, ventricular rate during atrial fibrillation/flutter, and detected arrhythmia episodes/therapies delivered. Signs and symptoms of heart failure and noncompliance with prescribed therapies were identified in approximately 85% of patients with a high-risk heart failure risk score.

NEGATIVE STUDIES

Not all studies have shown a favorable impact of remote monitoring. The MORE-CARE trial was a prospective trial in which 865 patients who underwent implantation of a *de novo* Medtronic CRT-D device were randomized to undergo remote checks alternating with in-office follow-up every 4 months or in-office follow-up every 4 months alone.[25] For patients in the remote arm, automatic alerts for system integrity, atrial tachyarrhythmias, and lung fluid accumulation were programmed. The primary endpoint was a composite of death and cardiovascular and device-related hospitalizations lasting greater than 48 hours. During a median follow-up of 2 years, there was no difference in either the individual components of the primary endpoint or the primary composite endpoint between the two groups. There was, however, a 38% reduction in health care use in the remote arm driven by a reduction in need for in-office visits.

Similarly, the REM-HF study randomized 1650 device patients (approximately two-thirds had either a CRT-pacemaker or CRT-D) with heart failure to active remote monitoring or usual care.[26] The primary endpoint was time to first unplanned hospitalization for a cardiovascular reason or death. Secondary endpoints included death from any cause, death from cardiovascular reasons, death from cardiovascular reasons and unplanned cardiovascular hospitalization, unplanned cardiovascular hospitalization, and unplanned hospitalization. During a mean follow-up of 2.8 years, no difference in any primary or secondary endpoint between the two groups was observed. A major challenge in using device-based alerts alone to identify high-risk patients is that many important determinants of heart failure decompensation cannot be precisely captured; these include, medication/diet nonadherence, socioeconomic factors, infection and pulmonary processes, worsening renal function, hypertension, arrhythmias, and ischemia.[27]

SUMMARY

Remote monitoring has become an essential component of the care of patients with a cardiac implantable electronic device, including those undergoing CRT-D implantations. It allows for earlier detection of battery- and lead-related issue, atrial and ventricular arrhythmias, and may facilitate early identification of patients at risk for developing an exacerbation of heart failure. The data for the clinical utility of remote monitoring have been mixed. Some randomized studies have shown no benefit in comparison with usual in-office follow-up, whereas other randomized and large observational studies have shown favorable benefits with respect to stroke, appropriate and inappropriate shocks, prevention of heart failure–related hospitalizations, overall health care use, and survival. Additional studies are ongoing to determine how best to detect heart failure in these patients and how best to manage these patients based on the information.

REFERENCES

1. Slotwiner D, Varma N, Akar JG, et al. HRS expert consensus statement on remote interrogation and monitoring for cardiovascular electronic implantable devices. Heart Rhythm 2015;2:e69–100.
2. Ypenburg C, van Bommel RJ, Borleffs CJW, et al. Long-term prognosis after cardiac resynchronization therapy is related to the extent of left ventricular reverse remodeling at midterm follow-up. J Am Coll Cardiol 2009;53:483–90.
3. Rickard J, Cheng A, Spragg D, et al. Durability of the survival effect of cardiac resynchronization therapy by level of left ventricular functional improvement: fate of "nonresponders". Heart Rhythm 2014;11: 412–6.
4. Mullens W, Grimm RA, Verga T, et al. Insights from a cardiac resynchronization optimization clinic as part of a heart failure disease management program. J Am Coll Cardiol 2009;53:765–73.
5. Crossley GH, Boyle A, Vitense H, et al, for the CONNECT investigators. The CONNECT (clinical evaluation of remote notification to reduce time to clinical decision) trial. J Am Coll Cardiol 2011;57: 1181–9.
6. Saxon LA, Hayes DL, Gilliam FR, et al. Long-term outcome after ICD and CRT implantation and influence of remote device follow-up: the ALTITUDE survival study. Circulation 2010;122:2359–67.
7. Hindricks G, Taborsky M, Glikson M, et al, for the IN-TIME study group. Implant-based multiparameter telemonitoring of patients with heart failure (IN-TIME): a randomized controlled trial. Lancet 2014; 384:583–90.

8. Varma N, Piccini JP, Snell J, et al. The relationship between level of adherence to automatic wireless remote monitoring and survival in pacemaker and defibrillator patients. J Am Coll Cardiol 2015;65: 2601–10.

9. Kurek A, Tajstra M, Gadula-Gacek E, et al. Impact of remote monitoring on long-term prognosis in heart failure patients in a real-world cohort: results from all-comers COMMIT-HF trial. J Cardiovasc Electrophysiol 2017;28:425–31.

10. Piccini JP, Mittal S, Snell J, et al. Impact of remote monitoring on clinical events and associated health care utilization: a nationwide assessment. Heart Rhythm 2016;13:2279–86.

11. Ploux S, Swerdlow CD, Strik M, et al. Towards eradication of inappropriate therapies for ICD lead failure by combining comprehensive remote monitoring and lead noise alerts. J Cardiovasc Electrophysiol 2018. https://doi.org/10.1111/jce.13653.

12. Nishii N, Miyoshi A, Kubo M, et al. Analysis of arrhythmic events is useful to detect lead failure in patients followed by remote monitoring. J Cardiovasc Electrophysiol 2018;29:463–70.

13. Upadhyay G, Steinberg JS. Managing atrial fibrillation in the CRT patient: controversy or consensus? Heart Rhythm 2012;9:S51–9.

14. Gasparini M, Leclercq C, Lunati M, et al. Cardiac resynchronization therapy in patients with atrial fibrillation: the CERTIFY study (cardiac resynchronization therapy in atrial fibrillation patients multinational registry). JACC Heart Fail 2013;1:500–7.

15. Ricci RP, Vaccari D, Morichelli L, et al. Stroke incidence in patients with cardiac implantable electronic devices remotely controlled with automatic alerts of atrial fibrillation. A sub-analysis of the HomeGuide study. Int J Cardiol 2016;291:251–6.

16. Koplan BA, Kaplan AJ, Weiner S, et al. Heart failure decompensation and all-cause mortality in relation to percentage biventricular pacing in patients with heart failure: is a goal of 100% biventricular pacing necessary? J Am Coll Cardiol 2009;53:355–60.

17. Kamath GS, Cotiga D, Koneru JN, et al. The utility of 12-lead Holter monitoring in patients with permanent atrial fibrillation for the identification of non-responders after cardiac resynchronization therapy. J Am Coll Cardiol 2009;53:1050–5.

18. Mittal S, Aktas MK, Moss AJ, et al. The impact of nonsustained ventricular tachycardia on reverse remodeling, heart failure, and treated ventricular tachyarrhythmias in MADIT-CRT. J Cardiovasc Electrophysiol 2014. https://doi.org/10.1111/jce.12456.

19. Ruwald M, Mittal S, Ruwald AC, et al. Association between frequency of atrial and ventricular ectopic beats to biventricular pacing percentage and outcomes in patients with cardiac resynchronization therapy. J Am Coll Cardiol 2014;64:971–81.

20. Ghosh S, Stadler RW, Mittal S. Automated detection of effective left-ventricular pacing: going beyond percentage pacing counters. Europace 2015;17: 1555–62.

21. Plummer CJ, Frank CM, Bari Z, et al. A novel algorithm increases the delivery of effective cardiac resynchronization therapy during atrial fibrillation: the CRTee randomized crossover trial. Heart Rhythm 2018;15:369–75.

22. Al-Chekakie MO, Bao H, Jones PW, et al. Addition of blood pressure and weight transmissions to standard remote monitoring of implantable defibrillators and its association with mortality and rehospitalization. Circ Cardiovasc Qual Outcomes 2017;10: e005087.

23. Boehmer JP, Hariharan R, Devecchi FG, et al. A multisensor algorithm predicts heart failure events in patients with implanted devices: results from the MULTISENSE study. JACC Heart Fail 2017;5: 216–25.

24. Virani SA, Sharma V, McCann M, et al. Prospective evaluation of integrated device diagnostics for heart failure management: results of the TRIAGE-HF study. ESC Heart Fail 2018. https://doi.org/10.1002/ehf2.12309.

25. Boriani G, Da Costa A, Quesada A, et al. Effects of remote monitoring on clinical outcomes and use of healthcare resources in heart failure patients with biventricular defibrillators: results of the MORE-CARE multicenter randomized controlled trial. Eur J Heart Fail 2017;19:416–25.

26. Morgan JM, Kitt S, Gill J, et al. Remote management of heart failure using implantable electronic devices. Eur Heart J 2017;38:2352–60.

27. Hawkins NM, Virani SA, Sperrin M, et al. Predicting heart failure decompensation using cardiac implantable electronic devices: a review of practices and challenges. Eur J Heart Fail 2016;18:977–86.

Explanting Chronic Coronary Sinus Leads

Theofanie Mela, MD

KEYWORDS

• Left ventricular lead • Coronary sinus lead • Extraction • Cardiac resynchronization therapy

KEY POINTS

- Most coronary sinus leads are generally easy leads to extract, but the operators need to be familiar with the technique.
- Laser application inside the coronary sinus should be avoided for the risk of perforation.
- The infrequently used active fixation coronary sinus leads pose a challenge for the operator of the extraction and risk for the patient.
- Reimplantation of a coronary sinus lead may present more challenges than with the primary implantation.

Cardiac resynchronization therapy (CRT) has become the gold standard for patients with systolic left ventricular (LV) function, LV ejection fraction (LVEF) less than or equal to 35%, wide complex QRS, and symptomatic heart failure.[1–4] A total of 374,202 CRT procedures were recorded in Nationwide Inpatient Sample database from 2002 to 2010 in the United States.[5] The annual implantation volume ranged from 43,000 to 57,000 implants, with most of them being CRT with defibrillator. This number has steadily increased in subsequent years because of the expanding indications for CRT and the improved ability to perform these procedures successfully. During the earlier years, most patients receiving CRT were in New York Heart Association functional class III-IV heart failure. In subsequent years, the expanding indications included patients with New York Heart Association functional class II. The improved survival resulted in many of these patients having their CRT devices for many years and eventually requiring an increased number of device-related procedures, including coronary sinus (CS) lead revisions and replacements following a CS lead extraction.

INDICATIONS FOR EXTRACTION

The indications for CS lead extraction are parallel to the general indications for lead extraction, as seen in the Heart Rhythm Society expert consensus document[6] and in **Box 1**. Infection is likely the most common indication, with a close second being the need for repositioning of the lead because of malfunction or inadequate response.

An important determinant of successful cardiac resynchronization is the position of the LV lead. For example, the position of the LV lead in the apical position was unfavorable in the MADIT-CRT subanalysis.[7] It is also known that the response to CRT is proportional to the LV electrical delay.[8,9] Therefore, when the lead is not placed at an optimal site and the patient does not respond to CRT, consideration should be given to the removal of the lead and the reimplantation of a new lead at a more favorable site.

Loss of response to CRT with additional battery drainage may also occur when the pacing threshold has increased beyond the point of consistent capture of the LV. That would be an indication for LV lead extraction and implantation of a new lead. Although a second CS lead could be introduced in the main body of the CS, it is usually not possible to place two leads in a secondary or smaller branch of the CS.

Some LV leads may also be more prone to electrical malfunction and/or internal conductor

Cardiac Arrhythmia Service, Massachusetts General Hospital, 75 Fruit Street, Boston, MA 02114, USA
E-mail address: tmela@mgh.harvard.edu

Card Electrophysiol Clin 11 (2019) 131–140
https://doi.org/10.1016/j.ccep.2018.11.014

Box 1
Indications for lead extraction

Infection

   Class I

   1. Definite cardiac implantable electronic devices (CIED) system infection (level of evidence B)

   2. CIED pocket infection (level of evidence B)

   3. Valvular endocarditis without definite lead involvement (level of evidence B)

   4. Occult gram-positive bacteremia (level of evidence B)

   Class IIa

   1. Persistent occult gram-negative bacteremia (level of evidence B)

   Class III (not recommended)

   1. Superficial infection without involvement of the device and/or leads (level of evidence C)

   2. Chronic bacteremia caused by a source other than the CIED, when long-term suppressive antibiotics are required (level of evidence C)

Chronic Pain

   Class IIa

   1. Severe chronic pain (level of evidence C)

Thrombosis or Venous Stenosis

   Class I

   1. Thromboembolic events associated with thrombus on a lead or a lead fragment (level of evidence C)

   2. Bilateral subclavian vein or superior vena cava (SVC) occlusion precluding implantation of a needed transvenous lead (level of evidence C)

   3. Planned stent deployment in a vein already containing a transvenous lead, to avoid entrapment of the lead (level of evidence C)

   4. SVC stenosis or occlusion with limiting symptoms (level of evidence C)

   5. Ipsilateral venous occlusion preventing placement of an additional lead with a contraindication to the contralateral side (level of evidence C)

   Class IIa

   1. Ipsilateral venous occlusion preventing placement of an additional lead, without a contraindication to the contralateral side (level of evidence C)

Functional Leads

   Class I

   1. Life-threatening arrhythmias secondary to retained leads (level of evidence B)

   2. Leads that, because of their design or their failure, may pose an immediate threat to the patients if left in place (level of evidence B)

   3. Leads that interfere with the operation of implanted cardiac devices (level of evidence B)

   4. Leads that interfere with the treatment of a malignancy (level of evidence C)

   Class IIb

   1. Abandoned functional lead that poses a risk of interference with the operation of the active CIED system (level of evidence C)

   2. Functioning leads that because of their design or their failure pose a potential future threat to the patient if left in place (level of evidence C)

   3. Leads that are functional but not being used (level of evidence C)

   4. To enable MRI when there is no other available imaging alternative for the diagnosis (level of evidence C)

   5. To permit the implantation of an MRI conditional CIED system (level of evidence C)

Class III

1. Functional but redundant leads if patients have a life expectancy of less than 1 year (level of evidence C)

2. Known anomalous placement of leads or through a systemic venous atrium or systemic ventricle (level of evidence C)

Nonfunctional Leads

Class I

1. Life-threatening arrhythmias secondary to retained leads or lead fragments (level of evidence B)

2. Leads that, because of their design or their failure, may pose an immediate threat to the patients if left in place (level of evidence B)

3. Leads that interfere with the operation of implanted cardiac devices (level of evidence B)

4. Leads that interfere with the treatment of a malignancy (level of evidence C)

Class IIa

1. Leads that because of their design or their failure pose a threat to the patient that is not immediate or imminent if left in place (level of evidence C)

2. If a CIED implantation would require more than four leads on one side or more than five leads through the SVC (level of evidence C)

3. To enable MRI when there a no other available imaging alternative for the diagnosis (level of evidence C)

Class IIb

1. At the time of an indicated CIED procedure in patients with nonfunctional leads (level of evidence C)

2. To permit the implantation of an MRI conditional CIED system (level of evidence C)

Class III

1. Patients with nonfunctional leads and a life expectancy of less than 1 year (level of evidence C)

2. Known anomalous placement of leads or through a systemic venous atrium or systemic ventricle (level of evidence C)

Adapted from Wilkoff BL, Love CJ, Byrd CL, et al. Transvenous lead extraction: Heart Rhythm Society expert consensus on facilities, training, indications and patient management. Heart Rhythm 2009;6:1095–6; with permission.

externalization (St. Jude Quick Site and Quick Flex, St. Paul, MN),[10] which may become an indication for a lead extraction. The recall on these leads was announced in 2012 and, even if those leads have not presented with overt electrical abnormalities, they are already older leads and may develop problems simply because of their age.

DECISION WHEN TO EXPLANT

Some decisions are easier than others. Infection of the CRT system (wound dehiscence, clearly inflamed pocket, or vegetations on the leads) or valvular endocarditis with gram-positive bacteremia are some definite indications.

Absolute lack of pacing from the CS lead, or the lead placed in an anterior or posterior branch of a nonresponder patient, are additional strong indications. However, even in this case, the patient should not be exposed to an unnecessary procedure, unless there is certainty that an optimal

branch exists and is accessible. In this case, computed tomography (CT) could be used to assess the venous anatomy and dyssynchrony and potential scar extension.[11] If an appropriate branch exists, it is targeted following the extraction of the existing CS lead. If an appropriate venous branch does not exist, the patient may be directly considered for an epicardial lead placement, His bundle pacing, or LV endocardial pacing, without exposing him or her to the additional risk of an extraction.

Hesitancy to proceed with a CS lead extraction may also occur when the patient is a nonresponder and the pacing threshold of a CS lead placed in an optimal branch has risen or the lead is not functional because of fracture. In that case, other modalities should again be considered, including the strengthening of optimal medical therapy and consideration of more advanced heart failure management solutions.

Diaphragmatic pacing used to be a frequent hurdle of CRT in the era of unipolar and bipolar CS leads. For some patients, the situation was intolerable and would make optimal LV pacing impossible. Therefore, diaphragmatic pacing used to be a reason for CS lead removal and reimplantation. In the current era of quadripolar LV leads and numerous pacing vectors, this problem has subsided considerably, and, even if it is present, it is corrected by the appropriate programming changes.

Finally, CS lead dislodgment used to be a more common problem, reaching up to 5.7% of the implants in the large clinical trials.[12] Some leads would present with subacute dislodgment months or years after the initial placement. In that case, the lead would have to be removed, occasionally with the use of mechanical or laser tools, before a new one was reimplanted. This problem has also diminished in the era of quadripolar leads with improved design. However, it continues to be a strong indication for lead removal, especially in the responder patient who requires a reimplantation.

BEFORE THE EXPLANT

Most of patients with CRT have advanced heart failure and require careful evaluation and preparation. In our institution all extractions that may potentially require the use of laser are performed in the operating room under general anesthesia in the presence of a cardiothoracic surgeon and all patients are evaluated by cardiac anesthesia before the procedure. Unless the lead has to be explanted urgently because of an infection, the patients come to an extraction when they are as close to euvolemic as possible and when they are hemodynamically stable. The patients are aware that they will not have CRT for a few days or weeks, in the case of infection, and this may affect them symptomatically and/or hemodynamically. The patients who do not have infection are aware of the risk that the CS lead may not be successfully repositioned in which case other options will be explored. Most patients consent to an epicardial lead placement during the same procedure, if the transvenous approach is not successful.

Another consideration involves pacemaker-dependent patients, who before losing biventricular pacing, if they are infected, they need a temporary pacemaker to receive pacing until they receive their new system a few days or weeks later. For those patients we use an externalized pacing lead that is connected to their removed CRT device, secured on their front chest. This system allows patients to have free mobility while they are in the hospital, although they are not allowed to be discharged to their home or a rehabilitation center.

FACILITY

The procedure is performed in the electrophysiology laboratory or the operating room under conscious sedation or general anesthesia. A cardiothoracic surgeon needs to be readily available and a surgical table with the appropriate instruments/equipment for the patient to be able to have a sternotomy and go on bypass in less than 5 minutes. In our institution we perform lead extractions in the operating room under general anesthesia. There is the cart with all the extraction tools and another cart with the implantation tools. We perform the procedures under transesophageal echocardiographic monitoring and fluoroscopy.

HOW TO EXPLANT

The CS lead is a small-caliber tined lead that is removed by gentle traction, in most cases, when the lead is less than 2 to 3 years old, and often when it is even up to 5 to 6 years old (author's personal experience). For those cases, the steps require to free the lead from the pocket; detach it for the device; insert a soft stylet; free the suturing sleeve from the pocket and cut the sutures keeping it tight on the lead; and, under fluoroscopy, pull the lead gently until it is removed. If there is resistance, a locking stylet (Lead Locking Device, Spectranetics, Colorado Springs, CO; or Liberator, Cook Medical, Bloomington, IN) is inserted with special care, and the stylet is not advanced passed the tip of the lead and into the venous structures, potentially causing perforation. An Ethibond 0 suture is also tied on the insulation and the conductors for an additional ability to put traction on the lead.

In our institution we use a 12F catheter excimer laser sheath (GlideLight, Spectranetics) to go over the LV leads. An outer sheath may also be useful to provide additional support and ability to mechanically disrupt the adhesions. If a 14F catheter sheath has already been used for another lead extraction previously in the case, we may consider using that larger diameter sheath. In general, however, we prefer to use the smallest diameter sheath that can accommodate the lead.

Mechanical dilatation sheaths may be also used successfully. Rarely, rotating threaded tip sheaths (Evolution, Cook Medical; TightRail, Spectranetics) may be helpful to further lyse fibrous binding points. The access site may most commonly be the implant vein, but successful extractions may be performed via the femoral vein, or the right internal jugular vein.[13]

Sufficient rail is continuously applied to the lead to provide a rail over which to advance the laser or mechanical sheath. Many times, after the disruption of the fibrous binding points under the clavicle and the first part of the subclavian vein, the lead may come loose. If not, on reaching the CS os, countertraction is applied with the laser sheath while traction is applied to the lead. Although, the sheath may be advanced into the CS for further countertraction, laser should almost never be applied inside the CS because the risk for perforation is high, caused by the thin walls and the complex angulation of the CS.[14]

Once the lead is free, it is pulled out of the sheath, and a stiff long wire is used to maintain venous access when reimplantation is planned. If the CS lead is pulled out just with gentle traction, access could be maintained via an angioplasty wire inserted through the lead.

OUTCOMES

A small number of single-center studies and a limited number of multicenter reports have shown a significant success rate for the CS lead extraction. A common observation throughout these studies is the high success rate for removal of the CS lead with gentle traction. That percentage was 91% in one of the studies of 125 leads with lifetime of the CS leads ranging between 0.26 and 98.9 months with an average of 18.5 months.[15] The complete success for removal ranges between 99% and 100%.[16–18]

PROCEDURAL CONCERNS
Difficult to Extract Leads

The LV leads enter a venous structure that is easier to perforate and therefore their extraction may be challenging. Certain fixation mechanisms may also add to the difficulty of the extraction.

One characteristic of CS lead that needs special mentioning because of the difference in design, behavior, and challenge in extraction is the (Medtronic, Minneapolis, MN) StarFix Model 4195. It is a unipolar lead with an outer push tube that allows for fixation within the body of the tributaries of the CS. This results in an extremely low dislodgment rate.[19] When the lead is to be extracted, the active fixation lobes should be retracted. This may be possible for leads implanted less than 6 months prior, but often not successful for older leads.

A single-center study reported 100% success extracting these leads with the use of a mechanical sheath. However, advancement of the sheath to the tip of the lead should be avoided.[20]

A multicenter registry[21] compared the extractability of 40 Model 4195 leads with 165 different models of CS leads. There were 37 successful Model 4195 lead extractions (92.5%) as compared with 98.8% successful extractions of the other leads, performed by these high-volume centers and experienced operators. Six of 40 patients (15%) with a Models 4195 lead experienced a major complication compared with 6.1% of the patients with other CS leads, but the complication rate was not statistically different between the two groups. The authors recommended the use of standard techniques for the extraction of the leads, including the use of locking stylets, mechanical or laser sheaths, but avoiding active laser inside the CS. They also concluded that these more challenging to extract leads should be extracted in high-volume centers by experienced operators.

Inability to Reimplant the Coronary Sinus Lead

When the procedure involves the extraction of a CS lead with reimplantation of a new CS lead, a reasonable concern involves the inability to place the new CS lead in the branch that the old lead occupied. This is a result of fibrosis or thrombosis of the branch in a significant number of cases. An older small study of 10 patients who had CS venograms after lead extraction showed that the CS branch that was originally used was not usable in half of the patients.[22] However, a later publication reported a 95.6% reimplantation success rate, when out of 90 patients only 4 had no available CS branches.[18] In a series of 173 patients explanted for infection, reimplantation was unsuccessful in 19 (17.2%), because of lack of appropriate CS branches.[23]

FUTURE DIRECTIONS

The ease of CS lead explant continues to improve, as new or improved explantation tools continue to be released and as the need for difficult to explant active fixation CS leads is decreased. His-bundle pacing and LV endocardial pacing may also substitute in the future a significant portion of the CS leads placed today. Those leads will create their unique needs for extraction.

CASE STUDY

The patient had a long-standing history of (h/o) mitral valve prolapse for which he underwent a mitral valve repair in 2001 at age 56. However, the mitral regurgitation (MR) reoccurred and he eventually underwent a mitral valve replacement with a St. Jude prosthesis in 2004. He also had a long h/o paroxysmal atrial fibrillation for which he had a surgical maze in 2001 and a subsequent surgical cryoablation in 2004. His LVEF was 75% with severe MR in 1993, ejection fraction 68% with severe MR in 2001 before his mitral valve repair, and 54% following the repair along with mild MR. His LV end diastolic diameter (LVEDD) decreased from 65 mm to 49 mm following the repair. He subsequently developed symptomatic sick sinus syndrome and he received a dual-chamber pacemaker in 2005 (Boston Scientific device with two Medtronic 5076 leads). In July 2007 a repeat echocardiogram showed LV dysfunction and ejection fraction drop from 45% in 2004 to now 30% with LVEDD of 59 mm, despite medications being optimized for his heart failure management (carvedilol and lisinopril). His pacemaker interrogation at the time showed premature ventricular complexes (PVCs), couplets, triplets, and non-sustained ventricular tachycardia ranging 100 to 135 bpm. He had atrial pacing 63% and ventricular pacing 72% of the time.

The increasing percentage of right ventricular (RV) pacing was believed to be one of the reasons he had worsening cardiomyopathy. He therefore had a CRT with defibrillator upgrade for the cardiomyopathy and the symptomatic nonsustained ventricular tachycardia (VT) in 2007. The patient received a Medtronic 4193 to 88CM Attain OTW LV lead to a posterolateral CS branch (**Fig. 1**) and a Medtronic 6947 to 65CM Sprint Quattro Secure with capping of the 2005 Medtronic 5076 RV lead. He received a Medtronic C154DWK CONCERTO implantable cardioverter-defibrillator (ICD). His LVEF in 2012 was 45% with LVEDD 62 mm and left atrial 64 mm. In 2015 his LVEF was 48% with inferoposterior akinesis. Cardiac

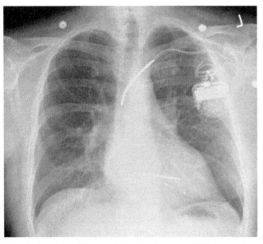

Fig. 1. Chest radiograph following the CRT upgrade.

CT scan on August 19, 2015, showed an atretic left circumflex artery, but right dominant circulation with no coronary lesions to explain the inferoposterior scar. He had multiple appropriate ICD therapies (antitachycardia pacing) for monomorphic ventricular tachycardia at 188 bpm in 2015. This VT could not be suppressed by sotalol and mexiletine. Thus, he underwent a VT ablation with substrate modification in September of 2015. A couple of weeks later, he called the office to report shortness breath with exertion, just walking across the room with a 10-lb weight gain. We asked that he take furosemide, 40 mg twice daily, until he reached his preprocedure weight. This was accomplished in 5 days. ICD interrogation showed that the LV lead had been off since the time of the ablation. He felt a great improvement in his symptoms once he was back at his goal weight and remained stable for 5 months.

He then presented to a local hospital with a headache and right-sided weakness after a fall at home. In the emergency department work-up was significant for international normalized ratio 8.1 and CT showed a large left frontoparietal and intraparenchymal hemorrhage with surrounding vasogenic edema, with a small subdural hematoma. Acetylsalicylic acid and warfarin were held and he was started on dexamethasone, sulfamethoxazole/trimethoprim, and levetiracetam. Neurosurgery recommended a cervical collar for C1-C2 subluxation and long-term physical therapy. He was able to recover from that and was restarted on warfarin approximately 6 months later.

He had an ICD generator replacement in February of 2017. On March 1, 2017, he had polymorphic ventricular tachycardia/ventricular fibrillation, successfully terminated by an ICD shock. He also had atrial tachycardia/atrial fibrillation (At/AF) episodes totaling 54.9%; longest in duration was 85 minutes. This was found to be caused by changes of his antiarrhythmic doses during his recovery from the intracerebral bleed. He did not have any further events after the reestablishment of his sotalol and mexiletine. He was admitted from April 14 to April 25, 2017, for progressive dyspnea and was diuresed. Transthoracic echocardiography showed decrease in LVEF to 37% from 48% with worsening RV hypokinesis, progressive inferior hypokinesis. He was able to recover and be stable for the subsequent year.

However, on ICD interrogation on March 29, 2018, his LV lead impedance was greater than 3000 Ω and lacked capture at 8v at 0.50 milliseconds. He was also having progressively increased "noise" on the atrial lead, which we had tolerated for some time. That led to inappropriate mode-switches because the device was confusing the noise for AF. We therefore programmed the device DDIR, and we scheduled the patient for an LV lead revision because of (likely) fracture and right atrium (RA) lead revision given the atrial lead noise caused by impeding fracture.

The decision making was not easy for this frail 72-year-old man with valvular cardiomyopathy and an LVEF 35%, class II heart failure, cerebral bleeding on warfarin, which he needed for the presence of a St. Jude mitral valve and ongoing atrial flutter and atrial fibrillation. This same patient had done remarkably well after he received CRT and had exacerbation of his congestive heart failure when the LV lead was turned off for 2 weeks.

The pros and cons of the procedure were calculated ahead of time. To support the safety of the lead extraction, he had prior sternotomy with two valve surgeries, which suggested that his pericardial space was fibrosed and the risk for perforation should be lower. However, in the rare possibility we had to emergently open his chest, the access would have been much more difficult. The cardiothoracic surgeon was prepared to do a lateral thoracotomy. On the positive side of the decision, the leads for extraction were pacing leads, and these are usually easier to extract than ICD leads. Thinking about the alternatives of the extraction procedure, would have been the addition of two more leads with abandonment of the two malfunctioning ones. The patient already had four leads. Adding two more leads without extraction would have been a major burden. We would also have less of a good chance to place the new LV lead in the same branch the previous one was located and therefore his response to CRT could be compromised.

We therefore went ahead with the extraction, booked in the hybrid operating room with the cardiothoracic surgeon present in the room. General anesthesia was provided and the patient had continuous transesophageal ultrasound monitoring. During the procedure, the left-sided ICD pocket was opened and the device was externalized, and the leads were dissected free. The generator and the leads were inspected visually. A break was visible in the LV lead at the edge of the pocket. A 6F catheter sheath was placed in the right femoral vein for rapid superior vena cava (SVC) access if needed during extraction. Both the atrial lead and LV leads were disconnected from the pulse generator. There was also an abandoned RV pacing lead in the pocket that was mobilized and prepared for extraction. The active fixation mechanism of the atrial lead and the abandoned RV lead were retracted while a

stylet was in place. First, the atrial lead was cut and locking stylet was placed inside the atrial lead. The RV lead was similarly prepared with retraction of the active fixation mechanism, the proximal end was then cut, and a locking stylet was advanced into the lead. Finally, the LV lead was cut proximal to the visible break and a locking stylet was placed inside the lead. Next, a 14F catheter laser sheath was advanced over the locking stylet and over the atrial lead. Under fluoroscopic guidance, the laser sheath was advanced slowly over the atrial lead. There was evidence of adhesions between the RA and RV leads in the subclavian vein adjacent to the SVC coil on the RV ICD lead. With gentle pressure and laser dissection, the sheath was advanced into the innominate vein. We transitioned between the RA and RV leads several times with the laser sheath to try to mobilize the leads. We were able to advance the laser sheath to the RA over the RV lead. Multiple attempts were made to free the RV lead but it would not mobilize. We externalized the laser sheath and realized it was no longer functional. Therefore, we exchanged for a second 14F catheter sheath and then the RV lead was freed. We then turned our attention to the LV lead, which had backed out somewhat with all the manipulation, and we extracted the LV lead easily. Finally,

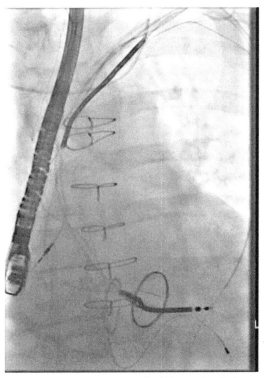

Fig. 2. Following the removal of the RV lead, the LV and atrial leads are still in place.

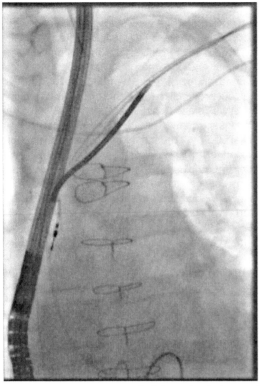

Fig. 3. Following the removal of the LV lead, the atrial lead is removed easily.

the laser sheath was placed over the RA lead and this was also extracted (**Figs. 2–4**). Throughout this process, the patient's blood pressure was continuously monitored via an arterial line, and the pericardial space was monitored with transesophageal echocardiography and no effusion developed. With extraction of the RV and RA leads, an Amplatz wire was placed to maintain venous access. There was an estimated blood loss of 800 to 1000 mL because of subclavian vein brisk bleeding despite holding constant manual pressure over the site the laser sheaths were inserting. Fresh frozen plasma was given. He also received 4.5 L intravenous fluid during the procedure. A venogram was performed that demonstrated a contained extravasation around the innominate vein (**Fig. 5**), which tracked up the left internal jugular vein. No evidence of continued mediastinal bleeding was noted.

New RA and LV leads were subsequently placed. The dilator of the 9F catheter introducer was removed, and a CS guide catheter was inserted via the hemostatic-valve sheath and the CS was cannulated using a diagnostic CS catheter. A CS venogram was performed via an occlusive balloon-tipped catheter. A subselector was then used to select a posterolateral LV branch and a bipolar LV lead was advanced over the wire into the branch (a quadripolar lead was not used because we would have had to then implant a new generator and his current generator had been placed the previous year). Endocardial potentials and stimulation thresholds were then determined, and found to be suitable. The LV lead had a capture threshold of 0.7 V at 0.5 milliseconds with a pacing impedance of 730 Ω. There

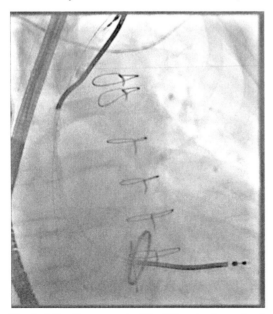

Fig. 4. After the removal of the RV pacing/sense lead, access was maintained with a guidewire, advanced to the inferior vena cava.

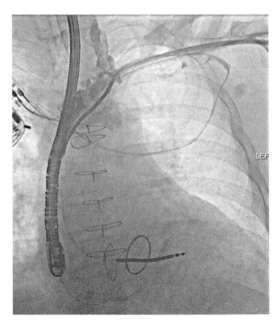

Fig. 5. A left subclavian venogram demonstrated a contained extravasation around the innominate vein, which tracked up the left internal jugular vein.

was diaphragmatic stimulation at 10 V; however, the output for LV capture was much lower. Next, the dilator of the 9F catheter introducer was removed, and a Medtronic CAPSUREFIX NOVUS 52CM 5076 to 52CM atrial lead was passed through the introducer and advanced to the RA. Under fluoroscopic guidance, the atrial electrode was then positioned in the RA cavity and tested repeatedly for stability. The active fixation mechanism was deployed and the lead parameters were found to be satisfactory (pacing threshold 0. 8V at 0.5 milliseconds and pacing impedance of 633 Ω).

With both leads in place, the 9F catheter introducer around the LV lead was split. Then the 9F catheter sheath around the atrial lead was split. There continued to be significant bleeding from the access site requiring manual compression and at this point both leads were anchored to the floor of the pocket. Next, a large purse-string suture was placed around the access site with 2–0 Vicryl to try to achieve some hemostasis. Then, further sutures were placed to anchor the leads to the pocket. The leads were again tested and then connected to the device and sealed in the prescribed manner. Appropriate function of the device was assured with the aid of a device programmer.

The wound was then flushed with vancomycin and closed using a double layer of 2–0 absorbable Vicryl sutures followed by a subcuticular running suture with 4–0 Monocryl and a layer of SteriStrips. Adequate hemostasis appeared to be present. A sterile dressing was then applied. The device was programmed as detailed next and the patient left the laboratory in good condition. The right femoral venous sheath was removed and manual pressure was applied. The patient was extubated by the anesthesia team in the operating room. However, he became hypotensive and required neosynephrine and so he was sent to the cardiac care unit for

monitoring. There he was rapidly weaned from neosynephrine. He was discharged with a stable left pectoral ICD pocket without hematoma. His final chest radiograph is shown in **Fig. 6**.

The patient was seen in October of 2018 and he was feeling well from a cardiovascular standpoint. His weight had been stable without any change. He denied dyspnea, orthopnea, pazoxysmal nocturnal dyspnea, chest pain, cough, or lower extremity edema. His ICD interrogation showed all measurements were within normal range. There was no VT/ventricular fibrillation. There were 1097 AT/AF detects totaling 17.3% (longest lasting 4 hours in duration); electrograms suggested AT/slow atrial flutter. Heart rate histograms showed good distribution. PVCs averaged 26.9 singles/hour. Total atrial pacing was 65.6%, biventricular pacing was 97.9%.

There are a few additional points to be made for this case. The LV lead extraction itself was not difficult, but the interference and common fibrosis with the other leads created most of the challenge. If this patient had not had cardiac surgery and a protected pericardium, we might have abandoned the effort to extract the leads from the left subclavian vein and we could have considered the completion of extraction from the right femoral vein. The extravasation of intravenous contrast around the subclavian, innominate, SVC did suggest microtears in the area. Because the intravenous contrast appeared contained and the patient was stable, we did not believe there was a need for any intervention. If there was evidence of expanding hematoma, the situation would have potentially called for the use of the Spectranetics Bridge occlusion balloon. This was not deemed necessary in this case. Finally, having a purse string around the laser sheath ready to control the bleeding, once

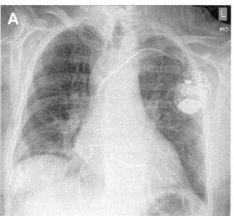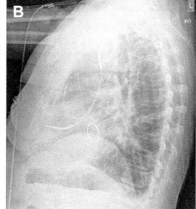

Fig. 6. (*A*) Posteroanterior view, final chest radiograph following the laser lead extraction and reimplantation of new leads and ICD generator. (*B*) Lateral view.

the extracted lead and sheath are removed is a good practice. It may be hard to do when there are multiple leads for extraction and the extraction sheath has to be moved from one lead to the other multiple times.

REFERENCES

1. Abraham WT, Fisher WG, Smith AL, et al. Cardiac re-synchronization in chronic heart failure. N Engl J Med 2002;346:1845–53.
2. Bristow MR, Saxon LA, Boehmer J, et al. Cardiac re-synchronization therapy with or without an implantable defibrillator in advanced chronic heart failure. N Engl J Med 2004;350:2140–50.
3. Cleland JG, Daubert JC, Erdmann E, et al, Resynchronization-Heart Failure (CARE-HF) Study Investigators. The effect of cardiac resynchronization on morbidity and mortality in heart failure. N Engl J Med 2005;352:1539–49.
4. Moss AJ, Hall WJ, Cannom DS, et al, MADIT-CRT Trail Investigators. Cardiac-resynchronization therapy for the prevention of heart-failure events. N Engl J Med 2009;361:1329–38.
5. Sridhar AR, Yarlagadda V, Parasa S, et al. Cardiac resynchronization therapy: US trends and disparities in utilization and outcomes. Circ Arrhythm Electrophysiol 2016;9(3):1–8.
6. Wilkoff BL, Love CJ, Byrd CL, et al. Transvenous lead extraction: Heart Rhythm Society expert consensus on facilities, training, indications, and patient management. Heart Rhythm 2009;6:1085–104.
7. Singh JP, Klein HU, Huang DT, et al. Left ventricular lead position and clinical outcome in the multicenter automatic defibrillator implantation trial-cardiac resynchronization therapy (MADIT-CRT) trial. Circulation 2011;123:1159–66.
8. Sing JP, Fan D, Heist EK, et al. Left ventricular lead electrical delay predicts response to cardiac resynchronization therapy. Heart Rhythm 2006;3(12):1515.
9. Roubicek T, Wichterle D, Kucera P, et al. Left ventricular lead electrical delay is a predictor of mortality in patients with cardiac resynchronization therapy. Circ Arrhythm Electrophysiol 2015;8:1113–21.
10. Available at: https://www.accessdata.fda.gov/scripts/cdrh/cfdocs/cfres/res.cfm?id=108651. Accessed May 3, 2012.
11. Truong QA, Hoffmann U, Singh JP. Potential use of computed tomography for management of heart failure patients with dyssynchrony. Crit Pathw Cardiol 2008;7(3):185–90.
12. Van Rees JB, de Bie MK, Thijssen J. Implantation-related complications of implantable cardioverter-defibrillators and cardiac resynchronization therapy devices: systematic review of randomized clinical trials. J Am Coll Cardiol 2011;58:995–1000.
13. Bongiorni MG, Soldati E, Zucchelli G, et al. Transvenous removal of pacing and implantable cardiac defibrillating leads using single sheath mechanical dilatation and multiple venous approaches: high success rate and safety in more than 2000 leads. Eur Heart J 2008;29:2886–93.
14. Cronin EM, Wilkoff BL. Coronary sinus lead extraction. Heart Fail Clin 2017;13:105–15.
15. Sheldon S, Friedman PA, Hayes DL, et al. Outcomes and predictors of difficulty with coronary sinus lead removal. J Interv Card Electrophysiol 2012;35(1):93–100.
16. Kasravi B, Tobias S, Barnes MJ, et al. Coronary sinus lead extraction in the era of cardiac resynchronization therapy: single center experience. Pacing Clin Electrophysiol 2005;28(1):51–3.
17. De Martino G, Orazi S, Bisignani G, et al. Safety and feasibility of coronary sinus left ventricular leads extraction: a preliminary report. J Interv Card Electrophysiol 2005;13(1):35–8.
18. Di Cori A, Bongiorni MG, Zucchelli G, et al. Large single-center experience in transvenous coronary sinus lead extraction: procedural outcomes and predictors for mechanical dilatation. Pacing Clin Electrophysiol 2012;35(2):215–22.
19. Crossley GH, Exner D, Mead RH, et al, Medtronic 4195 Study Investigators. Chronic performance of an active fixation coronary sinus lead. Heart Rhythm 2010;7:472–8.
20. Kypta A, Blessberger H, Saleh K, et al. Removal of active-fixation coronary sinus leads using a mechanical rotation extraction device. Pacing Clin Electrophysiol 2015;38:302–5.
21. Crossley GH, Sorrentino RA, Exner DV, et al. Extraction of chronically implanted coronary sinus leads active fixation vs passive fixation leads. Heart Rhythm 2016;13:1253–9.
22. Burke MC, Morton J, Lin AC. Implications and outcome of permanent coronary sinus lead extraction and reimplantation. J Cardiovasc Electrophysiol 2005;16(8):830–7.
23. Rickard J, Tarakji K, Cronin E, et al. Cardiac venous left ventricular lead removal and reimplantation following device infection: a large single-center experience. J Cardiovasc Electrophysiol 2012;23:1213–6.

CRT in Special Populations

Cardiac Resynchronization Therapy in Preserved to Mildly Reduced Systolic Function

Chance M. Witt, MD, Yong-Mei Cha, MD*

KEYWORDS

- Cardiac resynchronization therapy • Heart failure with preserved ejection fraction
- Heart failure with reduced ejection fraction

KEY POINTS

- Cardiac resynchronization therapy (CRT) is known to be beneficial in heart failure patients with a prolonged QRS and a left ventricular ejection fraction ≤35%.
- Patients with left bundle branch block and a mildly reduced ejection fraction have very poor outcomes, and most tend to worsen over time.
- Several studies have shown a beneficial effect of cardiac resynchronization in patients with a mildly reduced ejection fraction.
- Future prospective studies in these patients will be very important to further investigate the benefit of CRT in mild to moderately reduced EF to ensure that all patients who may potentially benefit from cardiac resynchronization are being treated with this therapy.

INTRODUCTION

The benefits of cardiac resynchronization therapy (CRT) for patients with heart failure and a prolonged QRS duration have been clearly demonstrated in several large randomized studies.[1–6] These studies, however, have only focused on those patients who were thought to be most likely to derive a symptomatic benefit. Thus, the patients with a current guideline-backed recommendation are those who have a low left ventricular ejection fraction (LVEF) of ≤35%.[7] This therapy has been of great benefit for this group with improvements in both mortality and quality of life.

However, there are many other patients who could potentially benefit from CRT. The 2 key groups in question would be (1) symptomatic heart failure patients with an LVEF greater than 35%, including normal LVEF; and (2) asymptomatic patients with an ejection fraction between 35% and 50%. In the latter group, this would be used as a preventive therapy similar to beta-blockers or angiotensin-converting enzyme inhibitors as recommended by the most recent American College of Cardiology/American Heart Association heart failure guidelines.[8]

The reasoning behind treatment of the first group is straightforward. These patients have symptomatic heart failure and a prolonged QRS. The only difference is that the LVEF is higher than 35%. It is understood that the LVEF is an imperfect measure of cardiac systolic function and that the 35% cutoff is arbitrary and varies significantly even within a single patient.

Disclosure Statement: No related disclosures or conflicts of interest to report.
Department of Cardiovascular Medicine, Mayo Clinic, 200 First Street Southwest, Rochester, MN 55905, USA
* Corresponding author. Division of Cardiovascular Diseases, Mayo Clinic, 200 First Street Southwest, Rochester, MN 55905.
E-mail address: ycha@mayo.edu

Card Electrophysiol Clin 11 (2019) 141–146
https://doi.org/10.1016/j.ccep.2018.11.012

Furthermore, some randomized trial-based evidence already exists that these patients may derive benefit from CRT, which will be discussed later.[9–11]

The second group likely requires more justification and evidence to determine if a benefit may truly be expected. This evidence comes in the form of population studies of left bundle branch block (LBBB) and pacing induced cardiomyopathy studies.

LEFT BUNDLE BRANCH BLOCK IS ASSOCIATED WITH POOR OUTCOMES IN PATIENTS WITH REDUCED EJECTION FRACTION

Several large population-based studies have demonstrated that patients with only an LBBB have worse outcomes than their counterparts with a non-LBBB electrocardiogram.[12–14] These studies are too broad to be useful in defining a need for therapy in patients with LBBB alone. Other studies have shown that LBBB is a negative prognostic marker in patients with heart failure and reduced systolic function,[15–19] but most of these patients are already offered CRT.

To identify a group that might benefit from "preventative" CRT, one would need to focus on a group that would have the most likelihood of progressing to significant symptoms associated with worsening LVEF. For an invasive therapy like CRT, the cost, time burden, and risk of complications require a patient to be at a high risk of poor outcomes to justify implantation of a device.

There have been studies suggesting a significant amount of dyssynchrony in patients with heart failure with preserved ejection fraction,[20] although there are others who have suggested this is no different from patients without heart failure.[21] It is certainly possible that patients with LBBB and heart failure with normal ejection fraction might receive a symptomatic benefit from CRT. However, many of the surrogate endpoints of prior CRT studies, such as LVEF and LV size, are normal to begin with and therefore could not improve with therapy. Studying this group is a reasonable endeavor but has not been significantly investigated at this point.

In a prior study by the authors' group, they focused on the group of patients with LBBB and an LVEF in the 35% to 50% range because these patients seem most likely to have progression to disease states meeting more traditional indications for CRT.[22] The authors compared these patients to a group with a similar LVEF but no LBBB on the electrocardiogram. The groups included both symptomatic and asymptomatic patients, although less than 10% were symptomatic at baseline. This study showed that the patients with LBBB and mildly reduced LVEF had much worse outcomes than the control group. Mortality was significantly higher (**Fig. 1**) as was the incidence of a clinically significant drop in LVEF and the need for an ICD.

At 5 years, almost 60% of the LBBB patients had either died or had a clinical change that would lead to a guideline-recommended indication of device implantation. Although these data are retrospective and do not demonstrate that CRT would change these outcomes, it shows that this group has a very poor prognosis that may justify the examination of the utility of preventative therapy.

It is also important in this discussion to clarify a key issue. It is not necessary to show that LBBB itself is a negative prognostic marker (although that has been shown in many studies as mentioned), or more specifically, that LBBB patients do worse than identical patients without LBBB. It is known that patients with a prolonged QRS, and even more so patients with an LBBB, are those who benefit from a CRT. Therefore, the fact that they have this dyssynchrony allows us a therapeutic opportunity. The authors would not withhold coronary revascularization if they were unable to prove that patients with ischemic cardiomyopathy had worse outcomes than patients with nonischemic cardiomyopathy. Physicians treat the issues in each patient that is treatable, regardless of that feature being a negative prognostic marker. For this reason, the most important feature of the aforementioned study is that it demonstrates the extremely poor prognosis of a primarily asymptomatic group of patient with a mildly reduced LVEF and LBBB.

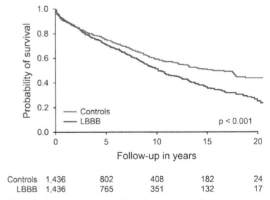

Controls	1,436	802	408	182	24
LBBB	1,436	765	351	132	17

Fig. 1. Long-term survival compared between patients with and without LBBB at baseline.

RIGHT VENTRICULAR PACING AS A SURROGATE FOR LEFT BUNDLE BRANCH BLOCK

Although there are many reasons that it may not be entirely accurate, the effects of right ventricular pacing are considered by many to mimic the dyssynchronous effects of LBBB. There have been many studies showing the adverse effects of right ventricular pacing, which has led to the increase of CRT devices and His bundle pacing in patients who will likely require frequent ventricular pacing.[23,24]

The BLOCK-HF study was perhaps the best demonstration of the prevention of the negative effects of right ventricular pacing with CRT.[25] This study compared the effects of biventricular pacing versus right ventricular pacing in patients with New York Heart Association (NYHA) class I–III heart failure and an LVEF of 50% or less. They showed that patients with biventricular pacing had a significantly lower rate of a combined endpoint of mortality, urgent heart failure–related visit, or LV size increase. The absolute difference in this endpoint was almost 10% and was statistically significant.

There are many reasons right ventricular pacing is not a perfect surrogate for the effects of LBBB. However, without a randomized prospective trial of CRT in patients with LBBB and mildly reduced EF, this trial provides us with some potentially useful information.

CARDIAC RESYNCHRONIZATION THERAPY BENEFITS SOME PATIENTS WITH LEFT VENTRICULAR EJECTION FRACTION GREATER THAN 35%

With the understanding that a large proportion of asymptomatic patients with a mildly reduced ejection fraction and LBBB will develop a heart failure syndrome, it is logical to predict that patients in this group who already have symptoms would be equally if not more likely to have progressive issues. However, demonstrating that patients will get sicker does not prove that CRT will be of benefit.

The authors are fortunate to have several large CRT studies in which patients were enrolled at peripheral study sites where they were thought to have an LVEF ≤35% (**Table 1**). On review at the core laboratory, however, the LVEF was deemed to be greater than 35%. These patients were then excluded from the study because they no longer met study criteria but they had already undergone CRT device implantation and were followed by the study team.

The investigators in MADIT-CRT demonstrated 696 (38%) patients enrolled in their trial had an LVEF greater than the cutoff, which was 30% in this study.[10] Although the median LVEF was 32% and thus still within current guideline recommendations, they demonstrated several pertinent points. Not only did CRT provide a benefit in this group of patients with an LVEF greater than 30% but also these patients demonstrated more remodeling with a greater reduction in LV and LA size than the patients with a lower LVEF.

These data corroborate the concept that there is likely a "sweet spot" for implementation of CRT. There is obviously a point when implementation of CRT is premature, mostly because it is not known if the patient will continue to progress. It also seems that there is likely a point of no return where cardiac resynchronization cannot help the LV systolic function to recover because the condition of the heart is beyond repair. Somewhere in between these 2 points and ideally closer to the former would be the ideal time for CRT implantation.

The REVERSE trial also noted a similar group with LVEF greater than 30% with a median LVEF of 35.1%.[11] They noted that in this group 74 (12.2%) patients had an LVEF greater than 35%. These study investigators showed that the benefits of CRT were seen regardless of LVEF with no significant interaction of LVEF with outcomes. The group with LVEF greater than 30% had an improvement in LV size and clinical outcomes.

Notably, many patients in both the MADIT-CRT and the REVERSE trials were NYHA class I and therefore *do* also represent a group whereby CRT may be considered a preventative therapy.

A substudy of the PROSPECT trial identified 86 (24%) patients whom the core laboratory deemed to have an LVEF greater than 35%.[9] These patients also had NYHA class III–IV heart failure and QRS duration greater than 130 milliseconds. In this group, more than 50% had an improvement in LV size and more than 60% had an improvement in a composite clinical outcome score. There was no statistically significant difference in these endpoints between the group with LVEF greater than 35% compared with the group with LVEF less than 35%.

CAN WE PROSPECTIVELY STUDY THIS GROUP?

One small prospective study by Fung and colleagues[26] evaluated the effect of CRT on 15 patients with NYHA class III heart failure, QRS greater than 120 milliseconds, and LVEF between 35% and 45%.[26] They compared this to a

Table 1
Comparison of analyses of cardiac resynchronization therapy trials accidentally including patients with left ventricular ejection fraction greater than 35%

Study	NYHA HF Class Included	QRS Duration Criteria (ms)	Median or Mean LVEF of Study Group	Number of Patients in Study Group	Important Outcomes Studied	Length of Follow-Up (mo)	Results	CRT Treatment Effect Compared with Low LVEF Group
MADIT-CRT 2013	I–II	≥130	31.8 (range 30.1%–45.3%)	696	1. First occurrence of HF episode or death 2. LV end-diastolic volume	12	Both outcomes improved	1. Improved similar to low EF group 2. Improved more than low EF group
REVERSE 2013	I–II	≥120	35.1 ± 3.9	177 (EF >30%) 74 (EF >35%)	1. Clinical composite score 2. LV end-systolic volume index	12	1. Trend toward improvement 2. Significant improvement	No difference between EF groups
PROSPECT 2010	III–IV	≥130	43.1 ± 7.2	86	1. Clinical composite score 2. LV end-systolic volume	6	Both outcomes improved	No difference between EF groups

Abbreviations: EF, ejection fraction; HF, heart failure; LV, left ventricular.

matched group with "conventional" CRT indications (ie, LVEF ≤35%). They showed an improvement in LV size, LVEF, and NYHA class in both groups. Improvements were similar between this group and the control group with the exception of a greater improvement in quality of life with the low EF group.

The obvious next step would be a randomized trial comparing CRT to no CRT in patients with a mildly reduced LVEF (36%–50%) and an LBBB. A trial of this design is exactly what was attempted in the MIRACLE EF study.[27] Unfortunately, the trial was stopped because of extremely slow enrollment after only enrolling 44 patients. The investigators cited several reasons for the failure of the study, which included a reluctance of physicians and patients to randomize to a long period with a device in place without therapy turned on.

Despite the failure of this trial, the importance of this issue has not waned. Future prospective trials must be designed to help answer this question, potentially with surrogate endpoints, shorter follow-up, or other adjustments that will improve the ease of recruitment to the trial. It is certainly inappropriate to provide expensive and potentially risky invasive treatments to patients who will not benefit. However, it is also unfortunate to prevent patients from receiving therapy proven to improve mortality and quality of life based on a labile number of uncertain significance (LVEF). Although even more difficult to prove for patients without heart failure, it is a shame to watch a large group of asymptomatic patients with LBBB and mildly reduced ejection fraction continue to worsen and develop symptoms before we are able to provide therapy.

REFERENCES

1. Abraham WT, Fisher WG, Smith AL, et al, MIRACLE Study Group. Multicenter InSync Randomized Clinical Evaluation. Cardiac resynchronization in chronic heart failure. N Engl J Med 2002;346:1845–53.
2. Cazeau S, Leclercq C, Lavergne T, et al, Multisite Stimulation in Cardiomyopathies (MUSTIC) Study Investigators. Effects of multisite biventricular pacing in patients with heart failure and intraventricular conduction delay. N Engl J Med 2001;344:873–80.
3. Cleland JG, Daubert JC, Erdmann E, et al, Cardiac Resynchronization-Heart Failure (CARE-HF) Study Investigators. The effect of cardiac resynchronization on morbidity and mortality in heart failure. N Engl J Med 2005;352:1539–49.
4. Linde C, Abraham WT, Gold MR, et al, REVERSE (REsynchronization reVErses Remodeling in Systolic left vEntricular dysfunction) Study Group. Randomized trial of cardiac resynchronization in mildly symptomatic heart failure patients and in asymptomatic patients with left ventricular dysfunction and previous heart failure symptoms. J Am Coll Cardiol 2008;52:1834–43.
5. Moss AJ, Hall WJ, Cannom DS, et al, MADIT-CRT Trial Investigators. Cardiac-resynchronization therapy for the prevention of heart-failure events. N Engl J Med 2009;361:1329–38.
6. Tang AS, Wells GA, Talajic M, et al, Resynchronization-Defibrillation for Ambulatory Heart Failure Trial Investigators. Cardiac-resynchronization therapy for mild-to-moderate heart failure. N Engl J Med 2010;363:2385–95.
7. Tracy CM, Epstein AE, Darbar D, et al. 2012 ACCF/AHA/HRS focused update of the 2008 guidelines for device-based therapy of cardiac rhythm abnormalities: a report of the American College of Cardiology Foundation/American Heart Association Task Force on practice guidelines. Heart Rhythm 2012;9:1737–53.
8. Yancy CW, Jessup M, Bozkurt B, et al, American College of Cardiology Foundation; American Heart Association Task Force on Practice Guidelines. 2013 ACCF/AHA guideline for the management of heart failure: a report of the American College of Cardiology Foundation/American Heart Association Task Force on practice guidelines. J Am Coll Cardiol 2013;62:e147–239.
9. Chung ES, Katra RP, Ghio S, et al. Cardiac resynchronization therapy may benefit patients with left ventricular ejection fraction >35%: a PROSPECT trial substudy. Eur J Heart Fail 2010;12:581–7.
10. Kutyifa V, Kloppe A, Zareba W, et al. The influence of left ventricular ejection fraction on the effectiveness of cardiac resynchronization therapy: MADIT-CRT (multicenter automatic defibrillator implantation trial with cardiac resynchronization therapy). J Am Coll Cardiol 2013;61:936–44.
11. Linde C, Daubert C, Abraham WT, et al, REsynchronization reVErses Remodeling in Systolic left vEntricular dysfunction (REVERSE) Study Group. Impact of ejection fraction on the clinical response to cardiac resynchronization therapy in mild heart failure. Circ Heart Fail 2013;6:1180–9.
12. Haataja P, Anttila I, Nikus K, et al. Prognostic implications of intraventricular conduction delays in a general population: the health 2000 survey. Ann Med 2015;47:74–80.
13. Schneider JF, Thomas HE Jr, Kreger BE, et al. Newly acquired left bundle-branch block: the Framingham study. Ann Intern Med 1979;90:303–10.
14. Zhang ZM, Rautaharju PM, Soliman EZ, et al. Mortality risk associated with bundle branch blocks and related repolarization abnormalities (from the Women's Health Initiative [WHI]). Am J Cardiol 2012;110:1489–95.
15. Abdel-Qadir HM, Tu JV, Austin PC, et al. Bundle branch block patterns and long-term outcomes in heart failure. Int J Cardiol 2011;146:213–8.

16. Huvelle E, Fay R, Alla F, et al. Left bundle branch block and mortality in patients with acute heart failure syndrome: a substudy of the EFICA cohort. Eur J Heart Fail 2010;12:156–63.

17. Imanishi R, Seto S, Ichimaru S, et al. Prognostic significance of incident complete left bundle branch block observed over a 40-year period. Am J Cardiol 2006;98:644–8.

18. McCullough PA, Hassan SA, Pallekonda V, et al. Bundle branch block patterns, age, renal dysfunction, and heart failure mortality. Int J Cardiol 2005; 102:303–8.

19. Stephenson K, Skali H, McMurray JJ, et al. Long-term outcomes of left bundle branch block in high-risk survivors of acute myocardial infarction: the VALIANT experience. Heart Rhythm 2007;4:308–13.

20. Wang J, Kurrelmeyer KM, Torre-Amione G, et al. Systolic and diastolic dyssynchrony in patients with diastolic heart failure and the effect of medical therapy. J Am Coll Cardiol 2007;49:88–96.

21. Menet A, Greffe L, Ennezat PV, et al. Is mechanical dyssynchrony a therapeutic target in heart failure with preserved ejection fraction? Am Heart J 2014; 168:909–16.e1.

22. Witt CM, Wu G, Yang D, et al. Outcomes with left bundle branch block and mildly to moderately reduced left ventricular function. JACC Heart Fail 2016;4:897–903.

23. Hussain MA, Furuya-Kanamori L, Kaye G, et al. The effect of right ventricular apical and nonapical pacing on the short- and long-term changes in left ventricular ejection fraction: a systematic review and meta-analysis of randomized-controlled trials. Pacing Clin Electrophysiol 2015;38:1121–36.

24. Weizong W, Zhongsu W, Yujiao Z, et al. Effects of right ventricular nonapical pacing on cardiac function: a meta-analysis of randomized controlled trials. Pacing Clin Electrophysiol 2013;36:1032–51.

25. Curtis AB, Worley SJ, Adamson PB, et al, Biventricular versus Right Ventricular Pacing in Heart Failure Patients with Atrioventricular Block (BLOCK HF) Trial Investigators. Biventricular pacing for atrioventricular block and systolic dysfunction. N Engl J Med 2013;368:1585–93.

26. Fung JW, Zhang Q, Yip GW, et al. Effect of cardiac resynchronization therapy in patients with moderate left ventricular systolic dysfunction and wide QRS complex: a prospective study. J Cardiovasc Electrophysiol 2006;17:1288–92.

27. Linde C, Curtis AB, Fonarow GC, et al. Cardiac resynchronization therapy in chronic heart failure with moderately reduced left ventricular ejection fraction: lessons from the Multicenter InSync Randomized Clinical Evaluation MIRACLE EF study. Int J Cardiol 2016;202:349–55.

Role of Atrioventricular Junctional Ablation and Cardiac Resynchronization Therapy in Patients with Chronic Atrial Fibrillation

Jonathan S. Steinberg, MD[a,b,c],*

KEYWORDS

- Atrioventricular junction ablation • Cardiac resynchronization therapy • Atrial fibrillation
- Biventricular pacing

KEY POINTS

- Patients with atrial fibrillation make up a significant minority of patients who may be eligible for cardiac resynchronization therapy.
- The benefits of cardiac resynchronization therapy may be muted in the presence of atrial fibrillation because conducted impulses compete with biventricular pacing capture. Current randomized clinical trial data in the subset of patients with atrial fibrillation have not shown benefit.
- If atrioventricular junctional ablation is performed in these patients, observational data suggest enhanced benefit although patients are rendered pacemaker dependent. Randomized trials testing the routine performance of this ablation procedure in patients with atrial fibrillation being considered for cardiac resynchronization therapy are warranted.

Cardiac resynchronization therapy (CRT) accomplished with biventricular (BiV) pacing is a demonstrably effective device intervention for patients with broad QRS and left ventricular systolic dysfunction. The clinical benefits of CRT include improved survival, functional status, and quality of life, and significant reductions in hospitalizations. CRT results in reversal of adverse pathologic remodeling, which is associated with increased left ventricular ejection fraction and autonomic function. The most recent heart failure treatment guidelines[1,2] classify CRT as a class I indication for patients in sinus rhythm, left brachial branch block (LBBB) (QRS >150 ms) and ejection fraction (EF) ≤35%.

The seminal clinical trials of CRT for advanced (class III–IV) heart failure (HF) regularly restricted enrollment to patients in sinus rhythm. The rationale was that BiV pacing required the presence of organized atrial activity to ensure synchronized and consistent delivery of the ventricular pacing impulse. Hence, current guidelines, and Food and Drug Administration indications, reflect the inclusion criteria of these trials and highlight the presence of sinus rhythm before CRT implantation. However, many patients with HF who are eligible for CRT are unable to maintain sinus rhythm. In addition, common clinical practice applies CRT to patients with persistent atrial fibrillation (AF).

Disclosure: Dr. Steinberg funded in part by a grant from the National Institutes of Health (5R34HL133526).
[a] Heart Research Follow-up Program, University of Rochester School of Medicine and Dentistry, 265 Crittenden Boulevard, Rochester 14462, NY, USA; [b] Department of cardiology, Hackensack Meridian School of Medicine at Seton Hall University, 340 Kingsland Street, Nutley, NJ 07110, USA; [c] SMG Arrhythmia Center, Summit Medical Group, 85 Woodland Road, Short Hills, NJ 07078, USA
* 85 Woodland Road, Short Hills, NJ 07078.
E-mail address: jsteinberg@smgnj.com

Card Electrophysiol Clin 11 (2019) 147–154
https://doi.org/10.1016/j.ccep.2018.11.013
1877-9182/19/© 2018 Elsevier Inc. All rights reserved.

PREVALENCE OF ATRIAL FIBRILLATION IN THE CARDIAC RESYNCHRONIZATION THERAPY POPULATION

Specifically in the population of patients with HF undergoing CRT, the prevalence of AF is substantial.[3–5] The 2011 US National Cardiovascular Data indicated that 36% of 87,692 patients with cardiac resynchronization therapy-defibrillator (CRT-D) had AF, and in 2012, 31% of 326,000 patients with an implantable cardioverter defibrillator (ICD) had AF.[6] The data are consistent and indicate that a substantial proportion of those patients who received CRT devices have underlying AF, despite little evidence to prove efficacy.

CURRENT GUIDELINES FOR CARDIAC RESYNCHRONIZATION THERAPY USAGE IN PATIENTS WITH ATRIAL FIBRILLATION

The 2012 published European Society of Cardiology (ESC) guidelines[1] state that patients with permanent AF "may be considered" for CRT if they have New York Heart Association (NYHA) class III-IV HF, QRS duration $\geq$120 ms, and an EF $\leq$35%, and are expected to survive with good functional status for more than 1 year, to reduce the risk of HF worsening. One of the following additional provisions are required: (1) the patient requires pacing for an intrinsically slow ventricular rate; (2) the patient is pacemaker dependent as a result of atrial-ventricular (AV) node ablation; or (3) the patient's ventricular rate is $\leq$60 beats per minute at rest and $\leq$90 beats per minute on exercise. These categories were awarded class IIb, IIa, and IIb indications with levels of evidence (LOE) C, B, and C, respectively. In 2016, ESC guidelines simply stated "CRT should be considered for patients with LVEF [left ventricular EF] $\leq$35% in NYHA Class III-IV despite optimal medical therapy in order to improve symptoms and reduce morbidity and mortality, if they are in AF and have a QRS duration $\geq$130 msec provided a strategy to ensure biventricular capture is in place or the patient is expected to return to sinus rhythm" (IIA, LOE B).

The 2012 update of device guidelines from the American Heart Association/American College of Cardiology/Heart Rhythm Society[2] awarded a IIa indication: "CRT can be useful in patients with atrial fibrillation and LVEF $\leq$35% on optimal medical therapy if (a) the patient requires ventricular pacing or otherwise meets CRT criteria *and* (emphasis added) (b) AV nodal ablation or pharmacologic rate control will allow near 100% ventricular pacing with CRT) (level of evidence, B)."

These guidelines reflect the consensus of expert opinion and are the basis for most clinical decisions in the real world. They illustrate the uncertainty that persists in the use of CRT in the patient with AF. Specifically, the guidelines stipulate that the patient must have very well controlled ventricular rate that will render the patient formally, or nearly so, dependent on a pacemaker for control of ventricular rhythm. Clearly these stipulations do not apply to the vast majority of patients with AF currently being considered for or receiving CRT in practice. That is, most patients do not have very slow conduction and thus, by definition, will have competition between intrinsic rhythm and the efforts to impose BiV pacing.

PROBLEMS OF CARDIAC RESYNCHRONIZATION THERAPY DELIVERY IN THE SETTING OF ATRIAL FIBRILLATION

Patients with AF have no AV synchrony, so coordinated AV pacing with appropriately programmed AV intervals is not possible. Thus, BiV pacing delivery, and more importantly capture, cannot be reliably ensured. Even when pacing is delivered, many ventricular complexes may be fused or pseudofused, making pacing capture percentages retrievable from the CRT device inaccurate and an overestimate of effective pacing capture.[7]

We examined 18 patients with implanted CRT devices and permanent AF who were maximally treated with medical therapy (digoxin, beta-blocker, and amiodarone) for rate control resulting in greater than 90% chronic BiV pacing by device interrogation.[7] The patients underwent 12-lead Holter recording, which permitted detailed QRS template matching and calculation of all paced beats as either fully paced, fused beats or pseudofused beats. Despite the maximal pharmacologic efforts to control ventricular rate, more than half the patients had approximately 40% ineffective pacing delivery, that is, substantial contribution by fused and pseudofused complexes. These patients demonstrated no response to CRT by any clinical measure, whereas the patients who were predominantly fully paced responded to CRT. This study supported the hypothesis that successful CRT delivery with effective BiV capture in the setting of AF is challenging and if not achieved, many patients will simply not respond. Furthermore, device diagnostics may suggest a higher ventricular pacing percentage is present, but when carefully analyzed, fusion beats or pseudofusion beats may represent a significant portion of ventricular pacing.

The amount of ventricular pacing is very important. It is generally believed that near maximal effective and complete BiV capture is necessary to ensure optimal CRT response. In a study of

1812 patients with CRT devices, patient freedom from death or HF hospitalization was analyzed relative to the prevailing pacing prevalence.[8] Pacing delivery was highly predictive of clinical outcome; those with pacing of less than 92% did poorly and those at 100% pacing exceeded all other groups. Groups with 92% to 97% and 98% to 99% had intermediate outcomes. Interestingly, patients with a history of atrial arrhythmia were more likely (P<.001) to be paced <92%. Using a manufacturer's remote monitoring database, Hayes and colleagues[9] also tested the importance of pacing prevalence to outcome in a study of more than 36,000 patients with 2 years of follow-up. There was a striking dichotomy in that pacing greater than 98.5% had much better outcomes than those with pacing ≤98.5% (**Fig. 1**). These data strongly support the notion that to maximize clinical response to CRT, pacing must be delivered nearly universally.

RANDOMIZED CLINICAL TRIALS OF CARDIAC RESYNCHRONIZATION THERAPY WITH PATIENTS WITH ATRIAL FIBRILLATION

As noted previously, none of the seminal clinical trials permitted enrollment of patients with AF and all required sinus rhythm, with 2 exceptions. In the MUSTIC study, patients were subdivided into those with sinus rhythm and those with AF.[10] The latter were required to have slow ventricular rates, "either spontaneous or induced by atrioventricular junction (AVJ) ablation." The study used a crossover design comparing 3 months of CRT with 3 months of right ventricular (RV) pacing. Only 43 patients with AF entered and only 37

completed both phases of the study. There were no differences by intention to treat in any of the defined endpoints of 6-minute hall walk (6MHW) distance, peak O_2 consumption on exercise test, or quality of life. There was a slight preference by patients for CRT. The neutral results of the study were attributed to small sample size and high dropout rates.

The recent RAFT study of patients with class II (80%) and class III (20%) HF provide the largest sample of patients with AF in a randomized clinical trial.[11] Enrollment was stratified based on the presence or absence of permanent AF. Permanent AF was defined as no evidence of sinus rhythm nor any plan to restore sinus rhythm. Patients with permanent AF were required to have a resting heart rate of ≤60 beats per minute and ≤90 beats per minute after a 6MHW to be eligible for the study. Of the 1798 patients in RAFT, 12.7% or 229 had permanent AF: 114 were randomized to CRT-D and 115 to ICD. The primary endpoint was HF hospitalization or death, and there was no difference in outcomes between the 2 groups (HR = 0.96, P = .82). Survival curves were super-imposable (**Fig. 2**). During a mean 40-month follow-up, 42.6% of patients with an ICD and 48.2% of patients with CRT-D had HF hospitalization or death. The 2-year event rate was approximately 33% even though 80% were in NYHA class II at baseline.

Importantly, patients in the CRT-D arm did not achieve substantial BiV pacing: during the first 6 months after randomization, only 34% had greater than 95% pacing and only 47% had greater than 90% pacing. These results would fall well below the levels of BiV pacing, which are believed to be required to generate a clinical

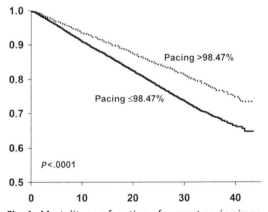

Fig. 1. Mortality as a function of percent pacing in patients with CRT. (*From* Hayes DL, Boehmer JP, Day JD, et al. Cardiac resynchronization therapy and the relationship of percent biventricular pacing to symptoms and survival. Heart Rhythm 2011;8:1472; with permission.)

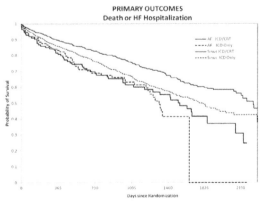

Fig. 2. Contrast between outcomes in RAFT for patients in sinus rhythm versus AF. (*From* Healy JS, Hohnloser SH, Exner DV, et al. Cardiac resynchronization therapy in patients with permanent atrial fibrillation; results from the Resynchronization for Ambulatory Heart Failure Trial (F-RAFT). Circ Heart Fail 2012;5:568; with permission.)

benefit (see previously), even though patients were preselected to have very well controlled ventricular rates. Of note, only 1 patient underwent AVJ ablation. These findings raise concerns regarding the value of CRT in patients with AF and/or the current management that prepares the patient for CRT, even though the study was not designed or powered to address AF specifically.

ATRIOVENTRICULAR JUNCTION ABLATION FOR CONTROL OF VENTRICULAR RATE IN ATRIAL FIBRILLATION

AVJ ablation should be considered when AF engenders a fast ventricular rate despite adequate doses of AV nodal active drugs or when such drugs are not tolerated or when antiarrhythmic medications are ineffective or contraindicated. This ablation procedure is relatively easy to accomplish and renders the patients pacemaker dependent. In the past, the His-bundle would be targeted, but contemporary practice focuses on the AV node, which results in a slow but stable intrinsic escape rhythm; nonetheless a pacemaker is generally required ("ablate and pace"). Many studies have confirmed the utility of this intervention with relief of symptoms related to excessive ventricular rates and simplification of medical therapy. As opposed to direct current energy ablation of the past, radiofrequency energy and AVJ ablation have not been associated with increased risk of sudden death. The PAVE study was a randomized comparison of univentricular RV pacing with BiV pacing in patients with uncontrolled ventricular rates due to AF and suggested modest benefit in the primary endpoint of 6MHW distance at 6 months.[12] In a post hoc analysis of patients with reduced EF, the benefits were more apparent.

OBSERVATIONAL COHORT STUDIES OF ATRIOVENTRICULAR JUNCTION ABLATION IN PATIENTS UNDERGOING CARDIAC RESYNCHRONIZATION THERAPY

Gasparini and colleagues[13] described the outcome of more than 600 prospectively followed patients treated with CRT at 2 European centers. Of the 114 patients with AF, a shockingly low proportion, 42%, achieved "adequate" biventricular capture (arbitrarily defined as >85% at 2 months) despite the usual pharmacologic and pacing programming efforts. Those who did not achieve adequate capture, by protocol design in a nonrandomized format, underwent AVJ ablation, resulting in near complete BiV capture. Reassuringly, patients with AF and patients with sinus

rhythm had similar benefits from CRT across multiple relevant endpoints. But it is within the AF group that the results yielded compelling and provocative data. Only the patients with AF who had undergone AVJ ablation demonstrated evidence of reverse remodeling (increased LVEF, decreased LV end-systolic volume [LVESV]) and functional improvement (**Fig. 3**). A substantial overall response rate (approximately two-thirds) was seen in the ablated patients, but a very poor response rate (~30%) was observed in the non-ablated patients. Mortality was also better in those who underwent AVJ, 4% versus 15%.[14] The investigators attributed this beneficial response to the imposition of AVJ ablation after CRT, resulting in predictable and consistent 100% ventricular capture versus the capture rate of 88% in the group that did not undergo ablation.

Certainly, explanations of this study's outcomes are plausible and further support the hypothesis that ablation renders the patient pacemaker dependent, thus ensuring that CRT is appropriately delivered without fusion or pseudofusion; inadequate rate control is removed from even an intermittent event; and the rhythm is regularized, imparting that additional benefit on ventricular performance.[15] The results of Gasparini and colleagues[13] suggest that even relatively high percentage BiV capture may be inadequate, and several recent large registries confirm the strong association of pacing prevalence and long-term outcome after CRT. Our own detailed Holter analyses[7] confirmed that approximately half of CRT patients with AF have inadequate pacing capture due to substantial pacing competition resulting in fusion and pseudofusion and that these patients respond poorly to CRT. In aggregate, these prior studies strongly support the uncertainty of benefit of CRT in AF and how it should be applied, and thus provide powerful justification for a randomized clinical trial.

Similar supportive findings have been noted by other investigators, and are detailed in **Table 1**. Two studies have reported favorable changes in LVESV in patients with AF with/without AVJ ablation or the equivalent high effective pacing capture.[7,13] At 1 year, comparing patients with versus without AVJ ablation, Gasparini and colleagues[13] noted a decline of LVESV of 18% versus 3% and we described a decline of 29.8% versus 6.2% based on effective versus ineffective capture.[8] In contradistinction, Dong and colleagues[16] observed an equivalent and slight improvement in LV end-diastolic dimension on echocardiogram of 2.1% in patients with and without AVJ ablation.

The large CERTIFY[17] multicenter observational study provides confirmation of the single-center

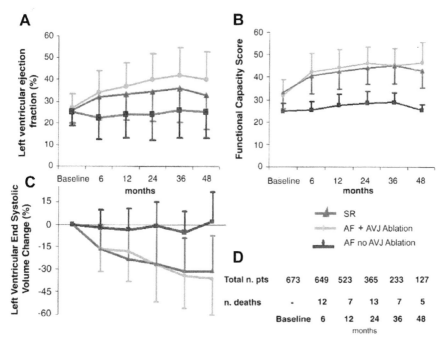

Fig. 3. Outcomes relative to AVJ ablation in patients with AF. pts, patients; SR, sinus rhythm. (*A*) Changes in left ventricular ejection fraction (LVEF). (*B*) Changes in exercise capacity. (*C*) Changes in left ventricular end systolic volume (LVESV). (*D*) Number of patients at follow-up visits. (*From* Gasparini M, Auricchio A, Regoli F, et al. Four-year efficacy of cardiac resynchronization therapy on exercise tolerance and disease progression: the importance of performing atrioventricular junction ablation in patients with atrial fibrillation. J Am Coll Cardiol 2006;48:740; with permission.)

studies. In comparison with a control group of 895 patients with AF not treated by AVJ ablation, 443 patients who underwent AVJ ablation had lower mortality (see **Table 1**) and more reverse remodeling, such that LVESV decreased by an additional 50 mL by 3 years.

These are important observational retrospective or cohort studies, but the results must be interpreted cautiously. In an editorial,[18] we suggested the results begged the question of whether all patients with advanced refractory HF and permanent AF should have AVJ ablation with CRT, but to

Table 1
Studies comparing outcome after CRT in AF

Author	Sample Size	HFH, %	AF + AVJ vs AF-AVJ 2-y Survival, %	CRT Response, %	Comments
Gasparini et al,[13] 2006	114/48	—	—	79/30	—
Gasparini et al,[14] 2008	118/125	—	96/65	—	—
Gasparini et al,[17] 2013	443/895	—	90/70	—	Absence of AVJ independently increased mortality
Dong et al,[16] 2010	45/109	16/20	96/75	—	AVJ independently predicted survival
Ferreira et al,[22] (Europace 2008)	26/27	15/41	95/62	85/52	AVJ independent predicted response
Molhoek et al,[23] (AJC 2004)	17/13	—	—	71/54	AVJ associated with better EF, 6MHW

Abbreviations: AF, atrial fibrillation; AVJ, atrioventricular junction; CRT, cardiac resynchronization therapy; EF, ejection fraction; HFH, heart failure hospitalization.

create pacemaker dependency in large numbers of patients with HF would require definitive results from a well-designed and powered randomized clinical trial.

Finally, one underrecognized benefit of appropriate CRT delivery in patients with AF is subsequent reversion to sinus rhythm. We have also reported that approximately 10% of CRT patients with permanent AF revert to sinus rhythm spontaneously, mostly in the first few months following implantation.[19] Four predictors of reversion were identified: smaller LV end-diastolic diameter, shorter QRS duration after CRT, smaller left atrial diameter, and notably, AVJ ablation. Patients with the spontaneous return of sinus rhythm showed an 87% reduction in mortality after 1 year.

Two recent meta-analyses attempted to understand the value of AVJ ablation in the setting of CRT given the limited published experience. When pooling 3 prior observational studies, Wilton and colleagues[20] concluded that there was a 40% increase in the response to CRT if AVJ ablation was used. The investigators opined that "routine use of AVN [atrioventricular node] ablation would ensure adequate BiV pacing in patients with AF. However, the potential benefits must be balanced against the risks associated with creating pacemaker dependency. The benefit reported with AVN ablation should be interpreted in light of the fact that patients were selected for this therapy based on clinical characteristics." Ganesan and colleagues in a recent article[21] observed that the pooled mortality was reduced by 42% if AVJ ablation was performed in patients with AF undergoing CRT ($P<.001$) (**Fig. 4**). The improvement in EF was greater if AVJ was used, but the difference was not statistically different.

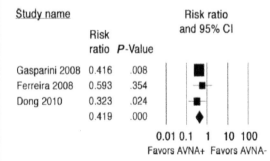

Fig. 4. Meta-analysis of AVJ in CRT for AF: mortality endpoint. AVNA, AV nodal ablation; CI, confidence interval. (*From* Ganesan AN, Brooks AG, Roberts-Thomson KC, et al. Role of AV nodal ablation in cardiac resynchronization in patients with coexistent atrial fibrillation and heart failure. J Am Coll Cardiol 2011;59:723; with permission.)

ONGOING STUDIES AND POTENTIAL IMPACT ON CLINICAL PRACTICE AND CLINICAL OUTCOMES

Data outlined in the preceding sections demonstrate that little evidence is available to support that CRT is effective in patients with permanent AF. Common practice includes patients with HF and AF who receive CRT devices, but the efficacy in these patients is unknown, especially without AVJ ablation. The uncertainty of using CRT in patients with AF is reflected in the most recent consensus guidelines, which place CRT intervention in patients with HF and AF as class II. A growing body of evidence, mostly based on single-center studies in small numbers of patients, support the hypothesis that AVJ ablation may increase the amount of BiV pacing in patients with AF, and thus may increase chances of a favorable clinical response. The literature is clear. What is lacking is prospective clinical trial data addressing this very important question to determine if AVJ ablation should be an obligate part of CRT application in this very important group of patients.

In clinical practice, many physicians are concerned that using AVJ ablation routinely will render many patients pacemaker dependent. Although there are no data suggesting long-term risk, this concern can override the best available evidence until and unless a large-scale randomized clinical trial provides guidance. Furthermore, safety concerns should be mitigated by the knowledge that CRT patients have back-up pacing leads (RV and LV), that an intrinsic escape rhythm usually exists, and that modern remote monitoring provides intensified surveillance. Finally, there is no certainty to whom to apply AVJ ablation, and real-world usage is quite variable, including subgroups of patients such as those with excessive rates, those who clinically do not respond, those with significant AVN disease and bradycardia, or patients with moderate rate control.

RANDOMIZED CLINICAL TRIAL OF JUNCTIONAL ATRIOVENTRICULAR ABLATION FOR PERMANENT ATRIAL FIBRILLATION IN PATIENTS UNDERGOING CARDIAC RESYNCHRONIZATION THERAPY

In 2016, we received National Institutes of Health funding to conduct a randomized clinical pilot study called Junctional AV Ablation for Permanent AF in Patients Undergoing CRT (JAVA-CRT) (NCT02946853). This trial was proposed as an unblinded randomized controlled longitudinal trial such that if the results were positive, a large-scale mortality trial would follow. Inclusion criteria were as follows: initial implantation of CRT-D or prior implantation of CRT-D within 1 year, ischemic or nonischemic cardiomyopathy, LVEF ≤35%, NYHA class II-IV (ambulatory) HF, QRS ≥120 ms for patients with LBBB and ≥150 ms for patients without LBBB, and continuous AF >3 months when no further efforts to restore sinus rhythm are feasible or pursued.

At enrollment, patients were randomized 1:1 to undergo AVJ ablation with CRT-D or no AVJ ablation with CRT-D. Patients were required to be on optimal medical therapy, including maximally tolerated doses of beta-blockers; angiotensin-converting enzyme inhibitors or angiotensin receptor blockers; aldosterone antagonists; and statins, digoxin, and aspirin as recommended by current guidelines. Warfarin or a novel oral anticoagulant was used for stroke prevention. Beta-blockers and digoxin were used for rate control of ventricular response. AVJ ablation was to be performed at the time of CRT implantation. Programming of implantable devices was by protocol and intended to provide maximal CRT pacing with attention to rate cutoffs and enhanced features. Patients were excluded from the trial if ventricular rates at rest were greater than 110 beats per minute despite optimal medical therapy or less than 50 beats per minute, or if they had heart block or symptomatic bradycardia that necessitated permanent pacing.

The primary aim of the study was to determine if patients with permanent AF who meet conventional criteria for CRT and undergo AVJ ablation have reduced ventricular remodeling (ie, echocardiographic improvement of LVESV), a potent marker of subsequent clinical deterioration, compared with patients who do not undergo AVJ ablation, over 6 months. This study was designed to test feasibility of enrollment and short-term improvement in surrogate endpoints, with anticipation of a full-scale large randomized clinical trial using hard outcome events (mortality and HF hospitalization) if this phase was promising.

The secondary aims were to examine (1) change in LVEF from baseline to 6 months, (2) LV end-systolic and diastolic volumes and change from baseline to 6 months, (3) HF hospitalization including repeated HF hospitalizations, (4) all-cause death; (5) ventricular tachycardia/ventricular fibrillation arrhythmic events requiring ICD therapy, (6) inappropriate ICD therapy, (7) percentage BiV pacing, (8) quality-of-life scores, and (9) complications related to AVJ ablation procedure.

The trial is currently ongoing at 25 centers in the United States. Additional international trials (eg, NCT01522898) are also in progress and focused on a similar population of patients to address the potential value of AVJ ablation.

SUMMARY

There remains a great deal of uncertainty about whether general application of CRT to patients with AF provides any benefit assuming all other eligibility criteria are met. Preliminary observations suggest that performing AVJ ablation can improve the results of CRT in patients with AF by rendering the patient pacemaker dependent. Ongoing randomized clinical trials may provide more definitive answers in the future.

REFERENCES

1. McMurray JJV, Adamopolous S, Anker SD, et al. ESC guidelines for the diagnosis and treatment of acute and chronic heart failure 2012. Eur Heart J 2012;33:1787–847.
2. Tracey CM, Epstein AE, Darbar D, et al. 2012 ACCF/AHA/HRS focused update of the 2008 guidelines for device-based therapy of cardiac rhythm abnormalities. Circulation 2012;126:1784–800.
3. Auricchio A, Metra M, Gasparini M, et al. Long-term survival of patients with heart failure and ventricular conduction delay treated with cardiac resynchronization therapy. Am J Cardiol 2007;99:232–8.
4. Dickstein K, Bogale N, Priori S, et al. The European cardiac resynchronization survey. Eur Heart J 2009;30:2450–60.
5. Medtronic, Inc. (internal data).
6. NCDR ICD Registry 2011-2 Data.
7. Kamath GS, Cotiga D, Koneru JN, et al. The utility of 12-lead Holter monitoring in patients with permanent atrial fibrillation for the identification of nonresponders after cardiac resynchronization therapy. J Am Coll Cardiol 2009;53:1050–5.
8. Koplan BA, Kaplan AJ, Weiner S, et al. Heart failure decompensation and all-cause mortality in relation to percent biventricular pacing in patients with heart failure: is a goal of 100% biventricular pacing necessary? J Am Coll Cardiol 2009;53:355–60.
9. Hayes DL, Boehmer JP, Day JD, et al. Cardiac resynchronization therapy and the relationship of percent biventricular pacing to symptoms and survival. Heart Rhythm 2011;8:1460–75.
10. Leclercq C, Walker S, Linde C, et al. Comparative effects of permanent biventricular and right-univentricular pacing in heart failure patients with chronic atrial fibrillation. Eur Heart J 2002;23:1780–7.
11. Healy JS, Hohnloser SH, Exner DV, et al. Cardiac resynchronization therapy in patients with permanent atrial fibrillation; results from the Resynchronization for Ambulatory Heart Failure Trial (F-RAFT). Circ Heart Fail 2012;5:566–70.
12. Doshi RN, Daoud EG, Fellows C, et al. Left ventricular-based cardiac stimulation post AV nodal

ablation evaluation (The Pave Study). J Cardiovasc Electrophysiol 2005;16:1160–5.

13. Gasparini M, Auricchio A, Regoli F, et al. Four-year efficacy of cardiac resynchronization therapy on exercise tolerance and disease progression: the importance of performing atrioventricular junction ablation in patients with atrial fibrillation. J Am Coll Cardiol 2006;48:734–43.

14. Gasparini M, Auricchio A, Metra M, et al. Long-term survival in patients undergoing cardiac resynchronization therapy: the importance of performing atrioventricular junction ablation in patients with permanent atrial fibrillation. Eur Heart J 2008;29:1644–52.

15. Daoud E, Weiss R, Bahu M, et al. Effect of irregular ventricular rhythm on cardiac output. Am J Cardiol 1996;78:1433–6.

16. Dong K, Shen W-K, Powell BD, et al. Atrioventricular nodal ablation predicts survival benefit in patients with atrial fibrillation receiving cardiac resynchronization therapy. Heart Rhythm 2010;7:1240–5.

17. Gasparini M, Leclercq C, Lunati M, et al. Cardiac resynchronization therapy in patients with atrial fibrillation. The CERTIFY Study (cardiac resynchronization therapy in atrial fibrillation patients multicenter registry). J Am Coll Cardiol 2013;1:1500–7.

18. Steinberg JS. Desperately seeking a randomized clinical trial of resynchronization therapy for patients with heart failure and atrial fibrillation. J Am Coll Cardiol 2006;48:744–6.

19. Gasparini M, Steinberg JS, Arshad A, et al. Resumption of sinus rhythm in patients with heart failure and permanent atrial fibrillation undergoing cardiac resynchronization therapy: a longitudinal observational study. Eur Heart J 2010;31:2677–87.

20. Wilton SB, Leung AA, Ghali WA, et al. Outcomes of cardiac resynchronization therapy in patients with versus without atrial fibrillation: a systematic review and meta-analysis. Heart Rhythm 2011;8:1088–94.

21. Ganesan AN, Brooks AG, Roberts-Thomson KC, et al. Role of AV nodal ablation in cardiac resynchronization in patients with coexistent atrial fibrillation and heart failure. J Am Coll Cardiol 2011;59:719–26.

22. Ferreira AM, Adragao P, Cavaco DM, et al. Benefit of cardiac resynchronization therapy in atrial fibrillation patients vs patients in sinus rhythm: role of atrioventricular junctional ablation. Europace 2008;10:809–15.

23. Moelhoek SG, Bax JJ, Bleeker GB, et al. Comparison of response to cardiac resynchronization therapy in patients in sinus rhythm versus chronic atrial fibrillation. Am J Cardiol 2004;94:1506–9.

Emerging Pacing Technologies
in Heart Failure

Left Ventricular Endocardial Pacing/ Leadless Pacing

Alan Hanley, MB, MSc, E. Kevin Heist, MD, PhD*

KEYWORDS

• CRT • Heart failure • LV endocardial pacing • WiSE-CRT

KEY POINTS

- Cardiac resynchronization therapy is an effective treatment for many patients with heart failure. Delivery is limited by coronary sinus anatomy and some patients fail to respond to therapy.
- Preclinical data show that pacing the left ventricular endocardium may be superior to traditional cardiac resynchronization therapy, which relies on epicardial pacing.
- In published cases of patients who have received left ventricular endocardial pacing, good clinical responses and improvement in surrogate markers have been seen.
- Early prospective studies of a novel leadless left ventricular endocardial pacing system have raised safety concerns; patients who received the therapy benefitted significantly.

INTRODUCTION: CARDIAC RESYNCHRONIZATION THERAPY

Several decades of work over the course of the twentieth century led to an expanded understanding of cardiac mechanical function and the relationship between electrical activation sequence and hemodynamics.[1] The global burden of heart failure and limitations of existing medical therapies precipitated several studies investigating the potential benefit of resynchronizing the heart using pacing. Cardiac resynchronization therapy (CRT) was first used clinically a quarter of a century ago.[2,3] Early studies included MUSTIC, PATH-HF, and MIRACLE.[4–6] The concurrent development and evidence of benefit for implantable cardioverter-defibrillators (ICD) meant that CRT could be combined with an ICD or not. These configurations were tested in a series of high-profile studies, including MIRACLE-ICD, COMPANION, CARE-HF, CONTAK-CD, MIRACLE-ICD II, REVERSE, MADIT-CRT, and RAFT.[7–14] This wealth of high-quality, multicenter, randomized data incorporating thousands of patients firmly established the superiority of CRT over optimal pharmacologic therapy alone in patients with heart failure, impaired left ventricular (LV) function and LV dyssynchrony.

CHALLENGES TO TRADITIONAL CARDIAC RESYNCHRONIZATION THERAPY

The earliest CRT systems were implanted with surgically placed epicardial LV leads and transvenous leads in the right atrium and right ventricle. The advent of entirely transvenous CRT, using the coronary sinus (CS) to deliver LV pacing, allowed the field to expand via the pivotal trials listed elsewhere in this article and lead to widespread availability of the technology, supported by society guidelines.[15] Transvenous CRT implant is a technically challenging procedure however, with long

Disclosure Statement: A. Hanley has no financial disclosures. E.K. Heist: Abbott: consultant, research grant. Biotronik: consultant. Boston Scientific: consultant, research grant. Johnson and Johnson: consultant. Medtronic: consultant.
Cardiac Arrhythmia Service, Massachusetts General Hospital, 55 Fruit Street, Boston, MA 02114, USA
* Corresponding author.
E-mail address: kheist@mgh.harvard.edu

Card Electrophysiol Clin 11 (2019) 155–164
https://doi.org/10.1016/j.ccep.2018.10.001

procedure times and, compared with standard permanent pacemaker or ICD implant, excessive exposure to ionizing radiation. Capture thresholds can be increased, limiting battery life and leading to requirement for frequent generator replacements.

The CS anatomy is also highly variable, often providing limited options in terms of an LV pacing site. Pacing from different locations in a single individual results in different degrees of hemodynamic benefit, although the site of optimal pacing is also different from person to person. The site dictated by CS anatomy may not provide the most favorable hemodynamic response.[16] Optimization of CRT can include finding an alternative LV lead position (which might not be feasible), pacing between different poles of a multipole electrode with variable results, or optimizing atrioventricular delays using electrical or echocardiographic indices of efficacy.[17,18] Despite optimization of CRT, up to 30% remain nonresponders to the therapy.[19,20] Considering that more than 300,000 CRT devices were implanted between 2006 and 2012, this represents a large unmet clinical need.[21]

Another concern is that epicardial LV pacing reverses physiologic activation of the ventricular wall, which is normally endocardial to epicardial. This change has downstream effects on repolarization, including earlier repolarization of the epicardium and increased transmural dispersion of repolarization, ultimately manifesting as QT prolongation, which may be arrhythmogenic.[22–26] In rare cases, CRT-associated ventricular arrhythmias may require treatment with catheter ablation to preserve delivery of CRT to patients who require it.[27,28]

These challenges have stimulated interest in alternatives to traditional CRT, including endocardial LV pacing. LV endocardial pacing could overcome constraints of the CS anatomy, provide more flexibility in terms of choice of pacing site, and allow for more physiologic endocardial LV activation.

LEFT VENTRICULAR ENDOCARDIAL PACING: EARLY EXPERIENCES (1998–2009)
First Cases

The first case report of intentional LV endocardial pacing is provided by Jaïs and colleagues.[29] A 73-year-old gentleman with end-stage heart failure and in whom a lead could not be placed in the CS received an LV lead via atrial transseptal access to good clinical effect; he improved from New York Heart Association (NYHA) functional class IV to NYHA functional class II and over 15 months of follow up, suffered no cerebral embolic events on oral anticoagulation. In 1999, Leclercq and colleagues[30] reported a series of 3 patients who received LV endocardial leads, also via a transseptal puncture. All three responded clinically with improved functional status and no thromboembolic events on anticoagulation. An editorial at the time by Gold and Rashba[31] cautioned regarding pursuing LV endocardial lead placement as a modality for delivering CRT in favor of using a tributary of the CS, on the basis that improved lead design would allow "routine access to left ventricular branches of the coronary sinus system."

In 2001, the French group that published the first case of LV endocardial pacing reported a series of 8 patients who received transseptal LV pacing leads for the indication of heart failure with a QRS of greater than 130 ms and unsuitable CS anatomy and compared them with 15 patients who received surgically placed epicardial leads for the same indication. All patients responded clinically; however, endocardial lead placement was superior to epicardial lead placement as assessed by echocardiographic indices of electrical resynchronization and hemodynamic performance.[32] The leads in this study were all placed on the anterolateral wall.

In 2004, Ji and colleagues[33] reported the first case of LV endocardial lead placement from the left axillary vein. The procedure required transseptal puncture from above and was facilitated by standard transseptal puncture from the groin to provide anatomic landmarks. Similar to the initial reports from France, the patient was in end-stage heart failure and had no CS options for implant of CRT. He also responded well clinically, recovering from NYHA functional class IV to NYHA functional class II status.

Follow-up of First Cases and Further Implants

Long-term follow-up (85 months) of 6 patients implanted between 1998 and 1999 in France was reported in 2007.[34] All patients had improved clinical status from NYHA functional class III or IV to II and had narrowed QRS to less than 120 ms on average. Two patients died of congestive 4 years after implant, 2 patients underwent cardiac transplantation at 2 and 4 years, and 2 patients were alive. Only one transient ischemic attack occurred when anticoagulation was interrupted. The same year, 10 further cases of LV endocardial placement were reported from the Netherlands in patients who required CRT but were not suitable for epicardial lead placement, and in whom a CS lead could not be placed.[35] The leads were delivered by a transseptal approach after puncture and dilatation from the groin. Successful deployment with good lead parameters was achieved in 9 patients.

A separate report of successful transseptal LV lead placement in a patient who required CRT and had no other options was reported in 2007.[36] This report was accompanied by a particularly strident editorial calling for caution as case reports of endocardial LV lead implantation had accumulated over the preceding decade. Kasai and colleagues,[37] while acknowledging that reports to date represented salvage of dire situations, highlighted several potential risks and the need for rigorous study of the approach. Particular concerns they raised include the implication of infection of a lead implanted in the LV, which could result in septic emboli to several organs including the brain and lead to more profound illness than infection of a right-sided implant.

In 2009, a series of 9 patients who received LV endocardial pacing was reported by Morgan and colleagues.[38] The procedure was atrial transseptal with puncture and dilatation from the groin first, as had been described by others. Procedural success was attained in 8 of the 9 patients, with resultant clinical improvement and no thromboembolic events up to 32 months after implantation. Also in 2009, a case of LV lead placement through a patent foramen ovale was reported, which obviated the need for transseptal puncture.[39] A method for crossing the septum from above without puncturing was also described by Lau.[40] In this case, transseptal puncture was performed from the groin, and a wire was positioned across the septum and used as a landmark to position a dilator from superior access at the transseptal puncture site. A wire could then be advanced across the septum without repuncturing.

PRECLINICAL STUDIES

In the early 2000s, the tranche of landmark CRT trials described elsewhere in this article were published and established CS lead placement with epicardial LV pacing as the standard of care in resynchronizing the sick heart. Apart from the early case reports, small case series, and 1 preclinical study discussed elsewhere in this article, interest in endocardial LV pacing would wane until later in the decade.

In 2003, Peschar and colleagues,[41] working in an open chest dog model, investigated the effect of pacing several different locations on cardiac pump function. In their model, pacing from the endocardial LV septum or apex provided pump function that was comparable with intrinsic conduction. RV pacing and epicardial LV pacing were all associated with varying degrees of lower LV pump function.

Mechanistic Studies

It would be another 5 years before the next preclinical model was reported. In 2008, Kavanagh and colleagues[42] replicated the findings of Peschar and colleagues using electrical indices. Of multiple sites tested, LV septal pacing provided transmyocardial activation closest to that seen with activation through the His-Purkinje system. In a comprehensive study by Mills and colleagues[43] in 2009, dogs received pacing at multiple different sites after atrioventricular nodal ablation. This study demonstrated the benefit of LV endocardial pacing compared with RV pacing or traditional biventricular pacing, both acutely and chronically. LV septal or apical pacing resulted in cardiac efficiency similar to that seen with native conduction. The same group simultaneously published data on the acute superior efficacy of LV endocardial pacing compared with traditional CRT in dogs with left bundle branch block.[44] Cardiac contractility and electrical resynchronization was improved with LV endocardial pacing. These findings are supported by later work from Xu and colleagues[26] in work in a canine model showing superior hemodynamics achieved by endocardial LV pacing compared with standard biventricular pacing, or multipoint epicardial pacing.

Additional evidence of the potential mechanism whereby endocardial pacing is superior to epicardial pacing was provided by Strik and colleagues[45] in a 2012 canine study. They used dense electroanatomic mapping of the endocardium and epicardium in canine models of heart failure, myocardial infarction and left bundle branch block to demonstrate that endocardial pacing results in faster endocardial and transmural conduction than epicardial pacing, with improved electrical synchrony and pump function resulting. A subsequent computational electrophysiological model by Hyde and colleagues[46] comparing endocardial and epicardial pacing and their effects on latest activation times supported these findings.

In 2016, Rademakers and colleagues[47] reported both canine and human data in their article evaluating LV septal pacing compared with epicardial pacing in CRT. The 12 patients in their study received CRT and had temporary LV septal pacing at the time of the procedure. In dogs, LV septal pacing decreased dispersion of repolarization. The hemodynamic benefits were similar to that seen with conventional CRT.

SECOND WAVE OF CLINICAL INTEREST

The compelling demonstrations of benefit with LV endocardial pacing in both animal models and humans prompted renewed interest in the technique.[48] In 2010, Spragg and colleagues[49] brought patients with preexisting RV pacing leads or traditional CRT leads to the laboratory for LV endocardial pacing to assess the effect on acute hemodynamic response (AHR). Biventricular pacing with endocardial LV pacing from any site was superior to RV pacing alone, whereas biventricular pacing with endocardial LV pacing from the best endocardial site was superior to traditional CRT. The following year, Ginks and colleagues[50] reported similar work comparing endocardial LV pacing with traditional CRT by measuring the AHR with a pressure wire in the LV.

The potentially proarrhythmic effects of standard CRT on repolarization was investigated in the context of LV endocardial pacing by Scott and colleagues.[51] Their cohort of 7 patients in whom LV endocardial leads had been placed were compared with 28 patients with CS leads and 8 patients with surgically placed epicardial leads. LV endocardial pacing was associated with less QT dispersion than epicardial pacing. This finding was subsequently investigated in a canine perfused LV wedge preparation by Xu and colleagues.[26] They tested pacing from endocardial, midmyocardial, and epicardial sites, and measured transmural dispersion of repolarization. Pacing from the endocardium and midmyocardium did not significantly increase transmural dispersion of repolarization, whereas epicardial pacing did so, resulting in ventricular arrhythmias in 2 of 8 preparations.

In 2012, the effect of LV endocardial pacing on cardiac hemodynamics was investigated invasively using pressure–volume loops in 10 patients undergoing traditional CRT implant.[52] Multiple LV endocardial sites were chosen for stimulation. The optimal site varied by person. In all cases, the optimal LV endocardial pacing site outperformed stimulation from a lead placed in the CS. Later the same year, a similar study was reported by Ginks and colleagues[53] demonstrating a superior AHR to pacing from the LV endocardium compared with conventional CRT. The same findings were reported in 2014 by Shetty and colleagues.[54] Sohal and colleagues[55] in an acute hemodynamic study of various pacing modalities demonstrated a superior effect of endocardial LV pacing compared with epicardial pacing, and an equivalent effect of biventricular endocardial pacing compared with LV-only endocardial pacing.

LV endocardial lead placement to this point had been used primarily for those who had failed CRT placement. Van Gelder and colleagues[56] enrolled 24 patients in an elegant hemodynamic study of the potential for LV endocardial pacing to benefit patients to were nonresponders to CRT. By pacing endocardially from different sites, AHR was achieved in 14 patients.

One of the more compelling demonstrations of superiority of endocardial pacing over epicardial pacing was provided by Behar and colleagues[57] in a 2016 report. Their group tested multiple endocardial and epicardial pacing sites in 8 patients with preexisting CRT devices and found that pacing the endocardium was superior with respect to an AHR than epicardial pacing. Furthermore, pacing at the same site endocardially was associated with a significantly shorter QRS and greater AHR than epicardially.

Two metaanalyses of LV endocardial pacing were published in 2018. In the first, Gamble and colleagues[58] analyzed reports of 384 patients who had received this therapy. Unsurprisingly, there was significant heterogeneity among the studies, but the authors noted overall response rates comparable with conventional CRT. In the second, Graham and colleagues[59] evaluated studies that included 362 patients. They identified improvement in functional class and LV function, but also a higher rate of stroke than in a comparable heart failure population.

TECHNIQUES
Transseptal Puncture

Atrial transseptal puncture from above has been described in many of the case reports and case series to date. This requires use of tools that were developed for transseptal puncture from a femoral approach. Novel methods designed specifically for LV endocardial lead delivery from above have been described. Lau in 2011,[60] and Patel and Whorley in 2013,[61] both describe a method of advancing a guidewire into the left atrium, which is snared from above and used as a rail into the left atrium over which a delivery catheter can be advanced.

Van Gelder and colleagues[62] report the technique of implanting a lead into the LV from femoral access, and then pulling the lead through the vasculature to the pectoral region. This procedure was performed in 11 patients with good lead parameters obtained and no thromboembolic events seen at the 6-month follow-up. An alternative method was described by Wright and colleagues.[63] They advanced the lead into the heart from above as in a standard implant, then snared the lead via a transseptal sheath from the groin, advancing the sheath, snare and lead across the septum into the left atrium. Moriña-Vázquez and colleagues[64] describe an entirely transfemoral system, with transseptal lead placement from the femoral vein and generator situated in the thigh.

Betts and colleagues[65] reported implant of an LV pacing lead via interventricular septal puncture in a series of patients. They used subclavian vein access and achieved good parameters and clinical response.

Transapical Implant

Transapical endocardial lead placement is feasible in patients undergoing epicardial lead placement with excessive pericardial adhesions.[66,67] This approach was tested against surgically placed epicardial leads in a small study by the group that first suggested it.[68] Both groups of patients responded to treatment, but the magnitude of improvement in functional status and LV function seemed to be greater in the group receiving endocardial pacing. Long-term follow-up (median, 40 months) in a group of 26 recipients.[69] Eleven patients had survived, with 2 suffering a stroke and 1 suffering a transient ischemic attack.

Leadless Left Ventricular Pacing

The preceding descriptions of LV endocardial pacing highlight several challenges facing the field. Endocardial pacing seems to be superior to epicardial pacing, both electrically and hemodynamically, and with good clinical success, albeit in very small numbers of patients. The appeal of traditional CRT is evident; however, implanting permanent hardware in the systemic circulation carries an attendant risk of thromboembolism and the placement of a lead across the septum and mitral valve that must then be connected to a generator that is traditionally prepectoral is a daunting task. The impetus for a solution to these problems lead to prospective studies to formally test the safety and efficacy of the approach, and the development of novel technology to address the challenges associated with it.

One solution consists of pacing the LV endocardially using a leadless system known as WiSE-CRT (EBR Systems, Sunnyvale, CA; https:// ebrsystemsinc.com/).[70] The system incorporates a standard pacemaker or ICD with leads in the right side of the heart, a subcutaneous ultrasound transmitter that synchronizes with RV pacing to emit a signal, a leadless receiver electrode in the LV that paces in response to the signal received, and a battery for the transmitter, also placed subcutaneously. The LV electrode is implanted via a retrograde aortic approach.

FOLLOW-UP

Long-term follow-up data on large numbers of patients who have received LV endocardial pacing

leads are lacking. Rademakers and colleagues[71] provide some midterm data. They reported 6-month outcomes on 51 patients (45 transseptal and 6 transapical) with LV leads, and noted 6 ischemic strokes, 2 transient ischemic attacks, and no worsening mitral regurgitation. All but one of the ischemic events occurred while anticoagulation was subtherapeutic. The 2-year follow-up of 20 patients who received LV endocardial-based CRT via a ventricular transseptal puncture was reported in 2018 by Gamble and colleagues.[72]

CLINICAL TRIALS
Alternate Site Cardiac Resynchronization (ALSYNC)

The first large multicenter study of LV endocardial pacing was ALSYNC[73] (**Table 1**). The study prospectively evaluated 138 patients with a minimum -p of 12 months. The implant technique involved atrial transseptal puncture from above and was successful in 89.4% of cases. Patients were taking coumadin with a target international normalized ratio of 2 to 4. Safety concerns were significant; 9 patients had transient ischemic attacks, 5 had nondisabling strokes, and there were 23 deaths at 6 months. The clinical response rate was around 60%. A subgroup analysis of 118 patients compared the outcomes in 90 failed standard CRT implant patients with 28 nonresponders to standard CRT.[74] At 19 months of follow-up, a greater proportion of patients who had failed standard implant had a reduction in LV end-systolic volume index of greater than 15% than those who had failed to respond.

Wireless Stimulation Endocardially for CRT (WiSE-CRT)

In 2013, Auricchio and colleagues[70] reported the first-in-man experience of implanting a wireless ultrasound-based LV pacing system. Three patients received the device, and all responded clinically. The patients were part of a trial evaluating the system, known as WiSE-CRT. The next report from the study in 2014 included data from 17 patients who had received the system.[75] Implant was successful in 13 patients, with significantly improved functional class and LV function at 6 months. Three patients suffered pericardial effusion.

Safety and Performance of Electrodes Implanted in the Left Ventricle (SELECT-LV)

Thirty-five patients received the WiSE-CRT system for this prospective, multicenter, nonrandomized trial.[76] Implant was successful in all but 1 patient. The indications included an inability to receive

Table 1
Prospective clinical studies of endocardial and leadless CRT

Study (Approach; Year of Publication)	Patient Population (Trial N)	Comparison	Endpoints (Mean Follow-up)	Findings
ALSYNC (transseptal; 2016)	Failed traditional CRT implant (n = 105) or nonresponder (n = 31)	Nonrandomized; baseline vs 6 mo follow-up	Primary: >70% freedom from complications at 6 mo after implant Clinical: LVESV (mL), LVEF (%), MR, NYHA functional class, 6MWT (m)	Primary: 82.2% freedom from complications at 6 mo Clinical: ↓ LVESV (29 ± 60 mL), ↑ LVEF (7 ± 10%), ↓ moderate to severe MR (41 vs 30%), ↓ NYHA functional class, ↑ 6MWT (47 ± 87 m increase)
WiSE-CRT (leadless; 2014)	Failed traditional CRT implant (n = 7), upgrade (n = 8) or nonresponder (n = 2)	Nonrandomized; baseline vs follow-up	Primary: BiV pacing on EKG at 1 mo; safety Secondary: safety; BiV pacing on EKG at 6 mo; efficacy	Primary: BiV pacing 82% of patients at 1 mo; 18% SAE Secondary: BiV pacing 92% of patients at 6 mo; 35% SAE; ↓ NYHA functional class (67% patients), ↑ LVEF (6%)
SELECT-LV (leadless; 2017)	Failed traditional CRT implant (n = 20), upgrade (n = 5) or nonresponder (n = 10)	Nonrandomized; baseline vs follow-up	Primary: BiV pacing on EKG at 1 mo; safety 0–24 h and 1–30 d Secondary: Composite clinical score, LVESV, LVESV, LVEF (%)	Primary: BiV pacing 97.1% at 1 mo; 8.6% SAE at 24 h, 22.9% SAE at 1–30 d Secondary: ↑ composite score (84.8% patients), >15%↓ LVESV (52%), >10%↓ LVEDV (40%), >5%↑ LVEF (66%), ↓ NYHA functional class (67% patients)

Abbreviations: 6MWT, 6-minute walk test; BiV, biventricular; CRT, cardiac resynchronization therapy; EKG, electrocardiograph; LVEF, left ventricular ejection fraction; LVESV, Left ventricular end-systolic volume; MR, mitral regurgitation; NYHA, New York Heart Association; SAE, serious adverse events.

conventional CRT because of anatomy or phrenic nerve pacing, or nonresponse to CRT. At 6 months, 28 patients improved clinically and 21 patients had improved LV function, as measured by echocardiography. Concerningly, 3 patients had a serious adverse event within 24 hours and 8 between 24 hours and 1 month. The events included ventricular fibrillation at the time of device implant, electrode embolization to the lower extremity, vascular complications, acute stroke, and death after ventricular fibrillation at the time of device implant.

Multicenter Registry

Five international centers contributed data from 104 patients with LV endocardial pacing to a registry from which the results of AHR were reported in an effort to identify characteristics of the optimal LV pacing site.[77] These included areas of electrical latency or late-activating tissue, and areas that are not scarred. Although areas of late-activating tissue provided a greater AHR than other areas, the areas of latest activation provided the best AHR in 62% of cases, highlighting again the variability in optimal pacing site between individuals. In a follow-up report, the group note that such targeted delivery of an LV electrode to the site of greatest AHR was achievable in almost all cases. Echocardiographic response was seen in 90% of patients and reverse remodeling in 71%.[78]

SUMMARY

CRT has been in use for a quarter of a century. Epicardial pacing of the LV from a tributary of the CS accounts for the majority of patients who have received and benefitted from this therapy, with surgical placement of an epicardial lead the preferred second-line approach. LV endocardial pacing has lagged, with a small handful of patients receiving the treatment since the first case was reported 20 years ago. The reasons for this are clear; the ready availability of an alternative, technical challenges with delivering the treatment, complications, and the subsequent need for anticoagulation. All currently available methods of pacing the LV endocardially involve either off-label use of pacing devices or investigational devices. There are abundant data supporting the concept of LV endocardial pacing however, and there remains a clinical need for patients with heart failure who require CRT but cannot receive it for one reason or another. The recent attempts at developing a system for delivering LV endocardial pacing are encouraging for this reason. With continued improvements in the technology, it is also possible that LV endocardial pacing could 1 day supersede traditional CRT.

REFERENCES

1. Leyva F, Nisam S, Auricchio A. 20 years of cardiac resynchronization therapy. J Am Coll Cardiol 2014; 64(10):1047–58.
2. Cazeau S, Ritter P, Bakdach S, et al. Four chamber pacing in dilated cardiomyopathy. Pacing Clin Electrophysiol 1994;17(11 Pt 2):1974–9. Available at: http://www.ncbi.nlm.nih.gov/pubmed/7845801. Accessed August 7, 2018.
3. Bakker PF, Meijburg HW, de Vries JW, et al. Biventricular pacing in end-stage heart failure improves functional capacity and left ventricular function. J Interv Card Electrophysiol 2000;4(2):395–404. Available at: http://www.ncbi.nlm.nih.gov/pubmed/10936005. Accessed August 7, 2018.
4. Cazeau S, Leclercq C, Lavergne T, et al. Effects of multisite biventricular pacing in patients with heart failure and intraventricular conduction delay. N Engl J Med 2001;344(12):873–80.
5. Auricchio A, Stellbrink C, Sack S, et al. Long-term clinical effect of hemodynamically optimized cardiac resynchronization therapy in patients with heart failure and ventricular conduction delay. J Am Coll Cardiol 2002;39(12):2026–33. Available at: http://www.ncbi.nlm.nih.gov/pubmed/12084604. Accessed August 7, 2018.
6. Abraham WT, Fisher WG, Smith AL, et al. Cardiac resynchronization in chronic heart failure. N Engl J Med 2002;346(24):1845–53.
7. Young JB, Abraham WT, Smith AL, et al. Combined cardiac resynchronization and implantable cardioversion defibrillation in advanced chronic heart failure: the MIRACLE ICD trial. JAMA 2003;289(20):2685–94.
8. Bristow MR, Saxon LA, Boehmer J, et al. Cardiac-resynchronization therapy with or without an implantable defibrillator in advanced chronic heart failure. N Engl J Med 2004;350(21):2140–50.
9. Cleland JGF, Daubert J-C, Erdmann E, et al. The effect of cardiac resynchronization on morbidity and mortality in heart failure. N Engl J Med 2005; 352(15):1539–49.
10. Higgins SL, Hummel JD, Niazi IK, et al. Cardiac resynchronization therapy for the treatment of heart failure in patients with intraventricular conduction delay and malignant ventricular tachyarrhythmias. J Am Coll Cardiol 2003;42(8):1454–9. Available at: http://www.ncbi.nlm.nih.gov/pubmed/14563591. Accessed August 7, 2018.
11. Abraham WT, Young JB, León AR, et al. Effects of cardiac resynchronization on disease progression in patients with left ventricular systolic dysfunction, an indication for an implantable cardioverter-defibrillator, and mildly symptomatic chronic heart failure. Circulation 2004;110(18):2864–8.
12. Linde C, Abraham WT, Gold MR, et al. Randomized trial of cardiac resynchronization in

mildly symptomatic heart failure patients and in asymptomatic patients with left ventricular dysfunction and previous heart failure symptoms. J Am Coll Cardiol 2008;52(23):1834–43.

13. Moss AJ, Hall WJ, Cannom DS, et al. Cardiac-resynchronization therapy for the prevention of heart-failure events. N Engl J Med 2009;361(14):1329–38.

14. Tang ASL, Wells GA, Talajic M, et al. Cardiac-resynchronization therapy for mild-to-moderate heart failure. N Engl J Med 2010;363(25):2385–95.

15. Daubert JC, Ritter P, Le Breton H, et al. Permanent left ventricular pacing with transvenous leads inserted into the coronary veins. Pacing Clin Electrophysiol 1998;21(1 Pt 2):239–45. Available at: http://www.ncbi.nlm.nih.gov/pubmed/9474680. Accessed August 7, 2018.

16. Derval N, Steendijk P, Gula LJ, et al. Optimizing hemodynamics in heart failure patients by systematic screening of left ventricular pacing sites. J Am Coll Cardiol 2010;55(6):566–75.

17. van Everdingen WM, Zweerink A, Salden OAE, et al. Atrioventricular optimization in cardiac resynchronization therapy with quadripolar leads: should we optimize every pacing configuration including multi-point pacing? Europace 2018. https://doi.org/10.1093/europace/euy138.

18. Chan WYW, Blomqvist A, Melton IC, et al. Effects of AV delay and VV delay on left atrial pressure and waveform in ambulant heart failure patients: insights into CRT optimization. Pacing Clin Electrophysiol 2014;37(7):810–9.

19. Auricchio A, Prinzen FW. Non-responders to cardiac resynchronization therapy: the magnitude of the problem and the issues. Circ J 2011;75(3):521–7. Available at: http://www.ncbi.nlm.nih.gov/pubmed/21325727. Accessed August 7, 2018.

20. Brugada J, Delnoy PP, Brachmann J, et al. Contractility sensor-guided optimization of cardiac resynchronization therapy: results from the RESPOND-CRT trial. Eur Heart J 2017;38(10):730–8.

21. Lindvall C, Chatterjee NA, Chang Y, et al. National trends in the use of cardiac resynchronization therapy with or without implantable cardioverter-defibrillator. Circulation 2016;133(3):273–81.

22. Fish JM, Di Diego JM, Nesterenko V, et al. Epicardial activation of left ventricular wall prolongs QT interval and transmural dispersion of repolarization: implications for biventricular pacing. Circulation 2004;109(17):2136–42.

23. Medina-Ravell VA, Lankipalli RS, Yan G-X, et al. Effect of epicardial or biventricular pacing to prolong QT interval and increase transmural dispersion of repolarization: does resynchronization therapy pose a risk for patients predisposed to long QT or torsade de pointes? Circulation 2003;107(5):740–6. Available at: http://www.ncbi.nlm.nih.gov/pubmed/12578878. Accessed August 8, 2018.

24. Fish JM, Brugada J, Antzelevitch C. Potential proarrhythmic effects of biventricular pacing. J Am Coll Cardiol 2005;46(12):2340–7.

25. Bai R, Yang XY, Song Y, et al. Impact of left ventricular epicardial and biventricular pacing on ventricular repolarization in normal-heart individuals and patients with congestive heart failure. Europace 2006;8(11):1002–10.

26. Xu T, Wang H, Zhang J-Y, et al. Effects of mid-myocardial pacing on transmural dispersion of repolarization and arrhythmogenesis. Europace 2012;14(9):1363–8.

27. Roque C, Trevisi N, Silberbauer J, et al. Electrical storm induced by cardiac resynchronization therapy is determined by pacing on epicardial scar and can be successfully managed by catheter ablation. Circ Arrhythm Electrophysiol 2014;7(6):1064–9.

28. Yamada T, Tabereaux PB, Thomas McElderry H, et al. Successful catheter ablation of epicardial ventricular tachycardia worsened by cardiac resynchronization therapy. Europace 2010;12(3):437–40.

29. Jaïs P, Douard H, Shah DC, et al. Endocardial biventricular pacing. Pacing Clin Electrophysiol 1998;21(11 Pt 1):2128–31. Available at: http://www.ncbi.nlm.nih.gov/pubmed/9826866. Accessed August 7, 2018.

30. Leclercq F, Hager FX, Macia JC, et al. Left ventricular lead insertion using a modified transseptal catheterization technique: a totally endocardial approach for permanent biventricular pacing in end-stage heart failure. Pacing Clin Electrophysiol 1999;22(11):1570–5. Available at: http://www.ncbi.nlm.nih.gov/pubmed/10598958. Accessed August 7, 2018.

31. Gold MR, Rashba EJ. Left ventricular endocardial pacing: don't try this at home. Pacing Clin Electrophysiol 1999;22(11):1567–9. Available at: http://www.ncbi.nlm.nih.gov/pubmed/10598957. Accessed August 7, 2018.

32. Garrigue S, Jaïs P, Espil G, et al. Comparison of chronic biventricular pacing between epicardial and endocardial left ventricular stimulation using Doppler tissue imaging in patients with heart failure. Am J Cardiol 2001;88(8):858–62. Available at: http://www.ncbi.nlm.nih.gov/pubmed/11676947. Accessed August 2, 2018.

33. Ji S, Cesario DA, Swerdlow CD, et al. Left ventricular endocardial lead placement using a modified transseptal approach. J Cardiovasc Electrophysiol 2004;15(2):234–6.

34. Pasquié JL, Massin F, Macia JC, et al. Long-term follow-up of biventricular pacing using a totally endocardial approach in patients with end-stage cardiac failure. Pacing Clin Electrophysiol 2007;30(s1):S31–3.

35. van Gelder BM, Scheffer MG, Meijer A, et al. Transseptal endocardial left ventricular pacing: an

alternative technique for coronary sinus lead placement in cardiac resynchronization therapy. Heart Rhythm 2007;4(4):454–60.

36. Nuta B, Lines I, MacIntyre I, et al. Biventricular ICD implant using endocardial LV lead placement from the left subclavian vein approach and transseptal puncture via the transfemoral route. Europace 2007;9(11):1038–40.

37. Kassai I, Szili-Torok T. Concerns about the long-term outcome of transseptal cardiac resynchronization therapy: what we have learned from surgical experience. Europace 2007;10(1):121–2.

38. Morgan JM, Scott PA, Turner NG, et al. Targeted left ventricular endocardial pacing using a steerable introducing guide catheter and active fixation pacing lead. Europace 2008;11(4):502–6.

39. D'Ivernois C, Blanc P. Resynchronization with left ventricle lead placement through the foramen ovale. Clin Cardiol 2009;32(6):E88–91.

40. Lau EW. A streamlined technique of trans-septal endocardial left ventricular lead placement. J Interv Card Electrophysiol 2009;26(1):73–81.

41. Peschar M, de Swart H, Michels KJ, et al. Left ventricular septal and apex pacing for optimal pump function in canine hearts. J Am Coll Cardiol 2003; 41(7):1218–26. Available at: http://www.ncbi.nlm.nih.gov/pubmed/12679225. Accessed August 8, 2018.

42. Kavanagh KM, Belenkie I, Duff HJ. Transmural temporospatial left ventricular activation during pacing from different sites: potential implications for optimal pacing. Cardiovasc Res 2007;77(1):81–8.

43. Mills RW, Cornelussen RN, Mulligan LJ, et al. Left ventricular septal and left ventricular apical pacing chronically maintain cardiac contractile coordination, pump function and efficiency. Circ Arrhythm Electrophysiol 2009;2(5):571–9.

44. van Deursen C, van Geldorp IE, Rademakers LM, et al. Left ventricular endocardial pacing improves resynchronization therapy in canine left bundle-branch hearts. Circ Arrhythm Electrophysiol 2009;2(5):580–7.

45. Strik M, Rademakers LM, van Deursen CJM, et al. Endocardial left ventricular pacing improves cardiac resynchronization therapy in chronic asynchronous infarction and heart failure models. Circ Arrhythm Electrophysiol 2012;5(1):191–200.

46. Hyde ER, Behar JM, Claridge S, et al. Beneficial effect on cardiac resynchronization from left ventricular endocardial pacing is mediated by early access to high conduction velocity tissue. Circ Arrhythm Electrophysiol 2015;8(5):1164–72.

47. Rademakers LM, van Hunnik A, Kuiper M, et al. A possible role for pacing the left ventricular septum in cardiac resynchronization therapy. JACC Clin Electrophysiol 2016;2(4):413–22.

48. Bordachar P, Derval N, Ploux S, et al. Left ventricular endocardial stimulation for severe heart failure. J Am Coll Cardiol 2010;56(10):747–53.

49. Spragg DD, Dong J, Fetics BJ, et al. Optimal left ventricular endocardial pacing sites for cardiac resynchronization therapy in patients with ischemic cardiomyopathy. J Am Coll Cardiol 2010;56(10):774–81.

50. Ginks MR, Lambiase PD, Duckett SG, et al. A simultaneous X-ray/MRI and noncontact mapping study of the acute hemodynamic effect of left ventricular endocardial and epicardial cardiac resynchronization therapy in humans. Circ Hear Fail 2011; 4(2):170–9.

51. Scott PA, Yue AM, Watts E, et al. Transseptal left ventricular endocardial pacing reduces dispersion of ventricular repolarization. Pacing Clin Electrophysiol 2011;34(10):1258–66.

52. Padeletti L, Pieragnoli P, Ricciardi G, et al. Acute hemodynamic effect of left ventricular endocardial pacing in cardiac resynchronization therapy: assessment by pressure-volume loops. Circ Arrhythm Electrophysiol 2012;5(3):460–7.

53. Ginks MR, Shetty AK, Lambiase PD, et al. Benefits of endocardial and multisite pacing are dependent on the type of left ventricular electric activation pattern and presence of ischemic heart disease: insights from electroanatomic mapping. Circ Arrhythm Electrophysiol 2012;5(5):889–97.

54. Shetty AK, Sohal M, Chen Z, et al. A comparison of left ventricular endocardial, multisite, and multipolar epicardial cardiac resynchronization: an acute haemodynamic and electroanatomical study. Europace 2014;16(6):873–9.

55. Sohal M, Shetty A, Niederer S, et al. Delayed transseptal activation results in comparable hemodynamic effect of left ventricular and biventricular endocardial pacing: insights from electroanatomical mapping. Circ Arrhythm Electrophysiol 2014;7(2): 251–8.

56. van Gelder BM, Nathoe R, Bracke FA. Haemodynamic evaluation of alternative left ventricular endocardial pacing sites in clinical non-responders to cardiac resynchronisation therapy. Neth Heart J 2016;24(1):85–92.

57. Behar JM, Jackson T, Hyde E, et al. Optimized left ventricular endocardial stimulation is superior to optimized epicardial stimulation in ischemic patients with poor response to cardiac resynchronization therapy. JACC Clin Electrophysiol 2016;2(7): 799–809.

58. Gamble JHP, Herring N, Ginks M, et al. Endocardial left ventricular pacing for cardiac resynchronization: systematic review and meta-analysis. Europace 2018;20(1):73–81.

59. Graham AJ, Providenica R, Honarbakhsh S, et al. Systematic review and meta-analysis of left ventricular endocardial pacing in advanced heart failure: clinically efficacious but at what cost? Pacing Clin Electrophysiol 2018;41(4):353–61.

60. Lau EW. Yoked catheter positioning in transseptal endocardial left ventricular lead placement. Pacing Clin Electrophysiol 2011;34(7):884–93.

61. Patel MB, Worley SJ. Snare coupling of the prepectoral pacing lead delivery catheter to the femoral transseptal apparatus for endocardial cardiac resynchronization therapy. J Interv Card Electrophysiol 2013;36(3):209–16.

62. van Gelder BM, Houthuizen P, Bracke FA. Transseptal left ventricular endocardial pacing: preliminary experience from a femoral approach with subclavian pull-through. Europace 2011;13(10):1454–8.

63. Wright GA, Tomlinson DR, Lines I, et al. Transseptal left ventricular lead placement using snare technique. Pacing Clin Electrophysiol 2012;35(10):1248–52.

64. Moriña-Vázquez P, Roa-Garrido J, Fernández-Gómez JM, et al. Direct left ventricular endocardial pacing: an alternative when traditional resynchronization via coronary sinus is not feasible or effective. Pacing Clin Electrophysiol 2013;36(6):699–706.

65. Betts TR, Gamble JHP, Khiani R, et al. Development of a technique for left ventricular endocardial pacing via puncture of the interventricular septum. Circ Arrhythm Electrophysiol 2014;7(1):17–22.

66. Kassai I, Foldesi C, Szekely A, et al. New method for cardiac resynchronization therapy: transapical endocardial lead implantation for left ventricular free wall pacing. Europace 2008;10(7):882–3.

67. Kassai I, Mihalcz A, Foldesi C, et al. A novel approach for endocardial resynchronization therapy: initial experience with transapical implantation of the left ventricular lead. Heart Surg Forum 2009;12(3):E137–40.

68. Mihalcz A, Kassai I, Kardos A, et al. Comparison of the efficacy of two surgical alternatives for cardiac resynchronization therapy: trans-apical versus epicardial left ventricular pacing. Pacing Clin Electrophysiol 2012;35(2):124–30.

69. Kis Z, Arany A, Gyori G, et al. Long-term cerebral thromboembolic complications of transapical endocardial resynchronization therapy. J Interv Card Electrophysiol 2017;48(2):113–20.

70. Auricchio A, Delnoy P-P, Regoli F, et al. First-in-man implantation of leadless ultrasound-based cardiac stimulation pacing system: novel endocardial left ventricular resynchronization therapy in heart failure patients. Europace 2013;15(8):1191–7.

71. Rademakers LM, van Gelder BM, Scheffer MG, et al. Mid-term follow up of thromboembolic complications in left ventricular endocardial cardiac resynchronization therapy. Hear Rhythm 2014;11(4):609–13.

72. Gamble JHP, Herring N, Ginks MR, et al. Endocardial left ventricular pacing across the interventricular septum for cardiac resynchronization therapy: clinical results of a pilot study. Heart Rhythm 2018;15(7):1017–22.

73. Morgan JM, Biffi M, Gellér L, et al. ALternate site cardiac ResYNChronization (ALSYNC): a prospective and multicentre study of left ventricular endocardial pacing for cardiac resynchronization therapy. Eur Heart J 2016;37(27):2118–27.

74. Biffi M, Defaye P, Jaïs P, et al. Benefits of left ventricular endocardial pacing comparing failed implants and prior non-responders to conventional cardiac resynchronization therapy: a subanalysis from the ALSYNC study. Int J Cardiol 2018;259:88–93.

75. Auricchio A, Delnoy P-P, Butter C, et al. Feasibility, safety, and short-term outcome of leadless ultrasound-based endocardial left ventricular resynchronization in heart failure patients: results of the Wireless Stimulation Endocardially for CRT (WiSE-CRT) study. Europace 2014;16(5):681–8.

76. Reddy VY, Miller MA, Neuzil P, et al. Cardiac resynchronization therapy with wireless left ventricular endocardial pacing. J Am Coll Cardiol 2017;69(17):2119–29.

77. Sieniewicz BJ, Behar JM, Sohal M, et al. Electrical latency predicts the optimal left ventricular endocardial pacing site: results from a multicentre international registry. Europace 2018. https://doi.org/10.1093/europace/euy052.

78. Sieniewicz BJ, Behar JM, Gould J, et al. Guidance for optimal site selection of a leadless left ventricular endocardial electrode improves acute hemodynamic response and chronic remodeling. JACC Clin Electrophysiol 2018;4(7):860–8.

Evolving Role of Permanent His Bundle Pacing in Conquering Dyssynchrony

Parikshit S. Sharma, MD, MPH[a],
Pugazhendhi Vijayaraman, MD[b],*

KEYWORDS

- Permanent His bundle pacing (HBP) • Ventricular dyssynchrony
- Cardiac resynchronization therapy (CRT) • Left bundle branch block (LBBB)
- Right bundle branch block (RBBB) • Heart failure (HF)

KEY POINTS

- Permanent His bundle pacing (PHBP) is a promising tool for patients who need ventricular pacing.
- PHBP can also overcome bundle branch blocks and thereby alleviate ventricular dyssynchrony.
- Several small studies have shown the clinical benefits of PHBP in patients with heart failure, depressed left ventricular function, and ventricular dyssynchrony.
- PHBP might provide an additional modality for cardiac resynchronization therapy in addition to conventional biventricular pacing.

INTRODUCTION

Permanent His bundle (HB) pacing (PHBP) was first described by Deshmukh and colleagues[1] in 2000. Over the past decade, with specific tools designed to enhance lead delivery, this technique has gained significant popularity. Several studies have shown improved clinical benefits of PHBP compared with conventional right ventricular (RV) pacing, particularly in patients with need for ventricular pacing.[2–5]

Cardiac resynchronization therapy (CRT) using biventricular pacing (BVP) is the cornerstone for patients with cardiomyopathy (CMP), heart failure (HF), and ventricular dyssynchrony.[6] Although not a new concept, more recently PHBP has been successful in overcoming bundle branch block (BBB), resulting in ventricular synchrony,

particularly in patients with more proximal His-Purkinje system disease. This development has allowed the use of PHBP for CRT, either as a primary strategy (PHBP as first line for CRT) or as a rescue strategy (when BVP fails because of inability to place the coronary sinus lead).

This article reviews the concept of PHBP for CRT and the available data on PHBP in various patient subgroups with an indication for CRT.

CONVENTIONAL CARDIAC RESYNCHRONIZATION THERAPY USING BIVENTRICULAR PACING

CRT using BVP (BVP-CRT) is as an integral part of the therapy for patients with HF with reduced left ventricular (LV) ejection fraction (LVEF) and BBB,

Disclosures: Honoraria and consultant for Medtronic, consultant for Abbott and Biotronik (Dr P.S. Sharma). Honoraria, consultant, and research for Medtronic; advisory board and consultant for Boston Scientific; consultant for Abbott, Biotronik, and Merritt Medical (Dr P. Vijayaraman).
a Division of Cardiology, Rush University Medical Center, 1725 West Harrison Street Suite 1159, Chicago, IL 60612-3841, USA; b Geisinger Commonwealth School of Medicine, Geisinger Heart Institute, MC 36-10, 1000 East Mountain Boulevard, Wilkes-Barre, PA 18711, USA
* Corresponding author. .
E-mail addresses: pvijayaraman1@geisinger.edu; pvijayaraman@gmail.com

Card Electrophysiol Clin 11 (2019) 165–173
https://doi.org/10.1016/j.ccep.2018.11.004
1877-9182/19/© 2018 Elsevier Inc. All rights reserved.

particularly left BBB (LBBB). Multiple prospective randomized studies have shown that BVP-CRT pacing yields improved quality of life, increased exercise capacity, reduced HF hospitalization, and decreased all-cause mortality.[6–11] BVP-CRT might also benefit patients who develop an RV pacing-induced CMP (PICM), which is another form of ventricular dyssynchrony.[12] The third group of patients who have an indication for BVP-CRT are patients with a low LVEF undergoing implantation of a new or replacement pacemaker or implantable cardioverter-defibrillator (ICD) with an anticipated requirement for a significant percentage (>40%) of ventricular pacing.[13]

However, despite a significant benefit and evolving indications, there are still limitations to BVP. First, up to a third of patients treated with BVP-CRT do not derive a detectable clinical or echocardiographic benefit, and some worsen after resynchronization.[6,8,14] Procedural factors such as the location of the LV lead may affect response rates. Anatomic limitations, including lack of suitable coronary sinus venous branches and unavoidable phrenic nerve stimulation at ideal anatomic LV lead positions, can limit the success of LV lead placement as well. BVP-CRT has also shown a lack of significant benefit in patients with a normal QRS duration (QRSd) and among patients with RBBB.[15]

THE EMERGING ROLE OF PERMANENT HIS BUNDLE PACING FOR CARDIAC RESYNCHRONIZATION THERAPY

The first description of PHBP by Deshmukh and colleagues[1] was for maintenance of interventricular synchrony in a series of 12 patients with atrial fibrillation (AF) and CMP undergoing atrioventricular node (AVN) ablation. Challenges including low success rates caused by lack of a targeted delivery system for PHBP, need for additional mapping catheters to help find the HB, and possible need for backup RV pacing were factors that contributed to lack of enthusiasm for PHBP in the early 2000s. Furthermore, the emerging benefit of BVP-CRT around the same time resulted in the overshadowing of PHBP for CRT. However, over the past decade, with improved and targeted delivery systems, interest has rekindled for PHBP and more data have become available on PHBP and ventricular dyssynchrony.

More recently, it has become a more attractive alternative to BVP for CRT with the demonstration of resynchronizing ventricular activation by various groups.[16–21] PHBP can also be used as a rescue strategy in cases where limited coronary venous anatomy limits the ability to place an LV lead. Other advantages include the lack of potential complications from LV lead placement, which include coronary sinus dissection, venous perforation, and reduction in proarrhythmia.

How Does Permanent His Bundle Pacing Result in Overcoming Ventricular Dyssynchrony?

There are several possible theories that have been proposed as a mechanism for overcoming ventricular dyssynchrony with PHBP.[22] These theories include (1) longitudinal dissociation in the HB with pacing distal to the site of delay/block, and/or (2) differential source-sink relationships during pacing versus intrinsic impulse propagation, and/or (3) virtual electrode polarization effect.[22]

The more popular theory is that longitudinal dissociation exists within the HB and intra-Hisian disease is often responsible for BBB or delay. Narula[23] first described this concept and postulated that delay or block within HB fibers could result in BBB. This work showed that pacing distal to the site of conduction delay could recruit fibers predestined to be the bundle branches and thereby narrow the QRSd. El-Sherif[24] showed similar findings in an experimental model. Understanding that BBB or delay can be within predestined HB fibers and that pacing distal to the site of disease/delay might overcome BBB patterns and narrow the QRS formed the basis for PHBP (**Fig. 1**). The authors have highlighted this concept in some of our reports[22,25] and a recent multicenter experience of 106 patients.[20]

However, it is important to realize that there may be multiple mechanisms at play in any given patient that help overcome BBB-induced dyssynchrony using PHBP. Even though disease is often discrete within the HB, there may be multilevel disease and multiple mechanisms (suggested earlier) may be responsible for overcoming dyssynchrony using PHBP. This concept is highlighted in **Figs. 2** and **3**, in which, at higher pacing outputs, the BBB is narrowed (recruited) and at lower outputs there is no narrowing. This finding might suggest that, despite mapping extensively and placing the PHBP lead in a distal HB location, there is still some disease distal to the lead tip, which results in output-dependent recruitment of various fascicles of the conduction system.

AVAILABLE DATA ON PERMANENT HIS BUNDLE PACING FOR CARDIAC RESYNCHRONIZATION THERAPY

The patients with low LVEF and HF that benefit from CRT can be categorized into 3 main groups:

1. Patients with BBB and resulting ventricular dyssynchrony.

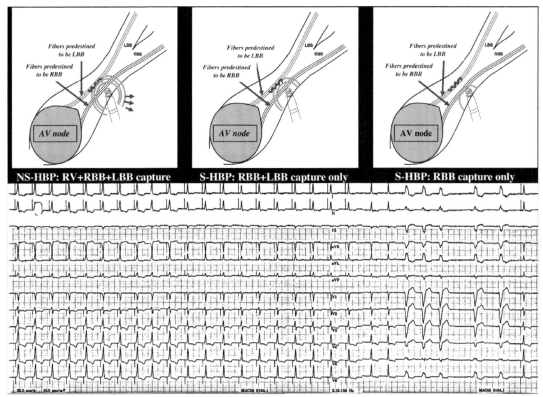

Fig. 1. Model for longitudinal dissociation within the HB. Conduction fibers within the HB are already predestined to become the right bundle branch (RBB) and left bundle branch (LBB) as depicted in the figure. If there is localized disease within the fibers predestined to be the LBB (shown in the figure) resulting in LBBB pattern, placing the lead at or distal to the site of delay/disease might overcome LBBB. Pacing at higher output of 3 V at 1 millisecond (*left panel*) results in capture of local ventricular tissue (RV) (*red arrows*) and His (both RBB and LBB fibers). Pacing at a lower output of 2 V at 1 millisecond (*middle panel*) results in selective His capture (both RBB and LBB fibers) with loss of RV capture, and pacing at a very low output of 0.5 V at 1 millisecond (*right panel*) shows capture of RBB fibers alone with LBBB pattern. AV, atrioventricular; NS-HBP, nonselective HB pacing; S-HBP, selective HB pacing. (*Adapted from* Sharma PS, Dandamudi G, Herweg B, et al. Permanent His-bundle pacing as an alternative to biventricular pacing for cardiac resynchronization therapy: a multicenter experience. Heart Rhythm 2018;15:413–20; with permission.)

2. Patients with RV PICM and pacing-induced ventricular dyssynchrony.
3. Patients with a narrow QRS undergoing AVN ablation and with need for significant ventricular pacing: prevention of ventricular dyssynchrony.

The available data on PHBP as a form of CRT are limited. Most of these studies are nonrandomized and have a small number of patients (**Table 1**). The available data on PHBP in each of these patient subgroups are reviewed in subsequent sections.

Patients with Left Bundle Branch Block and Resulting Ventricular Dyssynchrony

It is well recognized that the patients who derive the most benefit from BVP-CRT are patients with LBBB. Most of the data on PHBP for CRT focuses on this patient group.

Barba-Pichardo and colleagues[16] first described their experience with PHBP in failed CRT cases. They attempted HB pacing (HBP) in 16 patients with cardiomyopathy and failed CRT (ischemic cardiomyopathy in 7, idiopathic in 9). Temporary HBP corrected LBBB in 13 patients (81%) who were considered suitable candidates for CRT using PHBP. Successful CRT by PHBP was achieved in 9 patients, corresponding with 69% of the selected patients (ischemic 4, idiopathic 5). Mean QRSd decreased from 166 ± 8 milliseconds to 97 ± 9 milliseconds. New York Heart Association (NYHA) functional class improved from class III to class II and there was an improvement in LVEF and LV dimensions.

Lustgarten and colleagues[17] performed an elegant crossover study comparing PHBP versus BVP in patients with indications for CRT defibrillator (CRT-D) implants. Of the 29 patients enrolled,

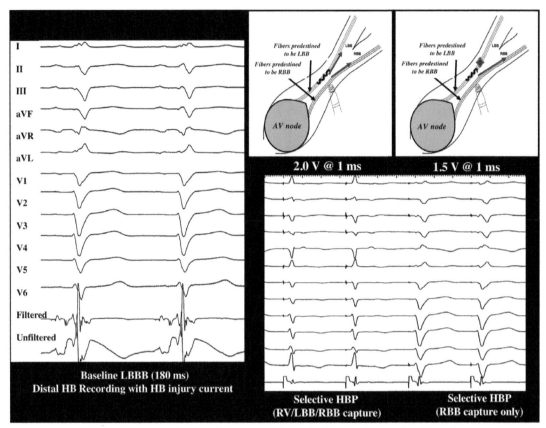

Fig. 2. PHBP in LBBB. A patient with a baseline LBBB and QRSd of 180 milliseconds with a distal HV interval of 50 milliseconds. Note the HB injury current on the unfiltered electrograms. PHBP results in selective His capture with LBBB recruitment at high outputs (2 V at 1 millisecond) resulting in paced QRSd of 96 milliseconds. At 1.5 V at 1 millisecond, there is selective His capture without recruitment and QRS morphology and duration identical to baseline (180 milliseconds). Site of LBBB with location of HB lead tip and red arrows representing conduction over different fascicles are shown above.

they were successful in showing electrical resynchronization in 21 (72%). All patients received both a coronary sinus LV lead and a PHBP lead connected to the LV port via a Y adapter. Patients were randomized in patient–blinded fashion to either HBP or BVP. Twelve patients completed the crossover analysis at 1 year. Both groups of patients showed significant improvements in ejection fraction, functional status, and 6-minute walk distance. PHBP was noted to have an equivalent CRT response to conventional BVP.

Su and colleagues[18] evaluated 16 patients undergoing successful CRT-D with PHBP lead in the LV port and 13 dual-chamber ICD implants (patients with permanent AF) with the HBP lead in the atrial port. They showed that incorporation of PHBP into a CRT-D/ICD system is feasible, and capture thresholds and R-wave sensing can be optimized using an integrated bipolar configuration with the RV lead.

Ajijola and colleagues[19] evaluated 21 patients with indications for CRT implant in lieu of a coronary sinus LV lead placement. PHBP was successfully performed in 16 of 21 patients (76%), with significant narrowing of the QRSd from 180 ± 23 milliseconds to 129 ± 13 milliseconds (P<.0001). During a median follow-up of 12 months, median NYHA functional class improved from III to II (P<.001), and mean LVEF and LV internal dimension in diastole improved from 27% ± 10% to 41% ± 13% (P<.001) and from 5.4 ± 0.4 cm to 4.5 ± 0.3 cm (P<.001), respectively. No dislodgments were observed, and only 1 patient lost nonselective capture, which resolved with increased pacing output.

The authors reported a multicenter experience on PHBP for CRT in 106 patients divided into 2 groups: PHBP as a primary (PHBP attempted first for CRT) or rescue strategy (PHBP attempted because of failed coronary sinus lead implant).[20] The overall success rate for PHBP was 90%.

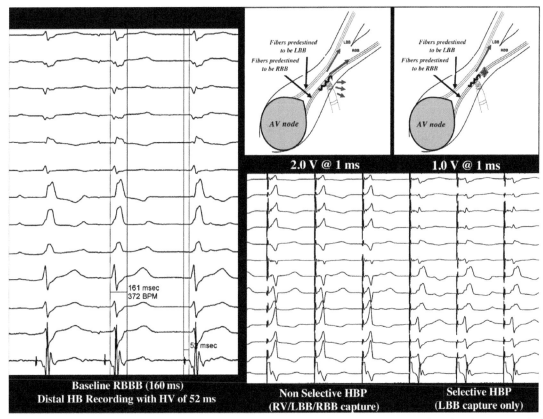

Fig. 3. PHBP in RBBB. A patient with a baseline RBBB and QRSd of 160 milliseconds with a distal HV interval of 52 milliseconds. PHBP results in nonselective His capture with RBBB recruitment at high outputs (2 V at 1 millisecond) resulting in paced QRSd of 110 milliseconds. At 1 V at 1 millisecond, there is selective His capture without recruitment and QRS morphology and duration identical to baseline (160 milliseconds). Site of RBBB with location of HB lead tip and arrows representing conduction over different fascicles are shown above.

BBB was noted in 45%, and paced rhythm in 39% of cases. His capture and BBB correction thresholds were 1.4 ± 0.9 V and 2.0 ± 1.2 V at 1 millisecond, respectively. During a mean follow-up of 14 months, both groups showed significant narrowing of QRS from 157 ± 33 milliseconds to 117 ± 18 milliseconds (P = .0001), increase in LVEF from 30% ± 10% to 43% ± 13% (P = .0001) and improvement in NYHA class from 2.8 ± 0.5 to 1.8 ± 0.6 (P = .0001) with HBP. Lead-related complications occurred in 7 patients.

Permanent His Bundle Pacing for Cardiac Resynchronization Therapy in Right Bundle Branch Block

It has been shown that BVP-CRT benefits patients with LBBB more than patients with RBBB or without LBBB. HF with RBBB is physiologically different from that with LBBB. In LBBB, the septum contracts first against a nonactivated free LV wall, resulting in dyssynchronous LV

contraction. In contrast, in patients with RBBB, it is the right ventricle that contracts asynchronously with mostly normal LV activation. Hence, BVP-CRT, in an attempt to synchronize contraction of the LV, may not improve outcomes in patients with RBBB. In contrast, in patients undergoing PHBP, synchronization of delayed RV activation and near-normal LV activation is feasible.

The authors recently reported a multicenter experience with PHBP in RBBB. PHBP was attempted in patients with a depressed LVEF, RBBB, NYHA class greater than or equal to II, and HF with an indication for CRT.[21] HBP was successful in 37 of 39 patients (95%), with correction of RBBB in 78% of cases. His capture and BBB correction thresholds were 1.1 ± 0.6 V and 1.4 ± 0.7 V at 1 millisecond, respectively. During a mean follow-up of 15 months, there was a significant narrowing of QRS from 158 ± 24 milliseconds to 127 ± 17 milliseconds (P = .0001), increase in LVEF from 31% ± 10% to 39% ± 13% (P = .004), and improvement in NYHA functional

Table 1
Studies on permanent His bundle pacing and cardiac resynchronization therapy

Study Name	Design	Study Population	Total Attempted Procedures	Success Rate (Recruitment of BBB) Using PHBP	Outcomes
Barba-Pichardo et al,[16] 2013	Prospective	PHBP attempted in pts with failed LV lead placement	16	9	Improvement in NYHA class; improvement in LVEF and LV dimensions
Lustgarten et al,[17] 2015	Crossover	PHBP and LV leads in all patients undergoing CRT	29	21	Significant improvements in ejection fraction, functional status, 6-min walk distance with both PHBP and BVP in 12 pts who completed the crossover
Su et al,[18] 2016	Prospective	PHBP in pts with indication for CRT	NA	29	Tested various pacing configurations and showed lower pacing thresholds using a bipolar HB lead and RV lead configuration
Ajijola et al,[19] 2017	Prospective	PHBP attempted in pts with failed LV lead placement	21	16 (76%)	Improvement in LVEF and dimensions
Sharma et al,[20] 2018	Prospective, multicenter	Failed LV lead placement (rescue CRT); primary HBP in pts with all indications for CRT	106	95 (90%)	Improvement in NYHA functional class; improvement in LVEF
Sharma et al,[21] 2018	Prospective, multicenter	PHBP in pts with RBBB and indication for CRT as a primary or rescue strategy	39	37 (95%)	Improvement in NYHA functional class; improvement in LVEF
Shan et al,[27] 2018	Prospective	PHBP for CRT in patients with chronic RV pacing	18	16 (89%)	Improvement in QRSd, LV dimensions, and LVEF

Abbreviations: NA, not available; NYHA, New York Heart Association; pts, patients.

class from 2.8 ± 0.6 to 2 ± 0.7 $(P = .0001)$ with HBP. Increase in capture threshold occurred in 3 patients.

Permanent His Bundle Pacing for Cardiac Resynchronization Therapy in Right Ventricular Pacing-Induced Cardiomyopathy and Pacing-induced Ventricular Dyssynchrony

It is well recognized that chronic RV apical pacing–induced ventricular dyssynchrony can lead to PICM. In patients with RV pacing burden greater than 20%, the incidence of this can be as high as 1 in 5 patients.[26] PHBP can help resynchronize ventricular activation, thereby resulting in resolution of cardiomyopathy.

In our multicenter experience on PHBP for CRT,[20] 31 patients with HF and high burden of RV pacing were evaluated. PHBP resulted in synchronous ventricular contraction in 25 of the 31 patients (81%). There was a significant decrease in QRSd from 177 ± 19 milliseconds to 125 ± 15 milliseconds $(P = .0001)$, and increase in LVEF from $32\% \pm 11\%$ to $45\% \pm 13\%$ $(P = .0001)$ with PHBP.

Shan and colleagues[27] recently published their experience on PHBP in 18 patients with chronic RV pacing. PHBP was successful in 16 patients (89%), 11 of whom had PICM, whereas the remaining 5 patients were CRT nonresponders. After upgrading to PHBP, QRSd decreased from 157 ± 22 milliseconds to 107 ± 17 milliseconds $(P<.01)$. At 1-year follow-up after PHBP, LV end-diastolic dimensions decreased from baseline 62 ± 7 mm to 56 ± 8 mm $(P<.01)$ and LVEF increased from baseline $36\% \pm 8\%$ to $53\% \pm 10\%$ $(P<.01)$.

Permanent His Bundle Pacing in Patients Undergoing Atrioventricular Node Ablation and Prevention of Dyssynchrony

PHBP might provide the best solution for maintenance of ventricular synchrony in patients with permanent AF and reduced LVEF undergoing an AVN ablation. As opposed to BVP-CRT, which creates a certain degree of ventricular dyssynchrony compared with baseline, PHBP preserves synchronized ventricular activation by pacing the intact native conduction system distal to the AVN.

The authors published our experience on AVN ablation and PHBP in 42 patients.[28] PHBP was successful in 40 of 42 patients (95%). PHBP threshold at implant was 1 ± 0.8 V at 1 millisecond and increased to 1.6 ± 1.2 V at 1 millisecond during a mean follow-up of 19 ± 14 months. LVEF increased from $43\% \pm 13\%$ to $50\% \pm 11\%$ $(P = .01)$ and NYHA functional status improved

from 2.5 ± 0.5 to 1.9 ± 0.5 $(P = .04)$. Patients with LVEF less than or equal to 40% at baseline showed a significant improvement in LVEF $(33\% \pm 7\%$ to $45\% \pm 9\%$; $P<.001)$, whereas those with an LVEF greater than 40% at baseline showed a preserved LVEF $(56\% \pm 5\%$ to $57\% \pm 7\%$; $P = .5)$ during follow-up.

Huang and colleagues[29] showed similar findings in a study evaluating PHBP with AVN ablation in 52 patients. PHBP and AVN ablation was successful in 42 patients (80.8%) and were followed up (median 20 months). About half of the patients had HF with reduced LVEF. There was no significant change between native and paced QRSd $(107 \pm 26$ vs 105 ± 24 milliseconds; $P = .07)$. LVEF increased from baseline $(P<.001)$, with a greater improvement in patients with HF with reduced ejection fraction $(N = 20)$ than in patients with HF with preserved ejection fraction $(N = 22)$. NYHA functional status improved 2.9 ± 0.6 to 1.4 ± 0.4 after PHBP in patients with a low LVEF and from a baseline 2.7 ± 0.6 to 1.4 ± 0.5 in patients with a preserved LVEF. After about a year of PHBP, the number of patients who required diuretics for HF decreased significantly $(P<.001)$.

Permanent His Bundle Pacing in Nonresponders to Cardiac Resynchronization Therapy Using Biventricular Pacing

Current data suggest that up to a third of patients treated with BVP-CRT do not derive a detectable clinical or echocardiographic benefit, and some might continue to worsen.[30] Limited data exist on PHBP in patients who have not responded to traditional BVP-CRT. In our multicenter experience on PHBP for CRT,[20] we studied 8 patients who were deemed nonresponders to BVP-CRT and who underwent successful upgrade to PHBP. Six of the 8 patients had an echocardiographic response with PHBP (75%), with an average increase in LVEF from $30\% \pm 10\%$ to $38\% \pm 13\%$ $(P = .07)$.

LEFT VENTRICULAR CONDUCTION SYSTEM PACING: THE NEW KID ON THE BLOCK

Despite adequate mapping of the HB, there may be 10% to 20% patients who have more distal or widespread conduction disease resulting in LBBB and PHBP, and it may not be possible to overcome LBBB with a reasonable capture threshold. A recent technique described by Huang and colleagues[31] shows the feasibility of pacing the left bundle branch immediately beyond the conduction block via an intraseptal approach to functionally restore the impaired His-Purkinje conduction system in patients with left BBB (LBBB) with an improved clinical outcome. More data are needed to assess the benefits of this technique; however, it does provide implanters with an additional option for patients with ventricular dyssynchrony.

FUTURE DIRECTIONS

BVP-CRT has a significant impact in cardiovascular morbidity and mortality in patients with ventricular dyssynchrony and HF. However, high nonresponder rates and inability to predict response remains a challenge. PHBP may provide a real alternative to BVP-CRT. It can be used as a rescue strategy for patients who fail coronary sinus lead implants before considering alternative options such as surgical epicardial or endocardial LV lead placement. There are also emerging data of its benefit as a primary strategy, although randomized controlled trials are needed before this can be recommended strongly. HBP may be the more physiologic primary option in patients with normal His-Purkinje conduction who develop RV PICM and in patients undergoing AVN ablation. PHBP may also be considered in patients with cardiomyopathy and underlying RBBB with or without prolonged PR intervals as an option for CRT.

Despite the data presented earlier, it is important to realize that there have been no published randomized trials assessing the effectiveness of PHBP compared with BVP-CRT. Although preliminary data from a small, randomized, crossover study suggest equivalent response, there are no large, long-term outcome data. Current studies have used a 20% narrowing in QRSd (from baseline BBB) as a marker of success for PHBP. However, what degree of correction is necessary to achieve electrical and mechanical resynchronization and clinical response remains unanswered. Are there patient or electrocardiogram characteristics preprocedure that can help predict which patients will achieve successful PHBP and will respond to this therapy? Larger, multicenter, randomized studies comparing PHBP with BVP need to be performed to evaluate the clinical efficacy of PHBP and help answer some of these questions.

SUMMARY

PHBP is a promising technique for patients who need ventricular pacing and might help maintain synchronous ventricular contraction. It might also have a role in overcoming ventricular dyssynchrony, and mounting data suggest the potential benefit of PHBP for CRT. It provides implanters with an additional tool to achieve resynchronization. More randomized data are needed to help understand the benefit compared with BVP-CRT.

REFERENCES

1. Deshmukh P, Casavant DA, Romanyshyn M, et al. Permanent, direct His-bundle pacing: a novel approach to cardiac pacing in patients with normal His-Purkinje activation. Circulation 2000; 101:869–77.
2. Sharma PS, Dandamudi G, Naperkowski A, et al. Permanent His-bundle pacing is feasible, safe, and superior to right ventricular pacing in routine clinical practice. Heart Rhythm 2015;12:305–12.
3. Abdelrahman M, Subzposh FA, Beer D, et al. Clinical outcomes of his bundle pacing compared to right ventricular pacing. J Am Coll Cardiol 2018; 71(20):2319–30.
4. Sharma PS, Ellenbogen KA, Trohman RG. Permanent His bundle pacing: the past, present, and future. J Cardiovasc Electrophysiol 2017;28:458–65.
5. Zanon F, Ellenbogen KA, Dandamudi G, et al. Permanent His-bundle pacing: a systematic literature review and meta-analysis. Europace 2018;20(11): 1819–26.
6. Cleland JG, Daubert JC, Erdmann E, et al. The effect of cardiac resynchronization on morbidity and mortality in heart failure. N Engl J Med 2005;352: 1539–49.
7. Bristow MR, Saxon LA, Boehmer J, et al. Cardiac-resynchronization therapy with or without an implantable defibrillator in advanced chronic heart failure. N Engl J Med 2004;350:2140–50.
8. Abraham WT, Fisher WG, Smith AL, et al. Cardiac resynchronization in chronic heart failure. N Engl J Med 2002;346:1845–53.
9. Young JB, Abraham WT, Smith AL, et al. Combined cardiac resynchronization and implantable cardioversion defibrillation in advanced chronic heart failure: the MIRACLE ICD trial. JAMA 2003;289: 2685–94.
10. Cazeau S, Leclercq C, Lavergne T, et al. Effects of multisite biventricular pacing in patients with heart failure and intraventricular conduction delay. N Engl J Med 2001;344:873–80.
11. Auricchio A, Stellbrink C, Sack S, et al. Long-term clinical effect of hemodynamically optimized cardiac resynchronization therapy in patients with heart failure and ventricular conduction delay. J Am Coll Cardiol 2002;39:2026–33.
12. Kiehl EL, Makki T, Kumar R, et al. Incidence and predictors of right ventricular pacing-induced cardiomyopathy in patients with complete atrioventricular block and preserved left ventricular systolic function. Heart Rhythm 2016;13:2272–8.
13. Tracy CM, Epstein AE, Darbar D, et al. 2012 ACCF/AHA/HRS focused update of the 2008 guidelines for

device-based therapy of cardiac rhythm abnormalities: a report of the American College of Cardiology Foundation/American Heart Association Task Force on practice guidelines. J Am Coll Cardiol 2012;60: 1297–313.

14. Singh JP, Klein HU, Huang DT, et al. Left ventricular lead position and clinical outcome in the multicenter automatic defibrillator implantation trial-cardiac resynchronization therapy (MADIT-CRT) trial. Circulation 2011;123:1159–66.

15. Moss AJ, Hall WJ, Cannom DS, et al. Cardiac-resynchronization therapy for the prevention of heart-failure events. N Engl J Med 2009;361:1329–38.

16. Barba-Pichardo R, Manovel Sanchez A, Fernandez-Gomez JM, et al. Ventricular resynchronization therapy by direct His-bundle pacing using an internal cardioverter defibrillator. Europace 2013;15:83–8.

17. Lustgarten DL, Crespo EM, Arkhipova-Jenkins I, et al. His-bundle pacing versus biventricular pacing in cardiac resynchronization therapy patients: a crossover design comparison. Heart Rhythm 2015; 12:1548–57.

18. Su L, Xu L, Wu SJ, et al. Pacing and sensing optimization of permanent His-bundle pacing in cardiac resynchronization therapy/implantable cardioverter defibrillators patients: value of integrated bipolar configuration. Europace 2016;18:1399–405.

19. Ajijola OA, Upadhyay GA, Macias C, et al. Permanent His-bundle pacing for cardiac resynchronization therapy: initial feasibility study in lieu of left ventricular lead. Heart Rhythm 2017;14:1353–61.

20. Sharma PS, Dandamudi G, Herweg B, et al. Permanent His-bundle pacing as an alternative to biventricular pacing for cardiac resynchronization therapy: a multicenter experience. Heart Rhythm 2018;15:413–20.

21. Sharma PS, Naperkowski A, Bauch TD, et al. Permanent His bundle pacing for cardiac resynchronization therapy in patients with heart failure and right bundle branch block. Circ Arrhythm Electrophysiol 2018;11(9):e006613.

22. Sharma PS, Huizar J, Ellenbogen KA, et al. Recruitment of bundle branches with permanent His bundle pacing in a patient with advanced conduction system disease: what is the mechanism? Heart Rhythm 2016;13:623–5.

23. Narula OS. Longitudinal dissociation in the His bundle. Bundle branch block due to asynchronous conduction within the His bundle in man. Circulation 1977;6:996–1006.

24. El-Sherif N. Normalization of bundle branch block patterns by distal his bundle pacing. Clinical and experimental evidence of longitudinal dissociation in the pathologic His bundle. Circulation 1978;57: 473–83.

25. Sharma PS, Ellison K, Patel HN, et al. Overcoming left bundle branch block by permanent His bundle pacing: evidence of longitudinal dissociation in the His via recordings from a permanent pacing lead. HeartRhythm Case Rep 2017;3:499–502.

26. Khurshid S, Epstein AE, Verdino RJ, et al. Incidence and predictors of right ventricular pacing-induced cardiomyopathy. Heart Rhythm 2014;11:1619–25.

27. Shan P, Su L, Zhou X, et al. Beneficial effects of upgrading to His bundle pacing in chronically paced patients with left ventricular ejection fraction <50. Heart Rhythm 2018;15:405–12.

28. Vijayaraman P, Subzposh FA, Naperkowski A. Atrioventricular node ablation and His bundle pacing. Europace 2017;19:iv10–6.

29. Huang W, Su L, Wu S, et al. Benefits of permanent His bundle pacing combined with atrioventricular node ablation in atrial fibrillation patients with heart failure with both preserved and reduced left ventricular ejection fraction. J Am Heart Assoc 2017;6 [pii: e005309].

30. Daubert JC, Saxon L, Adamson PB, et al. 2012 EHRA/HRS expert consensus statement on cardiac resynchronization therapy in heart failure: implant and follow-up recommendations and management. Heart Rhythm 2012;9:1524–76.

31. Huang W, Su L, Wu S, et al. A novel pacing strategy with low and stable output: pacing the left bundle branch immediately beyond the conduction block. Can J Cardiol 2017;33:1736.e1–3.

Printed and bound by CPI Group (UK) Ltd, Croydon, CR0 4YY

03/10/2024

01040371-0019